LIFE FORCE

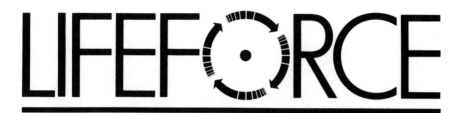

LIFEFORCE

THE SECRETS OF HIGH ENERGY
AND OPTIMAL HEALTH

JULIE CHRYSTYN

■

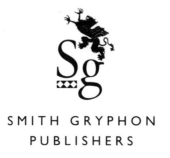

SMITH GRYPHON
PUBLISHERS

First published in Great Britain in 1994 by
SMITH GRYPHON LIMITED
Swallow House, 11–21 Northdown Street
London N1 9BN

A CIP catalogue record for this book is available from the British Library

ISBN 1 85685 065 X

Typeset by Computerset, Harmondsworth, Middlesex
Printed by Butler & Tanner Ltd, Frome

TO
GEORGE STANKOVICH

CONTENTS

ACKNOWLEDGEMENTS

I wish to express my deep gratitude to my publisher, Robert Smith of Smith Gryphon, and agent, Mike Sharland of the Sharland Organization, whose fantastic efforts have driven this book to life.

An exuberant thank-you is extended to my brilliant and unstoppable research assistant, Hannah J. Fox.

My thanks and appreciation also go to Nancy Duin, Helen Armitage, Alice Sharland, Ivanka Kapetanović, Major William Foxton, Mantósh Singh, R. J. Bear and the numerous gifted physicians, health professionals, researchers and writers who have made this vital information available for us all.

PREFACE

I stumbled upon an extraordinary realization several years ago – no one I knew was well. Some appeared healthy but, in reality, were not. The problems were not the common cold, a slight rash or hay fever, backache or a broken arm. The people I knew had cancer, heart failure, strokes. They had arthritis, chronic fatigue, debilitating allergies, recurring infections, frequent muscle spasms, episodes of depression. Others had developed osteoporosis, diabetes and other 'age-related' diseases – prematurely.

On further investigation, I also learned that virtually no one was satisfied with the health care they were receiving. Some have totally given up on the idea of consulting a doctor unless it is a matter of 'life or death'. Others trod along unenthusiastically and blindly, not having much faith in the medical services they were receiving. What truly amazed me, however, was how many people had sought *holistic* health care. The number of my friends who had taken their health concerns into their own hands surprised me. The more I prodded, the more I realised that their actions are becoming the norm.

It is incredible to imagine that most people in our society have never experienced optimal health. This does not have to be the case. Premature ageing, illness, stress and lack of energy are not things that just happen to you; these are things over which you can exert great control. By becoming aware of your environment, nourishment and lifestyle choices, you are empowered to practise considerable control indeed, and to possess the optimal health you deserve.

JULIE CHRYSTYN
FEBRUARY 1994

THE
MODERN
DIET MYTH

t was a fairy-tale wedding that took place in Bel Air, California on a sunny May afternoon between my beautiful 28-year-old friend Katherine and an entertainment industry mogul whom, she assured me, was absolutely perfect for her. You can imagine my surprise when, only six months later, a tearful Katie phoned me to say that her marriage was in ruins. Guiltily, she confessed that much of the problem was probably the result of her various ailments, which had cropped up during her short marriage. She claimed that she felt constantly fatigued, tense, irritable, short tempered and easily frustrated, and on occasion, she even reached near-hysteria because she was unable to breathe effortlessly.

At this point, being the motherly sort, I asked if she was getting enough sleep and eating properly. Katie said that, yes, she slept well enough – in fact, she usually slept late – but found that, once up, she had a hard time getting through the morning. Coffee and a sweet roll usually made her feel better and gave her the energy to make it through to lunch, when she grabbed a sandwich or slice of pizza or ate a quick salad. Come evening, she had a full meal with her husband.

Strangely enough, she continued, it was then that she felt her best all day – alive, happy, energetic and interested in activity and conversation. Her husband, however, simply wanted to wind down and relax in the evening. This irritated Katie terribly. He went to bed while she remained up late into the night, full of energy and exasperated that she had no one with whom to share it. Consequently, their lives were slowly being separated into two different worlds, and this realization had thrown her into a state of anxiety and depression which, consequently, kept her from having a decent relationship with her husband. Of course, I insisted that she go at once to a doctor.

Over the following months, Katie made the rounds of various physicians – from general practitioners to allergy specialists – but found no solution to her problems. Almost hysterical, she explained to me how, time and again, these 'specialists' had said they could find nothing physically wrong with her, and many of them had quickly grown impatient with her for insisting that all was not right.

Eventually, Katie was told to seek psychiatric help. Stunned, she informed that particular doctor that she was not a 'mental case'. Nevertheless, desperate for some cure for her ill health and becoming increasingly frantic over her declining marriage, she reluctantly decided to take the doctor's advice and seek therapy. She began to see a rare breed of psychotherapist, one who practised orthomolecular psychiatry – a type of holistic medicine based on treating patients' problems by determining their bodies' individual nutrient requirements.

Katie described to him her various ailments and severe level of stress, but blamed her husband for being emotionally unbalanced himself. After the doctor had examined both Katie and her husband and all the possible causes of destruction in their marriage, he came to the conclusion that neither had a psychiatric disorder. However, he pointed out that Katie was clearly the troubled one – and that at the root of her troubles was malnutrition.

Now, you can well imagine Katie's reaction: having previously been told that she was a head case, she was now being informed that she was suffering from malnutrition! Why, people who live in Bel Air and have live-in chefs don't suffer from malnourishment! Most of us would react with the same disbelief if we were told that we were malnourished. However, the plain fact is that an increasing number of people in Western societies today suffer what is known as 'affluent malnutrition'.

SUSTENANCE AND SURVIVAL

To understand why the citizens of the wealthiest and most industrialized and technological countries in the world are in this predicament, we must first understand the human body and its slow evolution over time. After all, despite our claims to superiority over other life forms on Earth, our bodies evolved through the effects of many of the same laws of nature that theirs did, and like it or not, we are organisms that require the same essentials if we are to continue to grow and evolve – air, water, sunlight and food being a few of the basics.

In our prehistoric ancestors' time, air, water and sunlight were taken for granted. It was the search for food that was a daily struggle. Since life centred around its availability, early humans sometimes travelled over large areas in search of sustenance. Their bodies' ability to store fat enabled them to maintain the energy to survive not only the highly strenuous day-to-day tasks of hunting and gathering but also periodic famines. Eating was solely a means of survival, and as with other animals, all members of a group were raised to be self-sufficient and to know where to find food.

Sustenance usually came from a wide range of foods including nuts, roots, fruits, beans, flowers, tubers and other plant parts, gums and, occasionally, lean red meat, fish and fowl. Of course, none of this food was processed before being eaten – at most, it was pounded, scraped, roasted or baked.

Most people are quick to point out that the lives of Stone Age humans were usually short. However, this was largely due to predators, violence between rival groups of people, natural accidents and some infectious diseases – not because of what they ate. Studies of skeletal remains and cave wall paintings indicate that our forebears were normally strong and lean and, due to their harsh lifestyles, either maintained a high level of endurance and fitness or succumbed to the stronger forces of nature. Survival of the fittest played a leading role in the lives of Paleolithic primitives.

Gradually, though, as prehistoric humans evolved, attitudes towards food changed. With the coming of agriculture approximately 10,000 years ago, people discovered that they could control their food production. Whereas their ancestors had been forced to rely on what the Earth gave them, they could now produce the fruits, vegetables and grains they wanted. Rather than having to follow herds of animals along their migratory paths or be forced to move on to 'greener pastures' in search of food, the humans of this new age could settle in one place and grow their means of sustenance around them.

As a result, human diets altered radically, and with this enormous change came a decline in overall human health. With people – and animals – living in closer proximity, epidemics of infectious diseases increased. In addition, more nutrient deficiencies surfaced. As well as a reduction in the range of food eaten (because fewer types were grown than were found in the wild), humans found that they could grow and eat only what they liked rather than instinctively eating what their bodies needed to be healthy. The resulting deficiency diseases, among them rickets and scurvy, reflected this new view of food.

Agriculture also brought traditions and rituals centred around food production, preparation and consumption – for example, feasting at harvest time and as a way of celebrating an occasion. Food no longer was simply a means of sustaining the life of an organism.

Although humans now had the ability to produce their food rather than relying solely on the hunting or gathering of it, they did retain the close relationship with the Earth that their ancestors had felt even more strongly. Because most people grew their own food, they understood farming methods, the seasons, the entire agricultural way of life.

BRUSSELS SPROUTS IN JULY

The arrival of agriculture may have changed human lifestyles drastically, but it took thousands of years to do so. Nothing has altered human beings' diets and view of food more rapidly or dramatically than the Industrial Revolution, which began little more than 200 years ago. With the advent of machinization and processing procedures, humans attained complete control over their food production.

Where once people relied on the produce of gardens and small farms, and perhaps went into town for such staples as salt, sugar and flour, they could now rely entirely on the well-stocked shelves of grocers' shops and, later, the local supermarket. Moving to towns and cities to find work and a new way of life, they lost touch with the land that had once been so much a part of their existence. It was no longer necessary for everyone to grow food or own land for agriculture. In fact, cultivatable land became either scarce or non-existent within or near cities, and so most people had no choice but to buy foods transported over increasingly large distances.

They also lost touch with the seasons and how they affect crops. Where, earlier this century, the availability of certain foods depended upon the season, now we can buy a lettuce in mid-December, Brussels sprouts in July, green beans in February and strawberries – previously the harbingers of June and Wimbledon tennis – all year round.

This dependency on food appearing as if by magic in supermarkets has continued for so many decades that some city dwellers now have no conception of where their food actually comes from. It has been said that, today, some children in the inner cities no longer realize that, for instance, mince comes from a cow or that there are many other varieties of lettuce than the type they find on their hamburgers. We have lost touch with our own personal food production to the point that there is now an entire adult generation that has never seen food grow.

The enormous chasm between modern human beings' and their ancestors' understanding of food probably becomes most obvious when you ask anyone the question: 'If you lost your way in a wilderness area, would you be able to find the food you would need to survive?' Today most people would answer: 'No.' Our prehistoric ancestors would most likely have replied, 'Of course.'

With the increasing use of machines also came a new fascination with speed. Suddenly society was expected to produce more, faster. Everyone, it seemed, had to be in the fast lane or they would be left behind, whether that meant owning a car, understanding computers or cooking a meal in a microwave in five minutes and eating at the speed of light.

Americans especially seemed to be affected by this new approach to food. Instead of viewing meals as a time for leisure and enjoyment, they became a nation whose motto, according to the French economist Michel Chevalier, was 'Gobble, gulp and go.'[1]

It would be difficult to convince many people today that our food and our attitudes towards it have not improved over time. It is wonderful to be faced with literally hundreds of food choices when you enter a supermarket. With such a startling variety from which to choose, the thought of eating nuts and berries and chasing down the odd rabbit is understandably quite unpalatable.

And the convenience! Walk into any modern supermarket and be dazzled by the shelf upon shelf of canned, homogenized, boxed, vacuum-packed, bagged, dehydrated, condensed, sealed, instant, chilled, frozen, dried, pre-cooked foods on offer. Grab a couple of boxes here, a couple of cans there, cook strenuously for 15 to 30 minutes and – *voila!* – dinner.

OUR ANCESTORS' HEALTH

Unfortunately, this glowing picture of modern convenience clashes with the reality of what our bodies require to maintain health. Instant food may fill a necessary niche in our push-button society, but are we more healthy today, with all our processed foods, than our grandparents of yesterday whose diets consisted of garden produce and the staples? Were our grandparents and great-grandparents much healthier than their Stone Age ancestors? Time and medical evidence is slowly giving us the answer, and it is a resounding 'No!'

The fact is that almost 99 per cent of our genetic material (e.g. DNA) actually developed many millions of years ago in our pre-human ancestors. The remaining 1 per cent evolved seven million years ago after the human and great ape lines separated. This means that the bodies of present-day humans are anatomically and physiologically almost identical to those of our ancestors of 40,000 years ago.

It takes thousands of years for organisms such as animals and humans (and their genetic material) to adapt to environmental changes such as new types of food. The many centuries that followed the introduction of agriculture saw a complete change in human lifestyles, including such a drastic alteration in people's eating habits that it resulted in widespread illnesses. But this was nothing compared to what the

Industrial Revolution perpetrated. Our bodies are programmed to respond to the conditions of 40,000 or more years ago, yet now, in the 20th century, we demand that they function under enormously different circumstances that promise to change still more rapidly in the immediate future.

The industrialized societies of the 20th century are suffering from the way they eat or, more pertinently, from the effects of over-consumption. We have too much food available to us and much of it is not what our bodies need to maintain health. Our prehistoric ancestors died of violence and infectious diseases. Those who lived during the introduction of agriculture also suffered from infectious diseases, but were also afflicted with illnesses caused by a lack of nutrients: vitamin C deficiencies led to scurvy; vitamin D deficiencies led to rickets. Now, in the post-industrial era, most wealthy nations are plagued not so much with infectious diseases or serious illnesses caused by nutrient deficiencies, but with the nutritional problems caused by the overeating of certain foods. Our bodies have simply not evolved quickly enough to handle the foods we eat today.

S. Boyd Eaton, Marjorie Shostake and Melvin Konner, authors of *The Paleolithic Prescription*[2], believe that it is the enormous difference between our diets and those of our ancestors that causes what they call 'discordance'. According to their hypothesis, many of the 'diseases of civilization' are the result of genetic maladaptation to environmental conditions. Diseases in this category – so common today in the West – include mature-onset diabetes, hypertension (chronic high blood pressure), chronic obstructive lung disease, clogging up of the arteries (atherosclerosis) and several different cancers, as well as obesity, osteoporosis (bone thinning), hearing loss, most dental problems, and alcohol-related conditions. These ailments are, in total, responsible for 73 per cent of the mortality in industrialized nations. The leading causes of death in both the United States and Britain are cancer, heart disease and stroke.

According to Eaton, Shostake and Konner, obesity is a prime example of how discordance can lead to disease. The bodies of prehistoric people were designed to store body fat. The strenuous tasks of hunting and gathering food, as well as surviving periodic famines, placed heavy demands on the energy to be derived from accumulated fat. Even regulating body temperature during seasonal extremes would drain internal energy resources. Hence the ability to store fat was a genetic advantage – those who could, survived, and those who could not, succumbed.

However, the domesticated animals of today are bred to produce meat that is at least 25–30 per cent fat, because fattier meats are considered more flavourful and tender. In addition, the fat of the wild game eaten by our ancestors was predominantly unsaturated, whereas our domestic beasts produce mostly saturated fat. Finally, fat made up only about 21 per cent of the diets of early humans – exactly half the amount of fat consumed by the average American.

Unfortunately, because the basic structure of our bodies has not changed for thousands of years, we still have the tendency to accumulate fat – all too easily – and unlike our early ancestors, our lifestyles are, for the most part, sedentary. Consequently, in North America 30 per cent of men and 20 per cent of women are obese (i.e. at least 20 per cent above the desirable weight). In Britain, the situation is not quite as bad, with 13 per cent of men and 15 per cent of women being described as 'obese' (up from 7 and 12 per cent, respectively, in 1986); however, 45 per cent of men and 36 per cent of women in the UK *are* considered overweight. All this extra poundage is the first step towards chronic health problems.

Other differences between prehistoric and modern diets abound. The calcium intake of early humans was approximately 1580 mg per day. Compare this to the 300–1200 mg recommended by the US government, and the even lower 350–1000 mg by the UK Department of Health[3], and the 740 mg and the 800 mg consumed by the average American and Briton, respectively. The difference between then and now is huge, especially when you realize that our ancestors derived their calcium from wild fruits and vegetables, not dairy products.

Sodium, the additive found in so many processed foods, was not a large part of early people's diet. Americans each consume as much as 6900 mg per day, whereas the daily intake of their predecessors totalled approximately 690 mg. To make matters worse, people in modern Western societies ingest far more sodium than potassium: a high-sodium, low-potassium diet is one of the leading causes of hypertension. The potassium intake of early humans was 16 times greater than their sodium intake.

Vitamin C consumption was approximately 440 mg per day due to the large amounts of wild plants, fruits and vegetables eaten. This is five times more than the average American consumes, and almost seven times more than the average Briton; the respective governments recommend only one-seventh (US) and – astonishingly – one-eleventh (UK) of that amount of vitamin C daily.

In the prehistoric diet, fruits and honey were the only sources of sugar, and the wide variety of unprocessed plant foods supplied a far greater amount of fibre. In addition – and most assuredly to the benefit of all prehistoric men, women and children – there were no soft drinks, coffee, alcohol or milk products.

The findings of modern nutrition research seem to be consistent with those of the authors of *The Prehistoric Prescription,* as are the current diet recommendations of the American Cancer Society and the American Heart Association. It is becoming increasingly evident that our diets have fallen into such an unnatural state that our very lives are being destroyed as a result. Many of us now suffer from constipation, varicose veins, venous thrombosis, haemorrhoids (piles), diverticular disease, bowel cancer, gallstones, peptic ulcers – all diseases that are directly related to diet.

THE BOTTOM LINE

Why do we eat what we do today despite the fact that we are becoming more aware that our diets are linked to ill health? Unfortunately, the answer is no longer a simple one.

Where once the food we ate was determined by where we lived and what the Earth would grow, now it is controlled by what the local supermarket will sell. And what the local supermarket will sell is influenced by sectors of society one would never expect to be involved in the food chain.

Manufacturers and marketing experts launch new products and new labels to gain our attention *and* our money. Scientists discover what various foods do to our bodies and then *create* new ones. Government agencies issue health advisories and argue over what information should be included on food labels. Psychologists tell us how social and environmental factors influence our food preferences. Consumer groups blow the whistle on food production practices deemed to be unhealthy or unethical. We are bombarded from all sides by information telling us what to eat, how to eat, why we should eat, where to eat and when to eat.

Information such as this would not be a source of problems if all the providers had the public's health in mind. But, unhappily, this is not usually the case. Much of the media, our most prominent sources of information, is dependent on – and thus controlled by – those with the money to spend on advertising. And today the average human stomach is the object of severe competition between food companies. The fact that the food that goes into the stomach affects human health is not of primary concern to them. The bottom line is profit.

It is an industry bent on selling at all costs. In the United States in 1989, nearly $5 billion was spent on food advertising, and in the UK in 1992, over £523 million was expended.[4] Ninety per cent of this money is poured into television advertisements that promote some of the least nutritional foods on the market – sugary breakfast cereals, sweets, soft drinks. How often do you see TV commercials advertising spinach?

Worse still, these companies target children with their advertising. It is estimated that the 30 million or so American children between the ages of 6 and 14 control a whopping $4.6 billion in food sales with their pocket money alone. It is hardly surprising that one British market research company has described children as 'an advertiser's dream'. As a result, food companies cram cartoon programmes full of advertisements for sweetened cereals, artificially flavoured fruit drinks and fast foods such as hamburgers and chips – all unhealthy foods, but exactly what children have developed a taste for.

Let's face it, food companies are out there to sell. When they persuade you to buy their products, they benefit, not necessarily your health. Simply ignoring this propaganda would seem to be the most logical way of avoiding the long tentacles of the food industry, but the reality is far bleaker.

Scientists – so long considered the sacred founts of knowledge that we, the unknowledgeable public, must rely on to light our way in nutritional and health matters – are not exempt from the control of these industries. The largest food manufacturers fund the nutrition studies carried out at the most prestigious universities, giving huge amounts of money to research, the results of which are presented to the public as supposedly unbiased information. We have just cause to wonder what the actual results of these multi-million-dollar/pound studies are.

The records of government agencies are no cleaner. Too often, they are pressured by special interest groups. An example of this happened in April 1991, when the US Department of Agriculture (USDA) announced that it would be issuing its long-awaited ' "Eating Right" Pyramid'. This new graphic was created to replace traditional food charts that presented the four 'basic food groups' as if each was of equal merit in a healthy diet; the new pyramid design placed more emphasis on the consumption of grains, fruits and vegetables than on dairy products and meat. When USDA board members and lobbyists of the National Cattlemen's Association were shown the new design, they were furious. They put pressure on the USDA and, needless to say, the pyramid design was yanked from distribution only weeks after it had been introduced to the public – even though it was the product of three years' research.[5] In Britain, the fact that the Ministry of Agriculture, Fisheries and Food (MAFF) is responsible for both the production *and* the consumption of food has led to numerous conflicts of interest – primarily, according to public watchdogs, to the detriment of consumers.

THE COMMERCIALIZATION OF FOOD

Yet the battles over the marketing of food would not be happening today if it weren't for food processing. While this in itself is not new, the commercialization of food is a relatively recent concept.

The beginning of agriculture and the consequent lifestyles that sprang up around the new methods of food production forced people to find ways of preserving their crops between harvests. Through the ages, different peoples have discovered different ways to prevent their food from spoiling and keeping its nutritional value over long periods: salting, drying and smoking meat; making wine from grapes; fermenting milk to make yoghurt; canning fruits and vegetables. These processes slowly became more sophisticated as societies evolved.

However, the commercial food processing we know today began in earnest only about 50 years ago, arising from needs different from those of small farmers. Armies in the field and other travellers required food that would be easy to carry and which could be kept without spoiling for a longer time than would be needed at home. Processed, packaged foods were the perfect answer. Institutions such as schools and hospitals quickly realized the benefits of buying foods in bulk and demanded processed foods as well. It wasn't long before even the public prized the convenience of readily usable foods, pushing up the demand for them still further.

Soon an increasing number of different foods was being packaged, given brand names and methodically stacked on shelves. We eagerly grabbed every new product that was handed to us, and now, years later, many of us can't imagine life without supermarkets and convenience foods. We have been conditioned to recognize and prefer only manufactured, artificial or modified tastes and textures, and have so absorbed processed foods into our way of life that, until recently, we never stopped to look at the negative aspects of having our sources of nutrition so altered by mechanical processes. Even today, most people view food processing as desirable and even healthy.

A growing number of illnesses have now been linked to the adulteration of our food – testimony that something is wrong with the way we view nutrition. If the people of industrialized nations are to regain the health that their ancestors had, it is crucial to dispel some of the myths and misconceptions that have sprung up about the food we eat.

TRUTHS, UNTRUTHS AND HALF-TRUTHS

Sorting the truths, untruths and half-truths from the tangled web of information surrounding processed foods can be a daunting experience. Food companies have not spent millions promoting their image without reason. It is important to their bottom line that you believe totally that their products provide you with safe, wholesome and attractive food. But, unbeknownst to many of us, most manufacturers have failed miserably in providing just that.

Of all the citizens of the Western world, Americans seem to have a particular obsession with the cleanliness of food. The open-air markets still found throughout the Third World – and in many European cities – are considered primitive and, in most cases, downright filthy. Food companies, understanding this paranoia, happily reinforce the American belief that packaged foods are sanitarily processed simply because they come in a package.

Most Americans would be horrified to learn that, according to the US Food and Drug Administration (FDA), there is no way to eliminate all food contamination. To provide some type of control over the amount of insect parts, rodent hairs, moulds and other tiny particles that can find their way into food but pose no real health hazard, the USFDA has set what are called 'defect action levels'.[6] However, these are designed only to prevent food from containing so many bugs, hairs and so forth that they become visible. Consequently, Americans inadvertently eat approximately 0.45–0.90 kg (1–2 lb) of (invisible) insect parts a year – ground up in their strawberry jam, peanut butter, spaghetti sauce, apple sauce . . . However, the occasional bug is only, as many people joke, 'added protein' and should be the least of our worries.

Food processing methods act as a double-edged sword. Sometimes unexpected and unwanted contaminants are added to the end product. But at the same time, food companies often eliminate the healthy, nutritious part of food in an effort to present their products in a way that is considered wholesome by the public. The result is that an estimated 80 per cent of American supermarket purchases can be classified as 'junk food' – devitalized food with little, if any, nutritional value.

A perfect example of this is bread. Wholemeal bread, which had come to be associated with the roughness of farm life and, in Britain, with rationing (as the 'National Loaf') during and after World War II, was no longer to the tastes of consumers. Food companies then gladly separated both the germ (the sprouting part of the whole grain, which contains protein, polyunsaturated fats, vitamin E and other important nutrients) and the bran (the outermost, vitamin B-rich fibre layer of the kernel) from the starchy endosperm of the wheat, to produce processed white-ish flour. Bleaching created the 'pure' white flour used to make America's all-time favourite – white bread. In Britain, manufacturers perform the same kind of elimination as their American counterparts, but are then required by law to *put back* some of the goodness they have taken away.

Another result of this needless processing is the totally bland taste of foods. It is no wonder that – when referring to the American restaurant fare he faced in his *Travels with Charley*, published as long ago as 1962 – John Steinbeck said, 'In eating places along the roads, the food has been clean, tasteless, colorless, and of a complete sameness.'

PEACE OF MIND?

Food manufacturers not only take out the nutrients – and usually tasty – part of a food during processing. As if that isn't bad enough, they also add substances that are actually detrimental to our health. It is fortunate that manufacturers are now required by law to label their products. In the US, over 80 per cent of consumers consult these labels when buying a product for the first time.

When the FDA began regulating labelling information in 1906, food companies were required to include only the name of the product, the name and location of the manufacturer, packer or distributor, and the net contents or net weight of the product. Today, this meagre amount of information would do little for any consumer's peace of mind. When trying to find healthy food, the important part of a label is the ingredient information.

However, there is still no law in either the US or the UK that forces manufacturers to list *all* the ingredients of a product. As a result, the label may reveal only a portion of what you are eating. For example, the USFDA has established 'standards of identity' or 'definitions' for the labelling of about 300 products presently on the market, which means that these products have specified mandatory ingredients that legally do not have to be identified on ingredient lists. Throughout the European Community, flavourings – the largest group of additives in the food chemist's kitchen – do not have to be listed separately by name, even though 3700 are in use in the UK alone.

In both the United States and Britain, regulations determine the minimum standards of composition for common foods, what additives need not be listed and when and what generalized terminology may be used in place of specific ingredients. The purpose of all this was ostensibly to simplify label reading, but it has instead resulted in more confusion for consumers and has given manufacturers a way to hide ingredients that buyers may consider unacceptable.

Of the ingredients that are listed, both the FDA and the UK's MAFF require that the one present in the largest amount by weight be listed first, the next largest second and so forth. Ingredients are also required to be listed by their 'common or usual names'.

In the US, nutritional information is required on a label only if one or more nutrients are added to the food or if a nutritional claim is made about the product. This section of the label must show the number of calories and the amount of protein, fat, carbohydrates and sodium in a specified serving of the product. Nutrition information must also show the percentage of the US Recommended Daily Allowances (USRDA) for seven essential vitamins and minerals in each serving.

The European Community has been trying to draft proposals to control food claims since 1981; they have already come up with some proposals to deal with food claims. However, in the absence of any agreement, the UK began to implement its own rules in April 1992. Now foods for which nutritional claims have been made must be 'labelled with an indication of the particular aspect of its composition or manufacturing process which gives it its particular nutritional characteristics.' In addition,

FOODS WHICH CLAIM TO PROVIDE ENERGY OR PROTEIN, CONTAIN VITAMINS OR MINERALS, AID SLIMMING OR WEIGHT CONTROL, TO BE SUITABLE FOR DIABETICS, OR WHICH MAKE CLAIMS RELATING TO POLYUNSATURATED FATTY ACIDS OR THE PRESENCE OR ABSENCE OF CHOLESTEROL MUST BE LABELLED WITH ADDITIONAL PARTICULARS SUPPORTING THE CLAIM.[7]

In addition, since October 1993 manufacturers making claims for their foods have had to provide nutrition information in tabular form. Until October 1995, they must tell consumers how much energy (i.e. calories), protein, carbohydrate and fat is in their product, plus details about any nutrient mentioned in the claim (e.g. saturates). After that date, they must give more detailed information: how much of the carbohydrate content is made up of sugars, how much of the fat content is made up of saturates, and how much sodium is present in the product.

Despite – or, perhaps, because of – the information provided, the majority of consumers today are still mystified by product labels. This is especially true of two of the most well-publicized yet unhealthy ingredients in processed foods: sodium and sugar.

BOWLING BALLS OF SALT

Many of us have felt a craving for a bag of potato crisps covered in salt (sodium chloride). Unfortunately it is cravings such as these that, added to the amount of sodium that manufacturers insist on including in their foods, cause the average American to eat about 6.8 kg (15 lb) of salt a year – an amount the size of a bowling ball.

Although sodium is a mineral essential for regulating body fluids and muscle function, excessive amounts may lead to hypertension, migraine headaches, abnormal fluid retention and potassium loss. High sodium consumption can also interfere with proper utilization of protein and increase the chances of heart disease. In addition, there is some evidence that the increased consumption of salt in the Western diet has led to an increase in the incidence of asthma.[8]

Some of the most persuasive evidence of the dangers of various types of diets comes from comparing different cultures that each have consistent rates of certain diseases that are associated with certain kinds of diets.[9] In the case of high sodium intake, we can compare the Japanese and the Americans. The former eat large amounts of salted and pickled foods and have high rates of stomach cancer. Although most Americans eat too much salt, their consumption of it is less than that of their Japanese counterparts – and their rate of stomach cancer is much lower.

Because of the bad press that sodium has received, many of us have consciously tried to cut down on the amount we consume. But it is almost impossible to escape it in the modern diet, as it is added in huge amounts to processed foods that we may never consider to be salty: cheese, soy sauce, pickles, olives, ketchup and even baked goods.

If you try to make sense of food labels in an effort to cut down your sodium consumption, you could easily become extremely frustrated. Labels are often written in 'manufacturese' – not 'consumerese' – specifically to benefit the company. When we think of sodium, we usually think of salt – sodium chloride – but it is the long-term consumption of sodium in high doses and *in any form* that can cause illness. Salt, 40 per cent of which is sodium, is the largest single source of the mineral in our diets, but there are some 70 other sodium compounds used in foods. It is no wonder that there is such confusion when it comes to finding low-sodium products at the supermarket. It is highly probable that many people who think they are eating low-sodium diets are actually consuming more than they should.

The FDA has required sodium content information on food labels since July 1986, but this hasn't entirely eased the difficulty that Americans have in finding low-sodium and sodium-free foods. US manufacturers normally use the following terms:
- 'sodium free, 'salt free' and 'no salt added' for products with less than 5mg of sodium per serving.
- 'very low sodium' for products with 35 mg or less per serving.
- 'low sodium' for products with 140 mg or less per serving.
- 'reduced sodium' if the normal level of sodium has been reduced by at least 75 per cent.[10]

In the UK, until the new regulations come into force in October 1995, MAFF rules on labelling in this area are much more general:

WHERE THE PRESENCE OR LOW CONTENT OF AN INGREDIENT IS GIVEN SPECIAL EMPHASIS, AN INDICATION OF THE MINIMUM OR MAXIMUM PER-CENTAGE (AS APPROPRIATE) OF THAT INGREDIENT IN THE FOOD MUST BE GIVEN NEXT TO THE NAME OF THE FOOD OR IN THE INGREDIENTS LIST CLOSE TO THE NAME OF THE INGREDIENT IN QUESTION.[11]

In any case, buyers should beware. 'Reduced sodium' may only mean lower sodium compared to another brand or an earlier version of the same product – it could still contain a substantial amount of sodium.

Manufacturers can further disguise the amount of sodium in a product by listing a serving size far smaller than you are likely to eat. The total amount of sodium can also be hidden behind a plethora of long, unpronounceable names or, in the European Community, behind 'E' numbers – e.g. monosodium glutamate (E622), sodium carbonate (E500[i]), sodium benzoate (E211), sodium propionate (E281), sodium stearoyl-2-lactylate (E481).

Because they realize that most people have a taste for salt, manufacturers have no intention of decreasing the amount of sodium in their products unless forced to – the FDA's request that the American food industry voluntarily reduce sodium was largely ignored. That leaves the problem of sodium reduction for us to solve. However, while this may at first appear next to impossible for someone born and raised on processed foods, it is not nearly as difficult as it may seem. Eat fresh foods and eliminate every packaged or canned food possible, take the salt shaker off your table, learn to be creative with herbs and spices when you cook – and you will be well on you way to a 'low sodium' diet.

HIDDEN SUGARS

Sugar, like sodium, is another ingredient that tends to sneak up on the consumer unawares. Because it is used not only as a sweetener but also to preserve food, to improve its texture and appearance and to absorb and retain moisture, sugar may be added to foods we wouldn't normally think of as sweet. Peanut butter, canned vegetables, tinned soups and even salt can contain sugar. The average American now eats almost 60 kg (130 lb) of 'natural' sweeteners annually; the average person in Britain consumes up to 22 teaspoonfuls every day, which, in a year, would fill a 40 litre (9 gal.) vat!

The problem begins with the fact that humans are genetically programmed to like sweet tastes. It seems that our prehistoric ancestors not only gained the energy to survive but also developed their larger brains because of diets that contained relatively high amounts of starches and sugars – that is, carbohydrates. Even today, this inborn positive response to sweets is so strong that it is sometimes termed an addiction, one as overwhelming as the craving for nicotine, alcohol or heroin.

Despite our biological response to sweets, the powers-that-be insist that sugar is bad for us. They have told us, along with our parents and our dentists, that eating it can lead to tooth decay and other health problems. Too much sugar, they say, can cause obesity, which in turn can increase the possibility of heart disease, mature-onset diabetes, hypertension, gallstones, back problems, arthritis. Some say it is responsible for personality changes and mood swings, and can cause the loss or imbalance of the body's essential nutrients.[12]

Because sugar is not good for our health when consumed in large quantities, many of us have tried dutifully to cut down. But identifying sugars on food labels is no easy task – they are perhaps even more hidden than sodium. Sodium is sodium whether it be sodium benzoate or sodium carbonate. Sugar, on the other hand, comes in a variety of forms, with names that are completely unidentifiable as sugar.

- *Fructose*, also known as laevulose. The sweetest sugar of them all; found in fruit. Since it is a 'natural' sugar, one might think it would be good for us, but in reality, it is utterly devoid of nutrients.
- *Glucose*, as well as a natural sugar found in most fruits, also the body's blood sugar. A monosaccharide, or 'single sugar', it is the simplest form of sugar.
- *Dextrose*, another monosaccharide that is chemically identical to glucose but made from cornstarch. Despite this difference, glucose is frequently referred to as dextrose.
- *Sucrose*, refined sugar, seen in its white granulated table form or as icing sugar; made from either sugar cane or sugar beets. It is a disaccharide, or 'double sugar', composed of both glucose and fructose. It also contains no nutritional value whatsoever.
  Demerara and other brown sugars may give the appearance of being less processed and therefore retaining some of their original nutrients. However, they are simply forms of refined white table sugar which have had molasses added for colouring.
- *Maltose*, a disaccharide made from the malting of whole grains. Although this may make it sound nutritious, it is no more so than any other sugar.
- *Lactose*, a milk sugar containing both glucose and another monosaccharide, galactose. While it is the least sweet, and may also appear nutritious because it comes from milk, it (like all refined sugars) lacks any nutrients. Lactose intolerance is common among people originating from Africa, Asia and South America.
- *Xylitol* (E967), produced commercially from xylose, or 'wood sugar'. Used mostly in products for diabetics, studies have linked xylitol (in large doses over long periods) with tumours and organ injury in animals. It is presently under review by the USFDA, and most US manufacturers have voluntarily stopped using it. However, it has been permitted throughout the European Community since 1 January 1993 (when food standards were harmonized), with the provisos that consumption should be limited to reduce its laxative effects, and that it may not be suitable for babies and young children.[13] In the EC, it is often used as a sugar substitute in the manufacture of sweets and chewing gum.

- *Sorbitol* (E420[i]), occurs naturally in fruits, berries, algae and seaweeds; made commercially by combining hydrogen and corn sugar. Because it raises the concentration of blood glucose more slowly and to a lesser extent than sucrose, sorbitol is used in many foods for diabetics. However, because the first product of its metabolism is fructose, some physicians doubt whether it is entirely safe to give to diabetics.[14] Because of its laxative effects, the EC has ruled that it should be not be used in foods or sweets intended for children under three.
- *Mannitol* (E421), occurs naturally in beetroot, celery and olives; also made industrially from hydrogen and corn sugar. No studies have been carried out to determine its possible negative side-effects to humans. However, it is recognized that, like sorbitol, mannitol is a laxative; yet the EC allows it in baby foods, but only when used as a carrier for other ingredients.

Any of these nine different types of sugar may, in their scientific disguises, grace packages of processed foods, leading people to believe that they are not eating sugar when they actually are.

There are other types of sugars that are far more simple to pick out and may seem to be nutritious at first glance. These include blackstrap molasses, black treacle, honey, maple syrup and golden syrup. However, of all of these, only blackstrap molasses and black treacle have any nutritional value, containing small but useful amounts of iron, calcium, potassium and B vitamins, particularly vitamin B_6.

According to current labelling rules in the EC, food producers have to list total sugars (i.e. separate from the blanket term 'carbohydrates') only if they have made a health claim such as 'low in sugar'. As a result, most don't list them. In any event, many of us trying to avoid sugar would rather not cope with the deciphering of labels and instead head straight for the packets branded 'no sugar added'. But even this label is deceiving – the term has no standing in law and usually refers to sucrose alone. Hence, your barbecue sauce that promises 'No sugar!' may be packed full of fructose. (Another ploy is for this label to appear on foods that *never* contain any sugar . . .)

Labels that say 'sugar-free' or 'sugarless' are slightly more honest. These products contain none of the common sugars such as glucose or fructose, but may include the sugar alcohols (xylitol, sorbitol and mannitol), provided the reason for the use of these is explained on the package – as an alternative to sugar in biscuits for diabetics, for example.

HEALTH KICKS

At this point, the farce that is today's commercialization of food becomes apparent. The games that manufacturers play with the consumer would be comical if it weren't for the fact that they're affecting public health.

Manufacturers let their labels reveal to you what they want you to know, not necessarily what you need to know. Nowhere has this become more evident than in the recent craze for 'added vitamins'. Because vitamins and minerals and their role in good health became a prominent issue and important to the public, manufacturers suddenly decided to go on a health kick and now add these nutrients to every conceivable food product. However, the mere fact that a package is plastered with 'shout lines' promoting the addition of these substances should make you stop and ask: 'Why was it necessary to add vitamins/minerals in the first place?' The claim of added nutrients may be just as deceiving as the cover-up of sodium and sugar.

These so-called 'fortified' foods may appear to be nutritious at the first quick glance. However, fortification is often the pumping of nutrients into foods that never contained those specific vitamins and/or minerals in the first place. The addition of calcium to orange juice makes it a fortified drink – but what's the point? The fortifying of white bread with the B vitamins thiamin and nicotinic acid and the minerals iron and calcium carbonate is demanded by law in the UK; breakfast cereals, too, are given extra vitamins and, sometimes, iron and protein. But in both cases, this fortification is required because the manufacturing process has stripped these foods of their natural goodness.

However, there is a bit of a silver lining in all this. The fact that the food industry is now touting the addition of vitamins and minerals in their products can be seen as something of a good sign, as it reflects people's growing awareness of food and its link to good health. First, certain illnesses became associated by the public with the overuse of sodium and sugar. Then they were informed of the benefits of various vitamins and minerals. This led to new concerns about too much fat and cholesterol and too little fibre in most diets.

But this new awareness of the inherent qualities of food has actually complicated the task of finding healthy products in the supermarket. While most shoppers may eventually learn how to pick out the sodium and sugar on labels, today's deceptive advertising regarding fat, cholesterol and fibre may leave many people completely confused or, worse, believing they're eating well when they're not.

FAT IS AN ISSUE

The fat content of food is one of the primary concerns of shoppers today. Yet we largely ignore the fact that fat is a necessary part of our diets, providing energy and carrying into the body the fat-soluble vitamins A, D, E and K and two essential fatty acids (linoleic and linolenic), as well as making many foods palatable.

It is the over-consumption of fat that can cause problems. Many of us have horrible visions of fat globules slowly settling around our waistlines and worry about fatty foods for this reason. However, research suggests that excessive fat in a person's diet may also lead to disease.

Animal studies, first conducted in the 1940s, revealed that rodents fed high-fat diets were more likely to develop mammary tumours than others fed normal diets.[15] Later, researchers began to notice that people who emigrated from countries where low-fat diets were the norm to places where high-fat diets were standard developed 'high-fat diet diseases'. The most widely cited comparison was again between the Japanese and the Americans. People in Japan eat much less beef and total fat than the citizens of the United States: little more than 40 g (1.4 oz) of fat a day – comprising only 23 per cent of an average individual's total energy (i.e. calories), compared with, for example, 42 per cent in Britain.[16] The Japanese also have much lower rates of breast and bowel cancer and heart disease than the Americans. However, the offspring of Japanese immigrants to the United States, after years of consuming the average American diet – which typically includes almost 150 g (5.3 oz) of fat a day – are far more likely to succumb to these diseases than their relatives back in Japan.

Further research has shown that countries such as the Netherlands and Denmark, renowned for national diets heavy in high-fat cheeses and cream, have even higher rates of death from breast cancer than the US.[17] And Britain – with its traditions of fish and chips and fried breakfasts, and its relatively recently acquired devotion to fast foods – has the highest death rate of all, with some 15,000 women dying of breast cancer every year, 45 every day.

With this type of information coming to light, it is no wonder that most consumers are concerned about their fat intake. But when they head down to the supermarket and scan the shelves for foods with little or no fat, they slowly begin to feel the confusion setting in. To understand label information concerning the fat content in foods, it is necessary to understand fats themselves.

The fats in foods are a mixture of *saturated* and *unsaturated* fatty acids. Those with a high proportion of saturated fatty acids are solid or nearly solid at room temperature and are normally found in foods of animal origin, such as lard and butter. Two vegetable oils are exceptions: palm oil, which is 86 per cent saturated fat, and coconut oil, which is 92 per cent. It is this type of fatty acid that is associated with atherosclerosis, the clogging of the arteries.

Fats with mostly unsaturated fatty acids are all of vegetable origin and remain liquid at room temperature. They may be either *monounsaturated* or *polyunsaturated*. Olive oil and groundnut (peanut) oil are especially high in monounsaturated fatty acids, while safflower, sunflower, corn, soya and grapeseed oils are high in polyunsaturated fatty acids.

Further misunderstanding comes from the labelling terms *hydrogenated* and *partially hydrogenated*. These refer to the process of adding hydrogen to an unsaturated fat to make it solid at room temperature and to increase its shelf life. Oils may be processed in this way to varying degrees to make them suitable for use in products such as margarine. The drawback to this procedure is that the more an oil is hydrogenated, the more saturated fatty acids (here called 'trans fatty acids') it contains. In a recent reassessment of the global evidence concerning the role of fat in coronary heart disease, Frans Kok, professor of epidemiology at Wageningen Agricultural University in the Netherlands, has concluded that trans fatty acids are as harmful as any saturates of animal origin. [18]

When checking labels, remember that ingredients are listed in descending order of predominance by weight. Therefore, if a fat or oil is one of the first ingredients in a list, it is safe to assume that the product has a high fat content! When fat is one of the main ingredients, the specific type must be listed. But in the US, when fat is less than 10 per cent of the product, the manufacturer is allowed to list several fats that the product may or may not contain. For instance, 'Oil (contains one or more of the following: soya, partially hydrogenated corn, palm or coconut)' could mean the oil is highly saturated ('palm or coconut'), technologically modified ('partially hydrogenated corn') or polyunsaturated ('soya'). In the UK, if such a compound ingredient comprises anything up to *25 per cent* of the finished product, the names of the ingredients making up the compound one do not have to be listed at all. [19]

Beware of manufacturers' buzz words. 'Made with 100 per cent vegetable oil' may mean that the product is made with palm or coconut oils – both vegetable oils but both high in saturated fats. 'Low in saturated fat' may describe a food that is still high in monounsaturated or polyunsaturated fats – therefore, the total energy (calorie) content will be quite high.

THE CHOLESTEROL TRAP

Cholesterol, a fat-like substance, is the next most worrisome diet issue for many people. Like fat, it is also essential to bodily functions, but unlike other nutrients, our livers produce all that our bodies need. After the age of five, there is no nutritional reason to include cholesterol in the diet, and so the amounts that many people consume often become excessive.

Cholesterol is found in foods of animal origin, such as red meat, poultry and dairy products, but not in foods from plants. Science has linked the presence of too much cholesterol in a person's blood to the development of heart disease. As most people in Western countries eat large quantities of meat and dairy products, it is not surprising that many have a problem with cholesterol. Manufacturers, aware of this new concern of their customers, try to use label information regarding cholesterol to their own benefit.

We've all seen 'NO CHOLESTEROL' emblazoned across packages of various foods. While the claims may be true, they can be deceiving. It is a fact that vegetable products do not contain cholesterol, but what these labels aren't shouting is that the product may be full of saturated fat which is far more likely to raise your blood cholesterol levels than eating cholesterol itself.

THE FIBRE BANDWAGON

The fibre content in food products, although not as vital to most shoppers as the sodium, sugar, vitamin, fat and cholesterol content, is fast becoming an important consideration. Studies have shown that the typical diets of most populations in industrialized countries consist of far too little fibre. Today, the British adult consumes a daily average of 22 g (0.8 oz) of fibre; a century ago, that figure was about 40 g (1.4 oz), and in prehistoric times, it was approximately 45 g (1.6 oz). This decrease in fibre consumption is now known to have led to higher rates of certain ailments and diseases: constipation, diverticulitis, gall-bladder disease and, especially, bowel cancer.

Dietary fibre is the part of plant cells that is not digested in the small intestine. Its health benefits first attracted attention in 1970 when the British researcher Dr Denis Burkitt published his findings.[20] He had discovered that certain African populations whose diets included large amounts of fibre had relatively few of the cancers and intestinal diseases that afflicted more affluent societies. The reason, scientists now believe, is that not only does dietary fibre increase the bulk and softness of stools and lowers high pressures in the bowel, it also reduces the time that cancer-causing substances reside in the gut and dilutes their concentration. The bulk of high-fibre foods actually carries toxins out of the body.

Bran and prune juice jokes aside, fibre is a very complex issue. Scientists cannot seem to decide what exactly constitutes fibre in food. Early studies (using what is known as the Southgate method) measured only the crude fibre, rather than making a distinction between the digestion-resistant starch and the digestible non-starch polysaccharides (NSPs) measured by the newer Englyst method.[21] Today, when researchers analyse the fibre content of food, they look at the total amount of fibre, as well as the proportion of soluble and insoluble fibre. The amounts of various types of fibre – such as hemicellulose, pectin, mucilage, cellulose and lignin – as well as the gum content for oats and barley, are also considered.

Not only is there confusion surrounding the different types of dietary fibres, but also what benefits these different types may have on health. For a long time, it was believed that dietary fibre merely provided bulk and helped normalize bowel movements. But recent studies seem to show that different fibres play various roles: water-*soluble* fibre may reduce the risk of heart disease and gallstones, and is helpful in the control of diabetes; water-*insoluble* fibre products the bulk that first comes to mind when we think of fibre.

Manufacturers, not ones to let promotional opportunities pass them by, have jumped on the fibre bandwagon as well. Unfortunately, labels advertising the fibre content of foods may be just as misleading as labels promoting other constituents of foods.

Some novel ingredients have cropped up in the manufacturers' quest for fibre in their products. One of the new forms actually used in foods meant for human consumption is purified wood pulp, an inexpensive by-product of the pulp paper industry. Semi-synthetic and totally artificial forms of cellulose have also been created. The dietary fibre craze and the consequent fibre substitutes have been a boon to food manufacturers. Rather than use relatively costly but nutritious food ingredients, they can fill their products with inexpensive non-nutritious ones – and still have the public flock to their labels simply because it says: 'HIGH FIBRE'.

Consumers are sometimes so blinded by the highly promoted health benefits of dietary fibre that they forget about the other things lurking in processed foods. For instance, that nutritious-looking, plump little bran muffin is probably also filled with sugar, sodium and saturated fat; the fibre in the bran may or may not be an equal trade-off. One British bread producer announces (in a wholesome Yorkshire accent) that its whole-meal bread has 'Nowt taken out' – but doesn't advertise what might have been put *in*.

HOW MUCH IS TOO MUCH?

'Over-consumption' is the watchword of our age. The link between obesity and disease is fairly well accepted in the scientific community. A more heavily debated issue concerns the link between dietary excesses and disease. For instance, most scientists believe that a diet high in cholesterol and saturated fats is likely to lead to heart disease, but how much of these fats is too much is still vigorously debated.

Meanwhile, other evidence of the link between diet and disease (or, in this case, the absence of disease) has come to light. Researchers have noted that obesity, mature-onset diabetes, hypertension and the other 'diseases of civilization' occur infrequently, if at all, in the modern hunter-gatherer societies that they have studied. Even when they live to advanced age, these people do not develop the conditions we consider a natural part of ageing. For example, in industrialized cultures it is considered quite normal for blood pressure and blood sugar levels to rise with age, yet these conditions do not occur among modern hunter-gatherers.

More startling is the fact that many young people in Western nations already show early signs of such chronic conditions as hypertension and atherosclerosis. Post-mortems on individuals in their late teens and early 20s, who have been killed in car accidents, have revealed that the early stages of these conditions sometimes appear at a very young age: many already showed signs of atherosclerotic plaques in their arteries. This is unheard of in hunter-gatherer societies.

Other research has demonstrated that – like the Japanese immigrants to the US – when people from hunter-gatherer societies move to industrialized settings, or when they simply adopt more Western lifestyles, the rates of chronic illness increase. Until the middle of this century, few Native Americans had diabetes. Now tribes such as the Pimas, found in the south-west United States, have some of the highest rates of this disease in the world. This rise in disease has also been documented in countries such as Ireland, Italy and Greece – and in Japan itself – as their populations changed their eating habits and lifestyles to fit a more Western model.

It has come to the point that, today, we can honestly say that we are literally eating ourselves to death. Why are we doing this? The answer may well be just as complex as the food industry itself, and buried beneath layers of custom and ritual, some of which have taken years to develop, while others have only surfaced within the last two decades.

WHO EATS WHAT?

The earliest rituals surrounding eating originated with the development of hunting among prehistoric humans. Communal eating became a way of sharing the spoils of the hunt, and was one of the first marks of civilization that set humans apart from animals. Before this, early peoples behaved like their ape cousins in their solitary and selfish consumption of whatever food they could gather.

As time passed, other factors came to determine what and how human beings ate. The geographic location, religious rites and social customs of a society all influenced the consumption of food. Many societies have retained the same eating habits for many decades if not centuries. It is the habits of the industrialized nations that have changed most radically, not only because of the foods the people eat, but also how they view food and the entire eating process itself.

Nowhere were these changes more drastic than in the United States. Since the 1960s, the food industry has witnessed – and, in part, helped to create – a major upheaval in the mealtimes of most families and individuals. But the changes have not been the same throughout American society. How an American consumer of the late 20th century eats basically depends on his or her income, age, type of work, level of education and cultural setting.

These underlying factors that determine the choice of food were reflected in a study carried out by the Pillsbury Company in 1988. After analysing the eating habits of 3000 American consumers over a 15-year period, researchers were able to separate them into five categories:

• *The 'chase-and-grabbits'* The largest and fastest growing group of consumers, comprising highly educated young urban singles and working couples without children. They have enough money to eat out and prefer this to cooking at home. Because of their busy lifestyles, they are the primary purchasers of convenience foods, consuming fast-food hamburgers, frozen dinners and microwavable *entrées* in huge quantities, with little thought of how this might affect their future health.

• *The 'careful cooks'* Usually upper-income, well-educated retired couples who have frequently had previous health problems, such as heart attacks, which have caused them to be careful about what they eat. Typical foods include wholemeal bread, skimmed milk, yoghurt, fresh fruits and vegetables, fish, skinless chicken and salads. Along with the 'chase-and-grabbits', this is the only group of eaters to increase during the Pillsbury study.

The remaining categories of consumers comprise people with the eating habits most often associated with traditional America.

• *The 'down-home stokers'* Usually modest-income, blue-collar (i.e. manual worker) families who staunchly prefer regional, often high-fat home cooking. Foods eaten by this group might include home-fried chicken, cornbread, sweet potato pie and vegetables cooked with bacon.

• *The 'happy cookers'* Normally grandmothers and younger mothers who enjoy baking and home cooking for their families. Foods common to this group might be homemade pies, cakes, meatloaves and casseroles.

• *The 'functional feeders'* Typically blue-collar, working parents over the age of 45, who tend to rely on traditional convenience foods such as canned soup, instant potatoes, frozen macaroni cheese.

Although this study separates and categorizes Americans by their lifestyles and the way they eat in general, it doesn't attempt to explain fully why people eat the way they do. It doesn't address the major social changes that have influenced all sectors of society, or give any indication of the effects these eating habits might have on the members of the different groups.

The 'baby-boomer' generation has seen a huge increase in the number of women working outside the home, and this has been one of the main reasons for changes in our way of eating. Now that more than half of all women hold down jobs, the image (still perpetuated by many advertisers) of Mum serving her adoring family a Mum-cooked dinner is well on its way to becoming extinct. Women no longer have the time to prepare elaborate meals. Convenience is a top priority, and if a meal takes more than 30 minutes to make, most women don't want to know. It has been said that, by the year 2000, cooking will have become a hobby, just like sewing is today.

Once the woman of the house determined what food was eaten, but this is no longer always the case. Although most women are still primarily responsible for the preparation of food, other members of the family will often shop and cook for themselves, and sometimes even eat by themselves. Increasingly, it's the individual who decides what and when to eat.

The fast pace of today's lifestyles has spurred industry – including food manufacturers – to accommodate our demands for convenience. Consequently, one of the most dramatic influences on our eating habits has been the introduction of microwave ovens and the pre-prepared foods to cook in them.

Over 75 per cent of American homes now have at least one microwave, and some even have two. Britain is slightly behind: the proportion of households owning a microwave increased from just 6 per cent in 1983 to 60 per cent in 1993.[22] When microwaves first became available to the general public in the 1970s, they were used only to cook single food items, such as baked potatoes, or to reheat leftovers. Foods such as stews, soups and roasts were still reserved for the cooker or the conventional oven. When, in the mid-1980s, food manufacturers finally realized the market potential of foods that could go from shelf to microwave to table, many replaced traditional foil serving trays for frozen foods with containers that were 'microwavable'. Result: no dishes, no pots and pans, no mess, virtually no time spent in the kitchen! Hundreds of products produced by manufacturers now have a microwave angle to them. You can buy microwavable vegetables, stews, lasagne, cakes and even individual cheeseburgers.

Those who simply want nothing to do with cooking and are satisfied with a cheap evening meal can turn to the typical fast-food restaurant. Pizzas, hamburgers, fried chicken and Indian and Chinese food are among the things on offer – to eat there, take away or, in some instances, to have delivered at home, often for free. For those who are tired of typical fast-food fare, more upmarket restaurants are now going into the take-away business. Practically anything that a restaurant serves can now be bought in convenient little containers and eaten at home (possibly after being reheated in a microwave).

In addition, the market for ready-cooked/prepared foods is the fastest growing part of the food industry. The no-cook, no-fuss meals now available from delicatessen counters at many supermarkets are a prime example of the popularity of these. Once convenience food meant a can of soup; today, a growing number of shops are providing their customers with freshly prepared foods: whole meals including appetizers, main courses, vegetables and desserts – and, in some cases, even salad bars. A portion of this lucrative market comprises independent gourmet take-away shops and fancy delis, where yuppie couples with money to burn and no time to spend think nothing of picking up their entire evening meal this way.

All this may sound terribly quick and easy, but the numerous negative results of surviving on such diets are seldom revealed. The most worrying aspect of this increased demand for convenience is that, where once perhaps only a portion of a meal came from a packet – for instance, instant potatoes – now whole meals are at the mercy of food manufacturers' decisions. Mum no longer has the time or inclination to ensure that her family eats fresh fruits and vegetables daily, and the manufacturer of the microwavable dinners she buys is the one who decides what she and her partner and her children eat.

The situation is made worse by the fact that children – notorious for eating what they want when they want it – are sometimes left to make meals for themselves. You could find your children living on a diet of jam doughnuts washed down with equally sugary squash or soft drinks. Unfortunately, it's your children's diet during the first 18 years of their lives that may determine their future health.

Fast-food restaurants provide no better sustenance. Most foods from these outlets are extremely high in saturated fats, cholesterol, sodium and sugar. Yet, despite warnings of the potential hazards of diets high in these ingredients, fast-food sales are growing. Restaurant and deli fare may give slightly more nutrition but even these alternatives have their drawbacks. How many restaurants produce truly edible vegetable dishes, and how many delis feature freshly cooked spinach?

AFFLUENT MALNUTRITION

The changes in Western society that have occurred over the last few decades, and the convenience products that have popped up to support them, indicate more than an increasingly profitable market for food, a demand for instant meals or alterations in lifestyles. That's the way these changes are perceived from the food industry's perspective. However, these eating trends actually reflect a public that has forgotten the link between food consumption and health.

Our food problems – 'affluent malnutrition', over-consumption, eating disorders – are connected to our lifestyles and diet. In the United States alone, a conservative estimate is that six of the ten major causes of death are diet related.

A large sector of society today views food preparation and even eating as disagreeable interruptions in the business of life. For instance, it is important to the 'chase-and-grabbits' – who see food only as substances that quell hunger pangs – to take care of this nuisance as quickly as possible, with whatever tasty edible happens to be at hand, so that they can return to their work or play. The nutrition – or, rather, the lack of it – that they derive from the foods they eat is of little consequence to them. As a result, their bodies continue to be deprived of the sustenance necessary for proper functioning until – one day – the symptoms of 'affluent malnutrition' appear and can no longer be ignored. Where will the typical 'chase-and-grabbit' be in 20 or 30 years? Probably in the 'careful cooks' category – struggling with various health problems.

At the other end of the scale, there is an equally large portion of society that is obsessed with food. Those who are extremely overweight try desperately to lose their excess fat through various 'foolproof' but dangerous diets. Blinded by their desire to slim, they also care little about the nutritional aspects of the food they eat, only that it is 'low calorie'.

Here again, the food manufacturers step in, their keen sense of profits telling them that there is money to be made. The soaring sales of low-calorie soft drinks and desserts, artificial sweeteners, calorie-reduced salad dressings and frozen diet dinners are testimony to the number of people who are (or think they are) suffering from weight problems, and the huge profits the food industry is making from this.

But industry – food manufacturers but also other sectors – not only profits from dieters: it is also a large part of the problem. Commercials portray slim, sexy young people (primarily young women), many of them promoting low-cal, low-fat, low-cholesterol foods. Dieters, trying to emulate these strong images, refuse to eat any foods that are not similarly low-cal, low-fat, low-cholesterol, but then, ravenously hungry because their bodies are not receiving the nourishment they need, they break their diets and are soon back where they started. Flip on the television and there is yet another slim, sexy young woman promoting both food and image. The vicious circle is complete.

Related to this are two serious (and sometimes fatal) eating disorders: bulimia and anorexia nervosa. Doctors who have studied and treated people suffering from these conditions contend that there is a wide variety of possible causes, including physical or sexual abuse during childhood, but most agree that deeply entrenched societal values are a major factor. The equating of thinness with beauty by the media puts pressure on young and vulnerable individuals to mould themselves to the image they believe is acceptable to society.

FOOD AS MEDICINE

What we have today is a public bombarded on all sides with nutrition information – some of it valid, some of it contradictory, some of it reflecting only the interests of the parties who will benefit from the public's response to it. We also have media that assume we desire to be or look a certain way and then mirrors our desires back at us through advertisements designed only to sell a product, with little thought as to how that product might affect our health. We lead hectic, pressured lives, push ourselves to keep pace and, at the same time, withhold the nutrition our bodies require to withstand the frantic daily activity. The bottom line is: we're a mess. And the best place to start pulling ourselves out of that mess is at the beginning, at Square One.

Science is telling us that the highly processed foods we eat are detrimental to our health. Studies comparing our diets with those of our prehistoric ancestors and of modern hunter-gatherers consistently point up the difference between their wonderful physical health and our lack of it. If the food we eat can damage our health and cause disease, then the converse would seem logical: the food we eat could also promote health and prevent disease. Ancient societies understood this. Why can't we?

Edmond Bordeaux Szchely, who carried out extensive research on the Dead Sea Scrolls, found that the Essenes, compilers of the Scrolls in the last centuries of the pre-Christian era, divided foods into categories based on what they perceived as their inherent energies. 'Biogenic' (from the ancient Greek meaning 'life-generating') foods are those that can be planted to produce more foods – e.g. seeds, whole grains, nuts and pulses. 'Bioactive' foods provide nourishment to the human body and sustain it, but cannot generate new life – e.g. fresh fruits and vegetables. 'Biostatic' foods are neither life-generating nor life-sustaining, and slow down life processes in the body – e.g. cooked foods and those that are not fresh. Finally, 'biocidic' ('life-destroying') foods are actually harmful to the body. In the modern diet, these would include foods containing additives and preservatives and those that have been refined and otherwise processed. Three quarters of the food in your local supermarket probably falls into this last category.

Other cultures went even further than the Essene community and used food specifically as medicine. It was the basis of medicine in ancient Egypt, Babylonia, Greece and China, and in Europe during the Middle Ages. It has been only within the last 100 years – and, particularly, the last 50 – that the industrial societies of the world have become dependent on artificially manufactured drugs to cure illnesses. These worked wonderfully against the infections that caused so many deaths in the past, but now, in the late 20th century, the main causes of mortality are chronic illnesses such as cancer and heart disease, against which drugs have been signally unsuccessful.

Today, researchers are beginning to look once more at the medicinal value of foods, and scientists have 'discovered' that various foods have the ability to heal. For instance:

- A chemical in barley is believed to control the production of cholesterol by the liver.
- Spicy hot foods, such as chilli peppers, appear to prevent and treat bronchitis and emphysema.
- Onions seem to be helpful in treating heart conditions, as they contain chemicals that thin the blood, retard clotting and raise a beneficial type of cholesterol.
- Rice bran apparently helps to prevent kidney stones.[23]

Although physicians from the establishment have only recently begun to look into the healing properties of foods, other sectors of the medical world have for some time understood the value of maintaining a proper diet centred around healthy food. Many of these latter doctors, who practise preventive medicine, believe that nutrition affects not only the physical body but the mind as well.

The doctor who finally diagnosed my friend Katie as malnourished is a perfect example: a practitioner of orthomolecular psychiatry. Linus Pauling, twice winner of the Nobel prize (for chemistry and peace), has described orthomolecular psychiatry as 'treatment of mental disorders by the provision of the optimum molecular environment for the mind, especially the optimum concentrations of substances normally present in the body.'[24]

The conclusion of researchers that schizophrenia is a physical illness caused by disturbances in the biochemical balance of the body established the field of orthomolecular medicine. Personalized diet plans and large doses of vitamins and minerals are prescribed along with therapy for psychiatric conditions, which include not only schizophrenia but also depression and anxiety. Even some over-eaters, alcoholics and drug abusers are being taught to control their cravings and self-destructive behaviour with adequate diets.

Proper nutrition is vital for normal brain function and good health. Research suggests that even a slight improvement in eating habits can:

- result in greater resistance to infection.
- reduce healing time.
- allow for better control of metabolic disturbances such as diabetes and hyperthyroidism.
- prevent minor mental deficiencies that can lead to a multitude of physical ailments, from common colds to cancer.

According to Dr Pauling:

THE AVAILABLE EVIDENCE INDICATES THAT, THROUGH IMPROVED NUTRI-
TION, THE AGE-SPECIFIC INCIDENCE OF DISEASE AND MORTALITY FROM
DISEASE CAN BE DECREASED TO ONE-QUARTER OF THE PRESENT VOLUME,
AND THAT OTHER HEALTH MEASURES TAKEN IN CONJUNCTION WITH THESE
COULD LEAD TO FURTHER DECREASE. THE LENGTH OF THE PERIOD OF WELL-
BEING OF MEN AND WOMEN MIGHT WELL BE INCREASED BY 16 TO 24 YEARS
THROUGH IMPROVED NUTRITION AND OTHER HEALTH MATTERS.

THE END OF KATIE'S QUEST

My friend Katie's quest for health had a happy ending. After being
diagnosed as malnourished, she was placed on a strict diet that avoided
sugar, salt, fat, caffeine, cholesterol, alcohol and processed foods as much
as possible.

She could no longer cheat and reach for coffee and a roll for breakfast
to 'jump start' her day. Instead, she was required to eat a full meal. Her
beverage choices for breakfast (and all other meals) now included fresh,
unsweetened juices, skimmed milk, herbal teas and water. Fresh fruit
and vegetables were encouraged. Rather than highly salted, fatty meats
such as bacon, ham and sausages, she could eat fish lightly sautéed in
olive oil. Whole-grain cereals without added sugar, and whole-grain
breads, muffins and pancakes replaced traditional white flour products.

Katie's lunches also changed dramatically. Rather than grab a quick
bite of pizza, she now had to choose from a selection of wholesome foods,
including pitta or whole-grain breads, tuna (low-salt, water-packed),
chicken, turkey, green leaf salads, natural cheese and yoghurt, and fresh
fruits and vegetables.

Dinner became a light affair rather than the heaviest meal of the day.
Katie could choose from a number of options, planning her meals around
pulses, poultry, fish or shellfish, or lean meats. Green leafy salads,
hearty non-creamy soups such as lentil or minestrone, a variety of fresh
vegetables (yellow, orange and green) and whole-grain breads or rolls
were also possibilities. Dessert, if desired, could consist of fruit or low-fat
yoghurt.

Initially, Katie was astounded by the volume of food her doctor
required her to eat. She was absolutely positive that she would gain
pounds and pounds and would never be able to shop in Rodeo Drive again!
However, the opposite proved true. She slowly learned to enjoy the taste
of wholesome, natural foods and, much to her surprise, even lost weight.
She found that she had enough energy to sustain her throughout the day,
and her mood swings, fatigue and irritability had disappeared.

The most important thing that Katie learned was that there was a
connection between what she ate and how she felt. Simple, nutritious

foods strengthened her body, while empty-calorie, processed foods, weakened her system and opened the door to all sorts of ailments. A return to a basic diet of lean meats, fresh fruits, mountains of vegetables and whole grains worked for Katie, and would benefit anyone whose sustenance is based primarily on processed foods.

It is ironic that the modern advanced societies are being urged to replicate the diet of their primitive ancestors. Unfortunately, what many advocates of this type of eating fail to point out is that, today, even our 'basics' are being defiled . . .

CHAPTER TWO

THE FOOD CRISIS

O ver the past half a century, doctors and psychologists have become somewhat dismayed by how much the equilibrium of the modern individual has become unbalanced. The gradual breakdown in our well-being – from weakened immune systems to mental dis-association – has caused some leading authorities to note a considerable gap between optimal health and just physical survival. This trend results in disease, discomfort, dissatisfaction and a general lack of 'wellness'. While experts are diligently and innovatively attempting to devise cures for such new-found ills, to some it has occurred that prevention should be the ideal to strive for.

A key problem that holistic physicians are faced with is that most people seek their assistance only *after* a problem has already taken its toll on their health. But if prevention is to be expected to work, it is our responsibility to get to grips with the root of our food supply problems – food adulteration. This includes processing, chemicalization, irradiation and, soon, biotechnology or food engineering.

The adulteration of the food supply for the past 50 years has allowed us not to starve but merely to be kept malnourished. Our doctors remind us to maintain a 'balanced diet', assuming that this will provide us with all the nutrients we need for good health: protein, carbohydrates, some fats, vitamins and minerals. But more than 12,000 chemicals contaminate our food during propagation, growth, harvesting, processing, packaging, shipping and preparation. The chemical brew that we consume in the guise of 'food' has, to a great extent, been the cause of much modern-day chronic ill health.

The 'balanced diet' theory is a dreadful injustice that has been palmed off on the general public by food manufacturers and the medical community. You are led to believe that, if you consume a wide variety of foods, essentially this will compensate for the 'junk foods' you eat. But this is clearly not the case: we consume about 68 kg (150 lb) of additives each year. It will take more than an apple a day – which, in any case, has more than likely been chemically treated – to ward off the harmful effects of this diet.

We shouldn't need the mind of an Einstein to eat well and healthily – after all, humans have been doing so successfully for eons. But such a mind may be required to dissect and understand the chemicalization that has drastically altered our entire food supply.

'HAZARDOUS TO YOUR HEALTH'

Strange things happen to food when it is processed. Proteins, fats and carbohydrates are isolated and then are eaten in pure form or are utilized in the 'enrichment' of laboratory-created 'foods'. Nature, however, does not provide any food in pure form. The nutrients are meant to be consumed together. Nevertheless, today we are able chemically to break down foods into any substance desired to create 'non-foods'. When robbed of all essential nutrients, these cannot be metabolized and will only be absorbed with the help of nutrients from proper foods – if they happen to be present. When this cycle occurs in your body regularly, there isn't much fuel left to support healthy tissues, organs, bones, brain . . . or to ward off diseases, especially when the immune system is weakened.

Besides the loss of vitamins and minerals through food handling, the most disturbing aspect of modern-day food processing is the abundant use of food additives. There are three basic reasons why so many are employed by food producers: (1) they enable food to be stored for very long periods; (2) artificial colourings make food look more appetizing; and (3) synthetic flavours can make food taste better after it has been processed from its natural state.

Much of what is sold to us in supermarkets and restaurants should carry warning labels – and some foods do. Saccharin – a petroleum-derived artificial sweetener that is absorbed but not modified by the body – was found to cause bladder cancer in laboratory rats. When, in 1977, the Food and Drug Administration (FDA) in the United States decided to ban it from foods and drinks, the US Congress stopped them. So a compromise was reached: saccharin was allowed to remain on the market, but a warning stating that ingesting a product containing it 'may be hazardous to your health' had to appear somewhere on the product's label. In the UK and throughout the rest of the European Community (where the sweetener is also known as E954), saccharin use is still widespread, and no warnings are required. It is specifically banned from ice cream, and is not permitted in foods specially prepared for children up to the age of three; the European Commission also recommends that children and pregnant women should 'limit their intake'. However, children ingest many foods and drinks that are not specially prepared for them and which also contain saccharin – e.g. soft drinks.

Saccharin is only one of numerous chemicals added to our food that have caused alarm bells to ring. For instance, the sulphites (E220–E228), used as preservatives in many drinks and foods, including squashes, wines and lettuce, can bring on asthma attacks and other allergic reactions. They also destroy thiamin, one of the B vitamins (*see* Chapter 5).

The flavour enhancer monosodium glutamate (MSG, or E621) has also been the subject of complaints for many years, but instead of this additive being eliminated, its use in food has actually increased ten-fold in the past decade. This known headache trigger was once confined to Chinese food and canned soups. It can now be found in a wide variety of restaurant foods – particularly sauces, soups and salad dressings – as well as in many tinned, frozen and prepared foods. The problem is that you can't always detect MSG by reading ingredient lists. In fact, most of the MSG found in foods is not identified by the words 'monosodium gluta-mate' or by its 'E' number, but by such diverse terms as 'hydrolysed vegetable protein' (HVP), 'hydrolysed plant protein', 'sodium caseinate', 'kombu extract' and, in the US, 'natural flavour', 'seasoning' and 'auto-lysed yeast flavouring'. In the EC, MSG might simply be swallowed up by the all-embracing 'flavouring'.

The headaches associated with MSG typically occur between 20 minutes and five hours after ingestion and often begin with facial flushing, fatigue, nausea and tingling of the tongue, hands and/or feet. If you're prone to migraine, eating MSG can lead to a full-blown attack.[1] However, it should be mentioned that researchers have been unable to duplicate 'Chinese restaurant syndrome', as it is known, in controlled experiments when MSG is used in normal amounts.[2]

SWEETENERS AND LABORATORY RATS

Well in the forefront of artificial additives – especially for dieters – are the chemical substitutes for sugar. As well as the previously mentioned saccharin, the two most widespread sweeteners on the market today are aspartame (E951) – commercially known as Nutrasweet – and acesulfame-K (E950), both of which are regarded with suspicion by many health experts.[3]

Controversy has surrounded aspartame ever since its availability to the public was first proposed. After anecdotal evidence suggested that a minority of people suffer from headaches and blurred vision after eating foods containing aspartame, it was reassessed by a number of authorities, including: the World Health Organization (WHO); the Expert Committee on Food Additives under the auspices of both WHO and the UN's Food and Agriculture Organization; the USFDA; and the EC's Scientific Committee for Foods. All approved it, with the sole proviso that it should be avoided by those suffering from phenylketonuria (PKU), a rare genetic disorder. In the US and France, all products containing aspartame must state on the label that they contain phenylalanine, the amino acid that accumulates dangerously in the bodies of those with PKU; in the UK, this information need be given only voluntarily.

However, some experts have criticized the manufacturers of aspartame for failing to conduct and report properly some of the key studies at the time of the safety assessment. There were protests against the additive after one study implied that aspartame might lead to brain tumours in rats, but independent researchers have never been able to duplicate these results.

Acesulfame-K – approved for use in the UK, the US and many other countries – is almost as controversial. Critics are unhappy with the tests that were done before approval, stating that the results were equivocal. For instance, the Washington-based Center for Science in the Public Interest claims to have evidence that, in some of the tests on which the FDA based its approval, the additive contributed to an increase in cancer in laboratory animals. In addition, the 34 references on which the UK's Committee on Toxicity (COT) based its approval were not publicly available, and therefore it was impossible for independent experts to assess the additive.

Two other artificial sweeteners currently approved for use in the European Community have not attracted such protests, but are not without their critics. Thaumatin (E957; also marketed under the name Talin) is a protein plant extract traditionally used in rural Sudan and Ghana. It has not been tested to modern standards, and some experts would like to see more large-scale studies carried out in countries where thaumatin has been in use for some time. Neohesperidine dihydrochalcone (NHDC; E959) has not been reviewed by either the WHO or the COT; the EC has examined it and concluded that there were no concerns about its safety, but the studies it used to reach this conclusion are – like those for acesulfame-K – unavailable to the public.

Finally, there is one artificial sweetener over which a battle was won – and then lost. The cyclamates were banned in both the UK and the US in the late 1960s when it was found that massive doses caused cancer in rats. Other studies showed that these substances enhance the cancer-causing effects of certain chemicals, and the COT admitted that there was evidence that a compound that results from cyclamate metabolism causes rats' testes to atrophy. Despite this, the cyclamates remained available in Germany, and with the harmonization of food standards within the EC as of 1 January 1993, they have been given an official 'E' number (E952) and are again approved for use in the UK.

Have the artificial sweeteners accomplished what they set out to do? Has this fake sugar reduced real sugar consumption and helped people to lose weight? During the past decade, the consumption of these additives has rocketed. In the UK, 61 per cent of people have artificial sweeteners as part of their daily diet. In 1988, the average American ate enough to equal 9 kg (20 lb) of sugar – almost treble the amount consumed ten years earlier. But oddly enough, the consumption of sugar per individual also increased over the same period by more than 3 kg (7 lb). In addition, a study in Britain in 1990 found that people who ate yoghurt sweetened with saccharin ate 200 more calories a day than other groups.

'The health benefits of low-calorie drinks with artificial sweeteners have never been demonstrated,' Mark Hegsted, professor emeritus of nutrition at the Harvard School of Public Health, told *American Health* magazine. 'The FDA has its hands tied, but sooner or later there will be a movement toward requirements in terms of the claimed benefit or truth in advertising . . . It seems to me that this issue will become more important.'

ARTIFICIAL FOOD

The Americans and the British have the dubious honour of consuming more 'non-foods' – which promote neither growth nor life – than any other nations in the world. Our intake of saturated, hydrogenated and dairy fats ranks No. 1 in the world. We also consume more additives and preservatives in one year than many people on earth consume food.

We may soon be confronted with a far greater range of synthetic food ingredients. Even the US government is trying to get into the act: scientists at the Department of Agriculture have come up with a zero-calorie substitute for flour.

Artificial fat is now being proclaimed by many as a godsend for fat lovers. One new product is sucrose polyester, which its manufacturer, Proctor & Gamble, is calling Olestra; it contains no calories and cannot be digested. In addition, the NutraSweet Company has created Simplesse, an 'all-natural fat substitute' made from egg white and milk protein. It contains a few calories but only a fraction of what is found in real fat.

Dr Michael Jacobson, executive director of the Center for Science in the Public Interest, protested for a long time against the introduction of Olestra in the US, demanding that more tests should be carried out before it was given approval. However, the FDA permitted Proctor &

Gamble to bypass tests on Olestra using laboratory animals. The fat substitute, classified as an additive in the EC, has still to gain approval from official nutrition and safety committees before it will be allowed on the European market. On the other hand, Simplesse – which is available only to manufacturers – was introduced into Europe in 1991.

One can't help but wonder why we rely on artificial foods when they have been shown not to reduce our waistlines or make us any healthier, and may actually be detrimental to our well-being. Dale Olds, a food scientist at the National Food Laboratory near San Francisco, provides a clue. 'People are conditioned to like artificial flavors,' he told *Harrowsmith Magazine*:

WITH NATURAL FLAVORS, YOU'LL OFTEN LOSE FRACTIONS OF THE FLAVOR DURING THE EXTRACTION PROCESS. YOU CAN ADD THEM BACK CHEMICALLY, BUT THEN YOU'VE GOT ARTIFICIAL FLAVORS. IT'S EASIER TO FORMULATE WITH ARTIFICIAL FLAVORS – YOU HAVE MORE CONTROL.

The food industry has succeeded in providing us with an endless supply of food at all times of the year. But what appears to be a magnificent convenience to the busy people that we all are today may, on closer inspection, prove to be just what is taking the richness out of our lives.

But it's all our own fault, food industry executives claim. If we didn't demand it, they wouldn't produce it. Every year, 3000 to 4000 'new foods' are created because industry says we ask for them. If these foods bear little or no resemblance to what Mother Nature produces, it's simply because we prefer heavy 'hedonics' – that is, things that give us pleasurable sensations: unusual flavours, incredible tastes. Not to mention convenience. As Michael McRae of *Harrowsmith Magazine* has put it:

GIVEN THE STATE OF THE FOOD ALCHEMISTS' ART, IF THERE ARE ENOUGH PEOPLE WHO WILL EAT A LOW-CALORIE, MICROWAVABLE CHICKEN-FRIED STEAK THAT COMES ON A STICK AND TASTES LIKE A CAJUN-STYLE PORK CHOP, THE FOOD INDUSTRY WILL SERVE IT UP.

However, this perceived process of supply and demand does not always take safety into consideration. This is particularly disturbing when you realize that our entire way of life – and all our eating habits – must be grounded in faith. If our faith in the safety of our food is diminished, this could have an enormous ripple effect, damaging our confidence, not only in food manufacturers, distributors and sellers, but also in government, agriculture, science and education.

POISONED CHICKENS

Nutrition is one area of our lives where technology does not help us but, instead, can cause great harm. Although it is not realistic today to expect everyone to hunt, fish and grow all their own food, it is not unrealistic to expect that food manufacturers will not poison us. Natural food is not that difficult to provide, although it is far less profitable for an industry that has become accustomed to high dividends and, in Europe, to agricultural policies that act against truly safe farming practices.

Such is the case with chicken production. Back in the mid-1980s, the headlines in the British press were screaming warnings about outbreaks of salmonella poisoning in chickens and eggs (and a junior government minister was forced to resign her post because she had admitted that there was a problem). The US government today estimates that nearly 80 per cent of chickens or chicken portions contain harmful bacteria.

The 26 May 1991 edition of the *Atlanta* (Georgia) *Journal & Constitution* told of a federal poultry inspector who had become so concerned about chicken not being wholesome that she had not served it to her family for more than a year. Sixty other inspectors interviewed agreed with her. 'Chickens we would routinely condemn ten years ago are now getting right through to the consumer,' one said. 'What's so bad is the people are paying taxes – $417 million [£278 million] a year – for us to do this job and we can't do it. We are not being allowed to protect the consumer.'

Scientists at the US Department of Agriculture (USDA), industry experts and consumer advocates claim that millions of the chickens leaving American processing plants each week are contaminated by unseen bacteria that results in serious food poisoning. The problem is severe. A USDA microbiologist who inspected ready-to-eat, store-bought chicken found that 98 per cent was contaminated by *Campylobacter*, a bacterium that causes twice as much food poisoning as salmonella. The US Centers for Disease Control estimate that, every year, millions of people become ill from eating contaminated chicken and thousands die. In the last 20 years in the US, salmonella poisoning alone has increased by 116 per cent.

In 1988, in England and Wales, there were about 25,000 reported cases of salmonella poisoning, and 50 people died. According to the Public Health Laboratory Service, by the beginning of 1991 new cases of *Salmonella enteritidis* were being reported at the rate of 500 per week. Many, many more people were affected by *Campylobacter*.

The American inspectors feel helpless to do anything about the problem. 'The oath I took to be an inspector said, if I ever saw anything wrong, like a problem with a bad product, I was supposed to report it,'

William Freeman told the *Atlanta Journal & Constitution.* 'But today I can't report anything. Today, if you blow the whistle, you're in trouble with the inspection service. I feel the oath I took is violated every day I work by the program we have.'

The reported cases of food poisoning are only the tip of the iceberg. Many more people suffer from salmonella or other types of poisoning under the mistaken belief that all they have is a bout of intestinal flu. Infections from improper food handling – at the production, storage and/ or preparation stage – are all too common. The chances of salmonella occurring and spreading are vastly increased by the excessive processing of foods, and not only chicken.

Molluscs such as oysters and mussels are often harvested at the seashore near sewage outflows, where they can be infected by bacteria. Poisoning also occurs from *Listeria monocytogenes* in soft cheeses (e.g. Brie and Camembert) and blue-veined types, plus pâté, cook-chill foods, salami, raw and cooked meats, ice cream, milk, fish and seafood, and salad vegetables. Reported cases of listeriosis in England and Wales rose from 115 in 1983 to 291 in 1988, when it contributed to or caused 52 deaths and 11 stillbirths.

The incidence of food poisoning is reaching epidemic proportions, according to some food safety experts. It is estimated that up to five million Americans suffer from bacterial food poisoning each year, many of them more than once, resulting in a total of 81 million cases of food-borne diseases annually. In England and Wales, a total of 41,196 cases of food poisoning were reported in 1988.

Such widespread food-borne poisoning is quite costly. In 1988, the *FDA Consumer* reported that, in the US, the direct cost of medical care for such illnesses was more than $160 billion a year, a figure that does not include the cost of absence from work and other indirect losses.[4] But industry officials say that it would be far too expensive to produce safer chickens. They assume that consumers would refuse to pay any more for poultry should prices need to be raised. However, chicken actually costs less today than it did 40 years ago.

THE RISKS OF PESTICIDES

It becomes increasingly difficult to have faith in our public officials when government departments permit products to be sold as food which clearly can have regrettable consequences. By now, most of us are aware that invisible dangers lurk in every aisle at the supermarket. We have been informed that packaged foods contain dubious additives, that chickens are loaded with bacteria, that fish and shellfish are infected via human and chemical wastes. To make matters worse, foods that are supposedly good for us – fruits and vegetables – are loaded with pesticide residues and other chemical poisons.

The US Environmental Protection Agency (EPA) ranks pesticides as one of the top environmental hazards. According to the US National Academy of Sciences (NAS), every third fruit or vegetable eaten by Americans has been treated with cancer-causing chemicals. One third of the American fruit and vegetable supply has been contaminated with a class of fungicide known as ethylene-bisdithiocarbamates (EBDCs). When sprayed on food that is later heated, stored for a long time or processed for canning, they break down into substances that could increase the risk of cancer and/or birth defects. In the US, 13.6 tonnes (15,000 tons) of EBDCs are used annually on half of the potatoes, on one third of the oranges, apples, tomatoes and spinach, and on vast quantities of melons, peas, carrots and peaches. Yet the FDA samples less than 0.2 per cent of domestic food production.[5]

In 1990, UK farmers and food storage companies employed 28 tonnes (31 tons) of chemicals. Of the approximately 3000 food samples tested by the Ministry of Agriculture, Fisheries & Food (MAFF) in 1990–91 – which comprised staples such as bread, milk and potatoes, as well as fruit and vegetables, cereal and cereal products, animal products, and miscellaneous items (e.g. bananas, Spanish strawberries, potato crisps) – 28 per cent contained detectable pesticide residues: a rise of 2 per cent from 1989–90. One per cent of samples contained more than the maximum residue levels legally allowed by the British government, the highest coming from pesticides applied to the surfaces of fruit, vegetables and wheat in storage.[6] But as Greenpeace UK has pointed out:

INDUSTRY AND GOVERNMENT CLAIM THEY HAVE SET SAFE LIMITS ON RESIDUES. BUT THE TRUTH IS THEY DON'T KNOW THE LONG-TERM EFFECTS – NOBODY DOES. THEIR LIMITS INCLUDE A SAFETY MARGIN THAT IS FAR TOO SMALL GIVEN THE VAST GAPS IN SCIENTIFIC KNOWLEDGE.[7]

In the US, more than 20,000 pesticide products containing 600 active ingredients are registered with the EPA. A total of approximately 385,555 tonnes (425,000 tons) of 325 active ingredients are used directly on food crops and livestock feed every year. But does it do any good? According to David Pimentel, professor of insect ecology and agricultural sciences at Cornell University, in the four decades that followed World War II, the volume of pesticides used in American agriculture increased ten-fold, yet crop losses due to insects rose from 7 to 13 per cent.[8] Nearly 500 insect species worldwide have developed resistance to at least one pesticide, leading farmers to use others that may be more toxic or kill a wider range of insects.

The NAS claims that many pesticides sold in the US have not been sufficiently tested for specific detrimental effects: cancer (71-80% of pesticides not tested), genetic mutations (21–30%), birth defects (51–60%) and adverse effects on the nervous system (90%). Besides cancer, medical researchers are especially concerned about the effects of pesticides on the nervous system.

Critics say that the laws of both the US and the UK favour the chemical companies, which, in the US alone produce $6.5 billion (£4.3 billion) worth of farm chemicals every year. In the UK, this favouritism is accentuated by the fact that full toxicological information is not available for public scrutiny due to the restrictions of commercial confidentiality.

Despite this – and primarily thanks to the US Freedom of Information Act – horrifying results continue to come to light. The NAS has reported that the pesticide residues in 15 common foods are directly to blame for an additional 20,000 cancers in the US every year. A study that focused on 28 of the 53 pesticides deemed carcinogenic by the EPA concluded that tomatoes, beef, potatoes, oranges, lettuce, apples, peaches, pork, wheat, soy beans, green beans, carrots, chicken, grapes and sweetcorn pose the worst risks. More than 80 per cent of the chemicals examined exceeded the EPA guidelines of 'acceptable' cancer risk.

The NAS concluded that 80 per cent of the total cancer risk from pesticides is caused by ten of the most commonly used chemicals: linuron, zineb, captafol, captan, maneb, permethrin, mancozeb, folpet, chlordimeform and chlorothanil. In actual use, they each exceed the EPA's acceptable risk standard hundreds of times.

Government and manufacturers' experts claim that there is nothing to be concerned about since the amount of pesticides we actually ingest is so low that it will not produce any ill-effects. The American FDA has taken care of such concerns by setting safety standards, but these are based on a most peculiar assumption of what the average American eats. Consider the cantaloupe melon, quite a popular food item. The FDA's 'average' diet assumes that Americans each eat no more than 215 g (7.5 oz) – about half a cantaloupe – per year. They also assume that they each consume annually only 1 avocado, 1 mango, 2½ tangerines, and the equivalent of 340 ml (12 fl. oz) summer squash, 400 ml (14 fl. oz) winter squash and 340 ml (12 fl. oz) Brussels sprouts. Eating anything over these levels will, therefore, put people over the 'safe' limit for cancer, birth defects, genetic mutation and nerve damage.[9]

Because of the expense, testing in Britain is limited. In 1989–90, for example, of all the bell peppers for sale in the UK, only 24 were tested (including only two British-grown ones), and only 48 pears. The relatively few items that are tested are examined only for what MAFF expects to find – i.e. only those chemicals approved for use in Britain. This is probably adequate for British-grown produce, but what about the increasing number of items imported from other countries, where the chemicals used on food crops might be completely different . . . and much more deadly? At least in Germany, citrus fruits are required to be labelled with the chemicals that have been applied to them during storage, and carry the warning: 'Skin not suitable for eating.'

In the US, where the lifetime risk of cancer for the general population is one in four, the ingestion of pesticide residues in food is the third leading cause of disease, according to the EPA. Proponents of pesticides say that they aren't of particularly serious concern since they cause less cancer than cigarette smoking. However, people have a choice over whether they will smoke or not; they do not have a choice over whether to eat or not.

Surveys have shown that 80 per cent of Americans view pesticide residues in food as a serious threat to their health. According to the Food Marketing Institute, two thirds believe that the government is doing 'too little' to ensure food quality. The head of the FDA's Center for Food Safety and Applied Nutrition still claims that 'The US food supply is the safest in the world.' MAFF in the UK blandly asserts: 'Ministers believe the approval arrangements for pesticides should not only be safe but should be *seen* to be safe.'

FRAUDULENT DATA

However, as the *Washington Post* has frankly noted, the debate about pesticides depends on whether you worry more about what scientists know about the risks or about what they *don't* know. For instance, experts hardly know anything at all when it comes to the long-term effects of exposure to low levels of cancer-causing chemicals. They also don't know much about the consequences of being exposed to a variety of chemicals from different sources – what is known as the 'cocktail effect'. The task of finding out is an immense and extremely difficult one: since cancer usually requires a couple of decades to develop after a person has been exposed to a carcinogen, it is quite a challenge to determine just what caused that person's cancer. But this task has been made almost impossible because of the quality (or lack of it) of the test data submitted.

In the UK, of the more than 400 active chemical ingredients found in pesticides, 250 were approved by MAFF more than 20 years ago using data that is now considered inadequate, and at a time when less was known about toxicology. Both the EPA and MAFF are 'reviewing' these chemicals (MAFF is not scheduled to finish for another ten years), but in the meantime, no action to restrict their use has been taken.

In addition, as far back as 1978, the EPA acknowledged that hundreds of pesticides had been registered on the basis of faulty or incomplete data. Manufacturers had simply submitted inaccurate and scientifically invalid results from health and safety tests. FDA investigators discovered that one of the largest testing laboratories in the world – Industrial Bio-Test Laboratories of Northbrook, Illinois – had for years been producing fraudulent data for industry. And still the EPA permitted the registration of more than 200 pesticides – 90 of which are used to treat food crops – to remain in force, even though these registrations were based on such worthless and misleading data.[10]

The American consumer organization Common Cause believes that chemical companies are determined to restrict the powers of the EPA as much as possible. In 1987 they reported that the industry had somehow persuaded the government to give them an indemnification programme that car manufacturers would kill for: a chemical manufacturer can sell a product to consumers without adequate safety tests, and then, if it is found to be a threat to health, the government will pay for the unsold stock – at market value. For instance, when the EPA decided to suspend sales of the weedkiller Dinoseb (with the ultimate intention of totally prohibiting it), the predicted cost of reimbursing the manufacturer for the unsold stock, hauling it away and disposing of it was between $60 and $120 million (£40–80 million) – at a time when the budget for the EPA's entire pesticide programme was $70 million (£46.7 million).[11]

Even if pesticides and other chemicals did not contain substances that could dramatically harm health, they would still affect the taste of the foods we eat. Odd smells and flavours are generally agreed to accompany the use of pesticides. Perhaps we are so accustomed to these unnatural tastes that we now don't recognize them as foreign. The roots of certain vegetables automatically absorb fat-soluble insecticides that, once inside the crop, derange the carbohydrate metabolism and nitrogen balance, leading to an odd taste and lack of aroma – sometimes only obvious when the vegetables have been cooked or canned. In addition, officials have stated that the use of a substance similar to paraffin used for weed killing among carrots leaves behind a paraffin flavour.

ATOMIC FOOD

Somehow food additives and pesticides can seem almost insignificant when you consider what we have in store for us: food irradiation. We must ask ourselves the following questions:
- Should the presence of carcinogens and free radicals (*see* Chapter 5) and the depletion of essential vitamins, polyunsaturated fatty acids, amino acids and enzymes be considered 'acceptable risks'?
- Is it really necessary to start a new nuclear industry – complete with the environmental risks involved in the transport, handling and storage of radioactive materials – simply to extend the shelf-life of food?

People who have been involved in this issue almost invariably answer 'No' to these questions, and they are certain that you would, too – *if* you were asked. However, government officials and industry have come to the conclusion that zapping food with gamma radiation from recycled nuclear waste products is the best food preservative on the market.

So what exactly is food irradiation? Well, imagine fruits and vegetables that can sit for weeks in your refrigerator without rotting, sprouting or going mouldy. Or chicken or seafood that is free of bacteria, especially salmonella. Imagine food that can be transported for days, be kept on sale for weeks and remain on the shelf for months, sometimes years, without spoiling. This is the picture that advocates of food irradiation offer us. It could, they say, be the biggest advance in food processing to date.

The technology is quite simple. Externally, a food irradiation plant is usually an unassuming warehouse-type building. Inside, however, you will find a room with concrete walls 1.8 m (6 ft) thick and a 7.6 m (25 ft) deep well of water containing radioactive isotopes: cobalt 60 or caesium 137. A conveyor belt carries food into this room, then the entry is sealed closed and the isotopes raised from the water to bathe the food with gamma rays. Anyone in that room would be killed instantly. The irradiation process lasts 3–30 minutes, after which the isotopes are replaced in their water storage and the food is moved on.

A few insects and bacteria will be killed and ripening will be inhibited at 1 kiloGray (kGy), the dose of radiation currently approved in the US for fruits and vegetables. This is equal to the radiation produced by nearly 10 million chest X-rays. A dose of 3 kGy is standard for poultry, which kills much of the bacteria, particularly salmonella; this dose is the equivalent of 30 million X-rays.

So what does this atomic food do to us once we eat it?

Critics allude to an increased risk of cancer, and some tests have shown reproductive damage in rodents and chromosomal damage in rodents, monkeys and children. Irradiation also reduces levels of essential nutrients in food, especially vitamins A, C, E and B complex. True, the industry admits the latter problem, but says it can be taken care of either by eating a 'balanced diet' or by taking vitamin supplements![12]

A frequently cited study, carried out in India, examined the effects of feeding irradiated food to children suffering from severe protein-calorie malnutrition. Fifteen children were divided into three equal groups; for six weeks, one group received a diet including wheat that had been freshly irradiated, another a diet with wheat that had been irradiated and then stored for some time, and the third ate wheat that had not been irradiated at all.

At the outset of the study and then at intervals of two weeks, tests were carried out on the children's leukocytes (white blood cells). Those receiving freshly irradiated wheat developed polyploid cells – i.e. those containing more than two sets of chromosomes in their nuclei – and other abnormal cells in increasing numbers for the duration of the study. Their blood gradually returned to normal after withdrawal of the irradiated wheat. In marked contrast, none of the children fed the unirradiated diet developed abnormal cells in any significant numbers. Although the biological importance of polyploidy is not clear, its association with cancer makes it imperative that the wholesomeness of irradiated wheat for human consumption be very carefully assessed.[13]

MUTAGENS AND GROWING CHILDREN

In an interview in 1988,[14] Dr George Tritsch, a cancer research scientist at the Roswell Park Memorial Institute and the New York State Department of Health at Buffalo, explained that what happens during the irradiation of food is unique. When high energy hits a molecule, you get a free radical.* That free radical will start a chain reaction by reacting with another stable molecule and forming another free radical and so on, until two free radicals react to produce a stable molecule. A number of these molecules (some of which have never been seen before) have been shown to be mutagenic – i.e. they can cause abnormal changes in DNA. All carcinogens are mutagenic.

The most abundant mutagen, said Dr Tritsch, is formaldehyde. By cross-linking with DNA, it causes all sorts of 'mutagenic insults'. Formaldehyde is produced by irradiating carbohydrate-containing food, and virtually every food contains carbohydrates, even those we think of as primarily protein, such as meat.

When food is irradiated, not only is there the creation of unique molecules – the effects of which are totally unknown – but also the formation of many other free radicals, in addition to formaldehyde. This is especially disturbing for young children, whose DNA repair system is not developed fully; as a result they are more susceptible to mutagenesis than adults. Chromosome abnormalities have been spotted in adults, too.

Dr Tritsch commented that it can take 10 to 30 years for a cancerous tumour to become big enough to be detected and diagnosed, and so the connection between diet and cancer may not be made. However, an association has already been made between diet and bowel cancer and, to a lesser extent, breast cancer. There is no doubt that bringing irradiated food on to the market will also place an added burden of carcinogens on the public – especially worrying in the case of growing children. If food irradiation is to become commonplace, say some experts, in a decade or

---

*See Chapter 5 for a full discussion of free radicals.

two we could see an enormous increase in leukaemia and lymphomas.

Advocates of food irradiation claim that this technology offers a means of decontaminating and disinfecting the food supply and retarding its spoilage.[15] But others will tell you that adequate cooking and hygienic preparation would accomplish the same goal. Irradiation is also supposed to reduce the need for toxic chemicals as post-harvest fumigants. However, some evidence indicates that irradiated foods are more, not less, subject to infection with certain fungi.[16]

The lack of safety evidence to support the introduction of irradiated food baffles all conscientious experts. When the FDA judged the safety of the process, they found – in a total of 441 available toxicity studies – only five animal studies that were 'properly conducted, fully adequate by 1980 toxicological standards and able to stand alone in support of safety'.[17] Yet when this remaining handful of studies was examined by the Department of Preventive Medicine and Community Health at the New Jersey Medical School, two were discovered to be methodologically flawed, either by poor statistical analyses or because negative data were disregarded.[18] In a third FDA-cited study, animals fed a diet of irradiated food lost weight and miscarried, almost certainly because of irradiation-induced vitamin E deficiency.[19]

Obviously, these five studies do not support the safety of food irradiation. This leaves one to wonder: if these were the *best* safety tests from which the FDA had to choose, what were the results of the remaining 436? While two of the five studies cited by the FDA appear to show that the process is safe, it is important to note that they examined the effects of diets consisting of foods irradiated at doses far below those actually approved for consumption by Americans.[20] Nevertheless, the FDA and the food industry continue to insist that irradiating food has been thoroughly tested and is absolutely safe.

As well as worries about the quality of food that has been irradiated, some consumer activists are concerned that we might not even be aware that our food has been processed in this way. According to Tim Lang and Tony Webb of the London Food Commission:

THERE IS NO METHOD CURRENTLY AVAILABLE TO ENABLE PUBLIC ANALYSTS TO DETECT WHETHER A FOOD HAS BEEN IRRADIATED AND, IF SO, WITH WHAT DOSES AND HOW MANY TIMES . . . CASES WHERE IRRADIATION HAS BEEN USED ILLEGALLY IN ORDER TO CONCEAL BACTERIAL CONTAMINATION OF UNFIT FOODS HAVE BEEN UNCOVERED, INCLUDING THE IRRADIATION OF CONTAMINATED PRAWNS AND MUSSELS IN THE NETHERLANDS. EVEN WHERE CONTROLS EXIST, THERE WILL ALWAYS BE A DANGER THAT THEY ARE NOT APPLIED TO FOOD FOR EXPORT OR RE-EXPORT, PERHAPS TO COUNTRIES WHICH HAVE NO CONTROLS. IN THE ABSENCE OF DETECTION METHODS,

THERE IS NO WAY THAT THESE AND OTHER ABUSES CAN BE EFFECTIVELY
CONTROLLED. [21]

With the passage of the Food Safety Act 1990, the UK's MAFF received
the power to regulate new food technologies, and has permitted food
irradiation. It has also specified that such foods must be listed on labels:

THE NAME USED IN ANY LIST OF INGREDIENTS FOR ANY FOOD WHICH HAS
BEEN IRRADIATED SHALL INCLUDE, OR BE ACCOMPANIED BY, THE WORD
'IRRADIATED' OR THE WORDS 'TREATED WITH IONISING RADIATION'. [22]

However, this seemingly blanket regulation does not apply to all ingredients. For example, if an irradiated herb or spice makes up less than 2
per cent of a product, it does not have to be labelled at all. The same thing
goes for other ingredients if they comprise less than 25 per cent of a
product – say, a jam tart containing jam made from irradiated
strawberries.

NUKING A JAYWALKER

It hardly seems justifiable to risk the health of people all over the world
simply to profit a small industry. However, in the US this small industry is
supported by a highly politicized bureaucracy.

The US Department of Energy (DoE), through its Byproducts
Utilization Program, is charged with the task of developing commercial
uses for radioactive waste products. According to Donald B. Louria,
writing in the *Bulletin of the Atomic Scientists*, the creation of a demand
for caesium – a waste product of both weapons production and civilian
nuclear power – has been one of the Department's expressed goals since
the early 1980s. DoE memoranda indicate that its plan has included
pricing caesium so low that it would drive Canadian cobalt out of the
market. [23]

Dr Louria, who heads the Preventive Medicine Department of the
New Jersey Medical School, goes further. He echoes the claim of certain
critics that the DoE has been even more devious, that it is less interested
in disposing of waste caesium than in overturning the ban on reprocessing
civilian nuclear fuel. According to these critics, the Department has
calculated that, when widespread food irradiation eventually depletes the
available supplies of caesium 137, the irradiation industry will begin to
lobby for the reprocessing of spent fuel; the DoE will then use this
demand to overcome the political and economic obstacles to nuclear fuel
reprocessing. Once this is permitted, the DoE could separate out the
plutonium from the spent fuel, which could then be used for weapons. [24]

Louria explains that, if irradiation is adopted prematurely, research into its effects on health will be hampered. Widespread use of the technology will make it impossible to detect any but the most obvious of adverse effects, because it will be impossible to find enough people who have not ingested this type of food to make up a control population for the purposes of study. This problem will be further complicated in the US if irradiation levels are increased to the proposed 1 million rad – equal to 100,000,000 chest X-rays.

In addition, there are great environmental concerns about the irradiation plants themselves. Allowing irradiation facilities to multiply like marigolds could pose a threat to both workers and the public, reported *Newsweek* magazine.[25] Radioactivity can leak; an accident can expose workers to cancer-causing and, possibly, more immediately lethal rays.

At present in the United States, there are about 40 plants suitable for food irradiation, which now mainly irradiate disposable medical equipment. Plant safety records are not encouraging. In New Jersey, where most of the plants are located, virtually every facility has a record of environmental contamination, worker overexposure and regulatory failures. In 1988, a dangerous accident happened at a plant in Georgia. The facility had to be shut down, clean-up costs have soared to $15 million (£10 million), and no conclusions have so far been reached as to the accident's cause.[26]

Dr Sheldon Morgan, a professor emeritus of public health nutrition at the University of California at Berkeley, told the *New York Times* that 'there are potentially serious concerns about the issues of waste disposal, engineering safety, transport of new isotopes, handling by poorly trained personnel, and others we haven't even thought of yet.'[27] But the public's concerns continue to fall on deaf ears. A plant was recently built in Florida only after the state government overrode local opposition to the presence of radioactive isotopes in the town.

We already know that food irradiation means serious nutritional depletion and reproductive and genetic toxicity, not to mention hazards to workers and the environment – but at the end of the day, the total risks remain unknown. Who then benefits from atomic food? Poultry producers might, since their chickens would no longer be smothered in salmonella. Yet introducing nuclear technology rather than insisting on more government inspection and tighter standards of hygiene is like nuking a jaywalker. Why can't we follow the lead of Germany, Denmark, Sweden, Australia and New Zealand, which all have prohibited the sale and distribution of irradiated food?

SUPER-CHICKENS AND SUPER-COWS

The most extraordinary innovation in food technology is about to dawn. It's what some scientists are calling 'Franken-food'. The latest 'advance' is genetically altered foods.

Genetic engineering – also known as biotechnology and recombinant DNA technology – involves adding characteristics to an organism or subtracting them, either by suppressing the action of a specific gene or by adding one from another plant or even an animal. A few years ago, scientists spliced a gene from a firefly into the DNA of a tobacco plant, and when the plant grew, it glowed in the dark.[28]

The British are already eating some cheeses and bread that have been made with genetically modified organisms – but you won't see this on any labels. And in one unprecedented and sweeping ruling, the FDA in the United States approved the use and sale of genetically engineered food without requiring toxicology testing or consumer labelling. To think that a genetically engineered food can be sold at random without any safety tests or a warning label is a horrifying prospect for consumers. Soon genetically engineered tomatoes, potatoes, apples, sweetcorn, soy beans and other foods will be sold throughout the United States and Britain. No one will know what the genes they are digesting will do to them since no pre-market testing will have taken place.

Dissent to the FDA's decision has come from an unexpected quarter. More than 100 world-class chefs – Rick Moonen, Wolfgang Puck and other culinary masters from renowned American restaurants including the Rattlesnake Club, the Red Sage, the Russian Tea Room and Club 21 – have banded together to protest against the US government's ruling. 'I'm appalled by this,' said Rick Moonen. 'If you want to shellac these products and put them in a window, that's OK. But if you want to cook with them and get nutritional value, leave them alone.'

The chefs are facing some impressive opponents. The biotechnology industry responsible for providing us with these 'new foods' includes a number of familiar names of both chemical and food companies: Monsanto, Upjohn, Eli Lilly, DuPont, Heinz, Campbell Soup, Dole Food, Hunt-Wesson, PepsiCo/Frito Lay. These huge corporations are investing billions because biotechnology offers them unprecedented potential to increase their profits and their control over food production.

Genetic engineering is a radically new technology, not simply an extension of traditional selective breeding methods. Gene splicing can combine genes from dissimilar species. In the years ahead, genetic engineers intend to transfer thousands of genes from bacteria, viruses, animals and plants into the food we eat. What, in theory, may be good for the new organism may not be good for us.

Already, antibiotic-resistant genes are incorporated into nearly every genetically engineered organism. The FDA has acknowledged that these genes and their products 'may reduce the therapeutic efficiency of [any prescribed] antibiotic when taken orally [by consumers] if the enzyme in the food inactivates the antibiotic.' Genetic engineering might also produce a counterfeit 'freshness' as certain fruits and vegetables sit for weeks on shelves, apparently fresh but not maintaining their nutrient quality.

Because they are alive, genetically engineered organisms are inherently more unpredictable than chemical products. These organisms can reproduce, mutate and migrate. Once released, it will be virtually impossible to recall them back to the laboratory.

Ethical questions have been raised over the crossing of species boundaries – inserting human genes into farm animals, and animal genes into other animals and plants. Many of the recent experiments appear to come straight out of science fiction. In the late 1980s researchers working for the US Department of Agriculture produced 'transgenic' pigs containing the gene for human growth hormone. Rather than the hoped-for leaner, faster-growing animals, the resulting pigs became lame, arthritic, sterile, skinny and excessively hairy.

A recent survey found that 53 per cent of Americans are morally opposed to animal genetic engineering. Many concerned individuals and organizations have pointed out that genetically altering animals is an issue of deep philosophical and spiritual concern. For some, it is appalling to consider animals as simply assemblies of genes that can be manipulated by people; others believe that it is only a matter of time before genetically altered animals lead to genetically altered human beings.

But most scientists view these biotechnically altered animals as human creations, inventions and commodities – nothing more. The US Supreme Court may have already opened a Pandora's box: in 1980, in the case *Diamond* v. *Chakrobatry*, they allowed the granting of the first patent for a living organism. Since then, many have come to believe that this decision was the first step towards the patenting of human genes. This was actually proposed by researchers working on the American end of the worldwide Human Genome Project, the attempt to identify all the genes that comprise human DNA; they wanted to secure the 'rights' to the gene sequences they had discovered, so that anyone else using their research would have to pay for it.

'Animal designers' – as bioengineers are sometimes called – have made enormous strides in recent years.
• In Britain, scientists at the Institute of Animal Physiology and Genetics Research at Edinburgh transferred a gene from sheep to mice, to add a protein to mice milk. They say that such a gene transfer into dairy animals should be viewed as a realistic approach for the production of

milk with enhanced nutritional value.

- USDA scientists have inserted genes from a virus into chicken eggs; these were then taken up by the developing embryos and incorporated into their own genes. The resulting chickens were then able to pass the new gene on to their chicks. Thus one super-chicken can have a multitude of such offspring. Eventually, we might have designer chickens that will produce larger eggs and resist disease and have other traits appreciated by chicken producers.
- Besides super-chickens, consider the possibility of super-cattle. Through artificial insemination, one super-bull can service 100,000 cows a year, and, through embryo transfer, the offspring of the latter can develop in surrogate cows.

The official rationale behind this biotechnical revolution is that food quality will be improved, livestock productivity will increase and the animals will be more disease resistant. Yet at what cost to the animals – and to us?

INVINCIBLE TOMATOES

Although well advanced, the technology for gene-tailored animals is not nearly as far along as it is for plants and microbes.

Very normal-looking tomatoes growing in fields now have the ability to fight off some destructive insects and viral infections, and can even handle certain lethal herbicides. The source of their power is found in the nucleus of every cell. Through the alteration of the plant's DNA, the tomato is well protected from its hazardous environment. Now, instead of simply not spraying tomatoes with deadly herbicides, the plants can be genetically altered so that they can withstand cheap, non-plant-specific herbicides.

Gene alteration is not a new phenomenon, but it was only in the 1980s that scientists were able to alter specifically a plant's DNA. By incorporating genes from evolutionarily distant organisms, genetic information is being blended in ways never imagined possible. 'Transgenic' plants number far beyond the tomato. The USDA has already allowed some 50 such plants to undergo limited field trials, with others soon to follow.

Even now, scientists can literally produce 'real' whole foods and other plant products artificially:

- A USDA geneticist has created orange juice in a laboratory.
- A pomologist (pomology=science of fruit-growing) at the University of California at Davis has grown cherries without pits.
- A researcher in Texas has grown cotton fibres in a tissue culture.

Consumers in the US and Britain are not eagerly embracing this rapid advance in technology in the same way that scientists are: in surveys in both countries, 85 per cent of people said they wanted genetically engineered foods to be clearly labelled, presumably so that they can be avoided. Possible health effects and environmental damage have not been properly assessed. Many are concerned about the irrevocable and unscrupulous disruption of the natural order of things.

Scientists actually have very few examples on which to base safety predictions, yet they confidently claim that plants that receive a gene for, say, a well-characterized protein from a known source will pose little if any health risk. The US government agrees, and has decided to promote this technology. Congress passed an ambitious five-year farm bill that established the National Genetic Resources Program, to be headed by the Secretary of Agriculture. His/her job will be to collect, classify, preserve and disseminate genetic materials of importance to American agriculture.

The day of totally artificial food production will soon be upon us, according to *Futurist* magazine. Scientists, they say, are now working on research that increases the likelihood of people being able to grow food without farms – a biotechnological dream that is much closer to being realized than, say, a cure for AIDS. These research scientists are modest about their achievements only because, according to the magazine, there is a certain amount of professional and political risk involved in being identified with a radical departure from traditional ways of doing things. Yet they are well aware that they are taking part in what could well prove to be the greatest change in food production since the beginning of agriculture itself.[29]

POOR COWS

So who decides about biotechnology? Do we consumers really want food additives and other chemicals, irradiated or genetically engineered foods that have not been proven safe or beneficial? And if it's not of benefit to us, who is it beneficial for?

Let's consider the case of milk – a basic, wholesome, nutritious food that science has decided to improve upon. Cows can now be injected with a genetically engineered hormone called rBGH. This is a synthetic analogue of the animals' natural hormone bovine somatotropin (BST), which induces milk production in the cows' mammary glands; adding rBGH is said to increase milk production by up to 25 per cent, each cow giving an extra 6 litres (11 pts) of milk every day.

What's odd about all this is that we in the West already have an abundance of milk. In the European Community, milk quotas – which have been in force since 1984 in an attempt to reduce production – haven't worked. In 1992, there was a surplus of over 92,000 tonnes (81,600 tons) of skimmed milk powder and over 168,000 tonnes (152,400 tons) of butter. Milk is sold off cheap to schools, and the EC continues to pour huge amounts of money into advertising, trying to persuade Europeans to drink more of the stuff.

In the US between 1987 and 1989, the government spent up to $1.3 billion a year buying up surplus milk under price-support legislation. At the same time as rBGH was being made available, dairy farmers were being paid $1 billion annually by taxpayers to slaughter one million cows to reduce these milk subsidy payments. The organization Consumers' Union estimates that if rBGH increases American milk output by a mere 10 per cent, it will cost the government (and, ultimately, consumers) an additional $1.8 billion.[30] The dairy industry counters these figures by stating that higher milk yield means, eventually, fewer cows, which, they claim, will then mean cheaper milk and dairy products for the consumer.

Set against this possible economic benefit is the distinct possibility of health risks to both human consumers and bovine producers. There is some evidence that rBGH negatively effects human growth hormone in both children and adults. According to Samuel Epstein, a professor of environmental and occupational medicine at the University of Illinois Medical Center, it has also been linked to premature growth in infants, excessive development of the mammary glands in male children and breast cancer in women.[31]

In her natural state, a cow's lifespan is anything between 25 and 40 years, and she gives each of her calves about 5 litres (9 pts) of milk a day. But life for her is very different in the industrial world of milk production. According to Professor John Webster of Bristol University:

THE COW IS OUR MOST OVERWORKED ANIMAL. FOR NINE MONTHS OF THE YEAR, SHE IS GIVING UP TO 44 LITRES (80 PTS) OF MILK EVERY DAY, AND EVERY SIX MONTHS SHE ALSO HAS A CALF. SO SHE IS LACTATING AND PREGNANT AT THE SAME TIME. IF WE WERE TO WORK AS HARD, IT WOULD BE EQUIVALENT TO JOGGING SIX HOURS EVERY DAY OF OUR LIVES.[32]

As a result of all her gruelling work, the modern dairy cow suffers constant hunger and exhaustion. Injections of rBGH will push up her milk yield far beyond her natural capacity, and may reduce her productive life. Samuel Epstein also claims that the higher metabolism induced in cows by rBGH may stress their immune systems. Already, cows injected with the synthetic hormone have to be treated with high levels of antibiotics to combat an increased number of udder infections, thus raising the level of antibiotics that remains in the milk. The effects of rBGH on cows' fertility and on calves born to rBGH cows are unknown.

From 1985, four companies conducted secret field trials of rBGH on 1000 dairy cows on ten British farms, under the authorization of MAFF.

The trials were carried out under the auspices of the Medicines Act 1968; because this guarantees commercial confidentiality, MAFF has refused to disclose any of the trial results. In addition, the milk produced by the cows in the trials was pooled with other milk and sold – unidentified – to consumers. However, in July 1990 the Veterinary Products Committee that advises the British government issued a report recommending that genetically engineered rBGH should not be licensed for use on diary cows. The committee was 'not completely satisfied with some pharmaceutical aspects of the product, or with aspects of the safety of treated animals'.

Subsequent to this, the European Community declared a moratorium on rBGH use. Four Scandinavian countries and three Canadian provinces have also banned the drug altogether. In the United States, the increase of biotechnology has resulted in a new wave of social activism. Congressional investigations, lawsuits, supermarket boycotts, leaks from FDA insiders, allegations that government regulators are controlled by industry – all have become a part of the biotechnological revolution.

However, as long as someone has a great deal to gain from them, the struggle for the acceptance of these new technologies will go on. *Technology Review* has assessed the involvement of one potential beneficiary of the new science, Monsanto. This huge chemical manufacturer has invested more than $800 million in agricultural biotechnology, of which rBGH is only the first of many biotech products to be unleashed on the public. Monsanto has projected that their biotechnology products will earn them $1 billion before the end of the 1990s.

DYING CELLS

With so much discussion being focused on food adulteration, chemical additives, food irradiation and the artificial creation of new foods, many of us have been left wondering about what lasting harm they can actually do.

Studies have been conducted to determine the *direct* toxic effects of some chemical additives, but scientists have not taken it upon themselves – nor has government funded any research – to analyse any possible untoward effects that are slight, delayed and indirect. Such subtle actions on the human body at the basic cellular level could result from any the hundreds or even thousands of substances biologically foreign to us, which we consume daily in our food. And it is impossible to guess what effects these substances might have in combination with the other chemical and physical factors we encounter – polluted air and water, pesticide residues, tobacco, drugs, alcohol, radiation.

Certain government officials and members of the scientific community would like us to believe that exposure to tiny amounts of toxic materials pose little or no risk. But the hidden danger is in the repeated small exposures over time with regular use. Nature does not provide the enzymes necessary to break down all these synthetic chemicals, nor can our bodies readily metabolize and excrete them.

The changes in our bodies can be very subtle, and it may take years before the harmful effects make themselves known. A keen pathologist might spot early signs of such endangerment to vital organs. The livers, kidneys and spleens of experimental animals have been found to become enlarged due to the stress put upon them to detoxify the body of foreign materials. These materials also interfere with the body's use of vitamins and minerals, thus impairing their performance of key functions such as cell repair. Further, enzymes – the thousands of substances produced by living cells, that act as catalysts, promoting chemical change – may be sent into a frenzy and not function as the chief agents of the entire life process. Every living cell constantly breaks down and, in a normal environment, is rebuilt. The introduction of chemical additives prevents this natural rebuilding, and when enough cells weaken and die, the body dies.

Symptoms of cell destruction can be seen in all of us to some degree. Fatigue, weakness, constipation, headaches, insomnia, indigestion, muscle ache and other bodily malfunctions are all too common. Take these complaints to your doctor and he or she will begin to question you about the amount of stress you have been under lately, instead of identifying the impairment of your body's vitamin/enzyme system.

Many frequently used enzyme destroyers can cause serious disorders. Additives such as sulphur dioxide (E220) and sodium nitrate (E251), food dyes, some hormones used to stimulate plant and animal growth, antibiotics, fluoride in water, and pesticides are all time-honoured enzyme robbers. And it doesn't take much of these chemicals to do serious harm. It only takes 0.4 parts per million of the now-banned pesticide DDT to negatively effect a crucial enzyme in human blood. Occasionally, detrimental chemicals can be measured in parts per *billion*.

Catalase is one enzyme that is frequently tampered with. Found in our bodies and all other living things, it is closely associated with cell respiration, which in part protects the cells from poisonous substances, infection by bacteria and viruses, radiation and cancer. In its normal state, the cell keeps the poisonous hydrogen peroxide within it to a very low level, using catalase to break down any excess into oxygen and water. But many chemicals destroy catalase, which then results in a rise in the level of hydrogen peroxide. This, in turn, causes the cell's electron-transport system to slow down or come to a complete halt. When this happens, cells are extremely vulnerable, and candidates for diseases such as cancer.

A physician specializing in catalase/hydrogen peroxide balance has said that, if this fundamental biological mechanism is interfered with for long enough by physical and chemical agents in the industrial environment of the West – whether in food, drink, drugs or the air we breathe – we shall see a progressive increase in the incidence of cancer. By contrast, in those so-called primitive communities where such agents are not common, the incidence will remain very low.[33]

Even when discussing these issues at length with open-minded, intelligent people, I still end up hearing the same well-worn rejoinder: 'Well, if certain chemicals are so harmful to us, surely the government would ban them?' But it is enlightening to examine in just whose interests government brings its might to bear.

In the United States, there is a government body called the Council on Competitiveness. Ah, competitiveness – industry's best friend! Set up by former vice president Dan Quayle, it hears industry appeals concerning federal regulations and intervenes if it decides that the rules are too cumbersome or place corporations at an economic disadvantage. The proceedings are held in secret, yet the council's rulings often usurp congressional legislation. One of its recent decisions forced the FDA to approve genetically engineered foods; another added massive loopholes to the Clean Air Act.

Government agency approval of certain chemicals and other products does not guarantee their safety. You simply have to look at the long list of currently banned – but once approved – chemicals to drive this point home. Unfortunately, the later banning of dyes, flavourings, pesticides and drugs only happens after they have been in widespread use, sometimes for decades. Adverse test results have often been ignored simply to rush a new chemical on to the market. The current trend is not much better. Now, rather than the elimination of dangerous substances, the allowable tolerance rates of toxic products have been lowered.

Additives that, at first, appear to have stood the test of time offer no comfort either. For 30 years, Americans ate breads and pastries that included a toxic flour bleach; for half a century, they consumed foods sweetened with the harmful dulcin, and seven decades saw the consumption of foods flavoured with coumarin, a vitamin K antagonist.

To complicate matters further, laboratory analysis of chemical food additives is not conclusive. US food and drug authorities admit that there is a current lack of data concerning reactions that certain chemicals can produce in the body. Yet experts have consistently assumed that, somehow, the body is able to detoxify foreign substances and, more, that the toxicity of chemical additives is reduced once in the body. In fact, just the opposite is true: chemical additives, once broken down through metabolism, become *more* toxic than in their natural state.[34]

Then we must consider something known as *synergism*. The poisonous effect of one additive can become more powerful when mixed with chemicals found in other foods. If you eat a wide variety of foods at each meal – in fact, if you eat the recommended 'balanced diet' – there is no telling how many chemical substances you will consume or what the overall effect these will have on your mind and body.

The European Commission has been reluctant to legislate on some of the more contentious issues in nutrition. It has limited itself to such matters as food additives, materials that come in contact with food, foods for particular nutritional purposes, methods of preservation, inspection of premises and enforcement of food law – all of which could be seen as steps in the right direction. However, issues such as the labelling of permitted residues, food irradiation and bioengineered foods have not yet been agreed at a European level. In contrast, the strict regulations governing agricultural pork and eggs are designed to promote trade rather than to protect the public's health. For example, meat regulations apply only when meat is exported to another member state and not when it is for the home market.[35]

However, it must be admitted that in 1991 the British government took some important steps forward in their policy on nutrition, with the publication of dietary reference values for food energy and nutrients[36] and the policy paper *The Health of the Nation*[37], which proposes population nutrition targets. According to the *British Medical Journal*, these are essential precursors to an integrated food and nutrition policy, but much remains to be done to find ways of helping and motivating people to choose a healthier diet. Among these will be, it is hoped, warnings concerning the dangers of food chemicalization, food irradiation and bioengineering.

The increasing growth in the power of the European Community (which on 1 December 1993, with the ratification of the Maastricht Treaty by all member states, officially changed its name to 'European Union') makes the reality of a single European market edge ever closer. This will undoubtedly make trade easier among member states, and larger enterprise will gain most.

As a result, the market for food may become even more concentrated in the hands of a few producers, and multinational companies may expand even further across the continent, all of them promoting similar products, especially processed foods with nutrient values ranging from nil to just adequate.

In the face of this, the European consumer will need to be educated about nutrition, food safety and food quality. If what has already happened to the food supply in the United States is any indication, European consumers – from the isles of Greece to John O'Groats – will have a great deal to learn.

Nearly 50 years ago, two respected British chemists stated: 'The chemistry of nature is being supplemented and even replaced with the chemistry of man.'[38] If only they could see how far we've come . . .

CHAPTER THREE

LIVING DANGEROUSLY

As human evolution slowly began hundreds of thousands of years ago, our ancestors lived as part of the Earth, a tiny link in the web of life, conscious each moment that one stroke of nature could abolish that life in an instant. Humans evolved by the sometimes harsh laws of the land, just as other creatures did. To survive and flourish, they became minutely attuned to their surroundings. Every bird call, every rustle of leaves could spell potential danger.

But as humans gradually changed, it was no longer as vital to listen to nature or to be so afraid of unseen forces lurking just beyond the range of vision. Instead, humans learned that they could tame the world. They could build on it, sail across its lakes and seas, even force the land to produce the food they wanted. Fresh air, clean water and fertile soil all played an extremely important role, allowing generation upon generation of humanity to develop and expand.

Then, thousands of years later, in the 17th century, the first spark of industrialization was ignited and with it, unbeknownst to humans, a Pandora's box of both good and evil was opened. People welcomed the new age with open arms, for their newly created machines and inventions allowed them to beat back their fears of the power of nature.

The industrial and technological revolutions allowed people to take the world – which had taken billions of years to evolve – and mould it like a piece of putty to their desires . . . in a blink of an eye. In their book *It's a Matter of Survival*[1] Anita Gordon and David Suzuki have put humanity's short time on Earth into perspective:

YOU CAN SEE JUST HOW [BRIEF A TIME HUMANS HAVE BEEN ON EARTH] IF YOU

USE A STANDARD CALENDAR TO MARK THE PASSAGE OF TIME . . . THE ORIGIN OF THE EARTH, SOME 4.6 BILLION YEARS AGO, IS PLACED AT MIDNIGHT, JANUARY 1, AND THE PRESENT AT MIDNIGHT, DECEMBER 31. EACH CALENDAR DAY REPRESENTS APPROXIMATELY 12 MILLION YEARS OF ACTUAL HISTORY. DINOSAURS ARRIVED ON ABOUT DECEMBER 10 AND DISAPPEARED ON CHRISTMAS DAY. HOMO SAPIENS MADE AN APPEARANCE AT 11.45 P.M. ON DECEMBER 31. THE RECORDED HISTORY OF HUMAN ACHIEVE-MENT . . . TAKES UP ONLY THE LAST MINUTE OF THAT YEAR.

Yet in that minute, we have drastically changed the world. Our excited embrace of technology has introduced increasing quantities of poisons and pollutants, some of which, although originally considered benign, are now beginning to show their darker side.

As recently as the 1930s the production of synthetic chemicals was an emerging field, at the forefront of science. Between 1950 and 1985, however, the annual output of chemical production in the US increased tenfold, from 11 billion kg (24 billion lb) to 102 billion kg (225 billion lb).[2] According to the United Nations Environment Programme, more than seven million chemicals have been discovered or created; 80,000 are in common use, and several thousand new ones are produced every year.[3] Where do they all go? At this rate, how can anyone keep track of them? How do they affect us as human beings?

Where once our forebears took for granted fresh air, clean water and rich soil and feared only nature's wrath, today our air, water and soil poison us, and we have only ourselves to fear. Horrendous environmental disasters – such as Chernobyl, the Exxon Valdez oil spill in Alaska and the chemical catastrophe in the Indian city of Bhopal, where about 2500 died in the first 24 hours – attract media attention and public outrage for a week or two and then fade quickly from the memories of all but those who must continue to endure their consequences. It is all too easy to watch, from our cosy position in front of the TV, these terrible accidents wreak havoc on others. 'Thank goodness we don't live next to that nuclear reactor/oil refinery/chemical plant!' we exclaim, glad that they're there and we're here.

BOILED FROGS

Such incidents are making it into the limelight with increasing frequency, but they are, unfortunately, only the tip of the iceberg. For instance, the US Environmental Protection Agency (EPA) estimates that there are more than 10,000 oil spills each year.[4] How many do we read about in the newspaper – three, four, maybe five?

Not only are environmental accidents increasing in number, but when they do occur, they affect large populations. In 1986, the catastrophic fire at the Chernobyl nuclear plant spewed over much of Europe 300 to 400 times more radioactive fallout than was released by the bombing of Hiroshima during World War II. Even today, the 830,000 people living within a contaminated radius of the plant must be continuously monitored, some 25 per cent of the land in the new state of Belorussia has been deemed unfit for agriculture, and sheep farmers in the uplands of North Wales are still prevented from selling their animals for food.

How do the many small chemical leaks and spills never reported affect us? If DDT from Africa and insecticides from the United States have been found in the once-pristine Arctic and in the livers of fish, seals, walruses and polar bears, if PCBs have been found in animals at depths of 3350 m (11,000 ft) in the Atlantic Ocean – then none of us is exempt from this chemical invasion.

What is especially frightening is that, despite all the evidence that shows how our bodies are being assaulted by chemicals, few of us are aware of the dangers posed by our environment. Again, Gordon and Suzuki have the perfect metaphor: the 'boiled frog syndrome'.

In an experiment carried out by particularly callous biologists, a frog was put in a pot of water and the temperature slowly increased from 20°C (68°F) . . . to 40°C (104°F) . . . to 90°C (194°F) – but the frog just sat there. Then, at 100°C (212°F), the water boiled and the frog, still motionless, suddenly died. This happened because the frog has no evolutionary experience of extremes of temperature; thus it has not evolved with thermal detectors in its skin, and so was unable to perceive as dangerous a gradual increase in temperature.

Just as the frog remained unaware of the disaster about to hit it, so are we ignorant of the threats we face from chemical toxins and radiation, undetectable by the sensory system we have evolved. We cannot taste most toxins in our food and water or feel pollution in the air, yet the chemicals that surround us are slowly killing us.

Once, what happened in Africa did not directly impinge on the lives of Europeans. This is no longer true. Every nation now has the ability to affect the rest of the world. Yet the question of whether the globally destructive power of human beings will ultimately affect all humanity is still debated by scientists – simply because there is no laboratory model with which to experiment and reach a solid conclusion. Slowly, over the years, the water in the pot has become hotter and hotter, and it is only now, because of human suffering, illness and death, that the scientific world is beginning to realize that once seemingly omnipotent species *Homo sapiens* may be as fragile as the frog.

WHITE MICE OF THE 20TH CENTURY

A neighbour's cancer and Grandma's Alzheimer's disease are each accepted as tragic but separate, unrelated events of daily life. But such illnesses are becoming more common. Science is gradually discovering the role that toxic chemicals play in the deterioration of human health. A person may be affected many years after the initial exposure – which may have even occurred before birth. We can no longer brush the threat of toxic chemicals aside and recklessly ignore the effects they may have on us: the health of future generations is at stake. A 1989 study of 285 four-year-olds in Michigan found DDT, a pesticide banned in 1972 (13 years before they were born), present in the blood of 70 per cent of them.[5] Their mothers' breastmilk was determined to be the principal source of the chemical.

Over the years, scientists have managed to agree that the hazard to health posed by a chemical after it enters the environment depends primarily on its toxicity and the extent of human exposure to it. It is also known that:

a Some chemicals are immediately toxic.
b Different chemicals have different levels of toxicity.
c When some chemicals react with each other, their toxicities are increased.
d Chemicals can accumulate in the human body, leading to disease.

These are proven scientific facts, yet chemical conglomerates continue to twist them to suit their own purposes. For example, soft drinks manufacturers have been known to say: 'A person would have to drink 5000 of our diet colas a day to experience any side-effects from our artificial sweetener.'

The risk of harmful side-effects from a single chemical in tiny, controlled amounts may be 1 in 1,000,000, but what happens when it accumulates within a person's body over years? Chemists might know exactly how a particular chemical reacts with another in a petri dish in a sterile laboratory, but what if this chemical comes into contact with other different chemicals in human tissue? The most horrifying aspect of all this is that, too many times, chemical companies appear not to care: profits and production schedules are everything; they are in the business of selling chemicals, not protecting society.

Of the approximately 49,000 chemicals that had been registered with the EPA by the late 1980s, companies supplied information regarding immediate toxicity to humans for only 21 per cent of them. What about the other 79 per cent? How are they affecting people today? What about the 30,000 chemicals that have been created and released on society since then? What about tests for chemical interaction and the effects of toxin accumulation in humans?

Carrying out these tests is not a simple matter. As one US government official bluntly put it, 'It takes a team of scientists, 300 mice, two to three years and about $300,000 to determine whether a single suspect chemical causes cancer.'[6] These costs increase exponentially when other chemicals are included. American scientists working in the National Toxicological Program have stated that a minimal study of the effects of a mixture of 25 chemicals would require more than 33 million experiments at a cost of more than $3 trillion. With the present recession, no country in the world – not even the United States – has this kind of money to spend on research, even if there was the political will to carry it out. Instead, people have become the white mice of the 20th century – and the results are slowly coming in.

TOXIC SOUP

For several decades, air pollution has been a topic that has risen and fallen in 'popularity'. Many of us spend little time thinking about what we're breathing. For those of us who live in cities, unfortunate experiences such as being stuck in heavy traffic or behind a fume-belching bus may jerk us momentarily back to reality, but once the choking and spluttering is over, the event is soon forgotten or simply regarded as an inevitable part of modern life.

In the past, air pollution such as the infamous 'pea-soupers' that once enveloped London – one of which, in 1952, killed 4000 people in the space of a week, and led directly to the passing of the 1956 Clean Air Act – were caused by domestic and industrial burning of high sulphur coal and were a visible enemy. Even today, most American cities have an ever-present smoky grey cloud above the rooftops, and cannot meet the clean air standards set by Congress more than 20 years ago. And in Britain now, pollution in most places continues to exceed the guide values set by the World Health Organization.

The difference today is that air pollution is no longer simply a mixture of smoke from coal and wood burning, but an invisible concoction of pollutants that are even more toxic. According to a recent estimate by the EPA, in one year American industry alone released 2.4 billion tonnes (2.7 billion tons) of hazardous pollutants into the air – and this figure does not include emissions from vehicles.[7] Once released, these pollutants combine to form a chemical potion that is further altered by the effects of the sun and moisture. Blown by the wind, the resulting smog affects not only city dwellers and suburbanites, but also people (and animals and plants) living sometimes hundreds of miles away.

However, unless we live in an area as polluted as Mexico City, whose inhabitants must drive with their headlamps on during the day, we almost never give a second thought to the air we breathe – despite the fact that air like it is slowly destroying some of the world's most famous monuments, from the Parthenon to the Taj Mahal. If the air we take for granted causes the acid rain that kills forests in Europe and maple trees in North America, it is only a matter of time before it kills us.

Although, for many people, the words 'air pollution' conjure up images of factories belching black smoke, many of the invisible pollutants emitted from road vehicles are as or even more harmful. Nitrogen dioxide (NO_2) and sulphur dioxide (SO_2) are known respiratory irritants that exacerbate asthma and may lead to chronic lung disease such as emphysema; they also both contribute to acid rain. Carbon monoxide (CO) may cause chronic bronchitis. Airborne particulates, emitted mainly by diesel vehicles and visible as black smoke, carry volatile organic compounds such as benzene, a substance known to cause cancer in humans. Ozone (O_3) at ground level, produced by the effects of sunlight on traffic fumes, can make people more susceptible to infections and may lead to impaired lung function. There is even some evidence that the increase in the air pollution emitted by motor vehicles over the past 40 years could be responsible for the increase in the number of asthmatics admitted to hospital and of deaths following asthma attacks.[8]

Although vehicle emissions cause a variety of health problems and the griminess associated with city life, there are other forms of air pollution that are even more dangerous, if less well known. The toxic fallout generated by industry and agriculture consists of invisible gases and fine particles of synthetic chemicals. PCBs, dioxin and radioactive materials are only a few of the ingredients of the toxic soup we may be breathing.

CHEESE-LIKE DISCHARGES

Polychlorinated biphenyls (PCBs) are among the most poisonous substances ever created. Contact with them may produce such symptoms as skin rashes, darkened skin, cheese-like discharges from the eyes, loss of hair and libido, fatigue, numbness in the arms and legs, stomach ache, headaches, nausea, dizziness, forgetfulness, menstrual disturbances, and bone and joint deformities, as well as miscarriages and stillbirths.

PCBs were originally used in electrical capacitors and transformers, electrical insulants, hydraulic fluids, coatings for ironing board covers, flameproofing for synthetic yarns, laminates of ceramics and metals, and adhesives in the manufacture of brake linings, clutch faces and grinding wheels. In 1978, due to overwhelming evidence of their toxicity, the US government banned the manufacture, sale and use of PCBs in anything but capacitors and transformers.

However, this ban did nothing to recover the approximately 343,800,000 kg (758,000,000 lb) of PCBs being used in the US at the time, the 131,500,000 kg (290,000,000 lb) in dumps and landfills or the 68,000,000 kg (150,000,000 lb) in the soil, water and air.[9] As PCBs are still employed by the electrical industry and are virtually non-biodegradable, the threat they pose is as real today as it was in 1978.

DEAD BIRDS FALLING OUT OF THE SKY

Although PCBs are very high up the scale of toxicity, the dubious honour of being the most poisonous compounds ever developed in a laboratory must go to the dioxins: an amount one-hundredth as large as a grain of salt can kill a guinea pig in an instant. The dioxins comprise a group of 210 chemicals, 17 of which may be dangerous. However, only one – 2378-TCDD – has been studied in any depth.

Dioxins are by-products of chlorine bleaching and waste incineration; they are also found in some herbicides and pesticides. The effects of 2378-TCDD on animals include suppression of the immune system, liver damage, skin disorders, cancer, miscarriage and birth defects. In humans, the most common effect is chloracne, a severe form of acne that appears wherever the chemical has touched the body. The problem is a chronic one and can leave behind severe scarring. Doctors have also found that those exposed to dioxins may develop malaise, lack of appetite and abnormal lipid biochemistry.[10]

It had been known for some time that some dioxins are the most potent cancer-causing substances in rats and mice, but it wasn't until 1991 that there was solid evidence as to their potential for causing cancer in people. A study was carried out on 5172 workers in 12 American factories producing weedkillers, insecticides and disinfectants, all of which contained traces of dioxins. It showed that those who had been exposed to the compounds for as long as 20–30 years ran a 15 per cent higher risk of dying of cancer than workers who had not been exposed.[11]

In 1976, we found out just how deadly dioxins could be when a reactor malfunctioned at the Swiss chemical firm of Givaudan, sending a cloud laced with 2–3 kg (4.5–6.5 lb) of 2378-TCDD over the northern Italian town of Seveso. In the weeks that followed, leaves withered on trees, birds fell dead out of the sky and people developed a multitude of symptoms, including headaches, nausea and chloracne on legs, faces and arms. They were the lucky ones. In others exposed to the toxic cloud, there was an increased incidence of liver and kidney problems, and an increased susceptibility to infectious diseases and circulatory troubles. Greater than average numbers of miscarriages and deformed babies were also reported.

But we don't have to wait for an industrial accident to be exposed to dioxins: they are around us all the time. Minute amounts are present in anything that has been subjected to chlorine bleaching: coffee filter paper, milk cartons, tea bags, toilet tissue, make-up pads – the list goes on. A Canadian study found that milk sold in cardboard cartons contained a concentration of dioxins that was ten times higher than milk sold in bottles. Although many manufacturers, reacting to the bad publicity surrounding dioxin, are looking for alternatives to chlorine bleaching, the UK government has consistently stated that dioxins in paper products do not pose a risk to human health. The National Chemical Inspectorate of Sweden disagrees, and has recommended that all personal hygiene products should not be chlorine bleached.

A MAJOR MELTDOWN

Radioactive materials are an extremely hazardous by-product of the nuclear industry, and they are also produced by coal-fired power plants. This toxic waste may, just like chemicals, be transported great distances by air and water from its origin, posing an increased risk of cancer and genetic defects to all creatures in its path. Daily emissions are known to cause hideous deformities in farm animals born in areas surrounding plants; small accidents have, at times, proved fatal. At least 17 of the 108 nuclear power plants in the United States have caused radioactive pollution in their vicinity.[12]

Dr John Gofman, one of the scientists who helped create nuclear power, has stated that 'Nuclear power is unacceptable because it unavoidably inflicts cancer and genetic injury on people . . . It is mass, random, premeditated murder.' If this is true, why is it still being used?

The most publicized examples of what can happen when these huge plants seriously malfunction remain Chernobyl and Three Mile Island – a nuclear power station in Pennsylvania where, in March 1979, an accident resulted in the release of radioactive gases, and clean-up costs of $1 billion. But the severity of the problem is not merely the possibility of a freak accident. The looming danger of these plants is that many are ageing rapidly and are either fast approaching their 30-year design lifetime or have already passed it. In some cases in the US, millions of dollars have been poured into patching up the structures in an attempt to prolong their use. To compound matters, many of these time bombs have been built in earthquake zones, directly over fault lines.

It is amazing that we are so concerned with the threat of nuclear war and the devastating radiation that it could leave in its wake yet we allow nuclear reactors to be built in our midst. In May 1986, James Asseltine, head of the US Nuclear Regulatory Commission, said on BBC TV, 'I have had to advise Congress that there is a 45 per cent chance of another serious nuclear accident' – that is, another Chernobyl, a major meltdown of a reactor – 'within the next 20 years.'[13] If this should happen, it would cause immediate fatalities within a ten-mile radius of the plant. Conservative figures estimate that land would be contaminated at least 200 miles downwind of the reactor, and that radiation-contaminated milk would cause later cancer deaths in people within a 1000-mile radius. To put such a disaster into perspective, picture this scenario: If the Palo Verde power plant near Phoenix, Arizona had a major meltdown, almost all of the United States west of the Mississippi would be affected.

What we tend to forget is that, once an environment becomes heavily contaminated with radioactive wastes, it remains contaminated for hundreds of years. The Chernobyl accident grabbed the public's attention for several weeks, then slowly faded from the media. Yet today, years afterwards, the deformed farm animals still being born in areas near the abandoned plant, the child leukaemias and the mutant crops provide potent reminders that the danger has not faded. To get an even longer view, consider this analogy by the British writer Judith Cook: 'If the Romans had invented nuclear power, we would still, 2000 years later, have armed militia guarding their dumps of high-level waste.'[14]

Most people living in the British Isles might be surprised to know that the nuclear plant once named Windscale and now called Sellafield, on the Irish Sea in Cumbria, is the largest commercial producer of plutonium in the world. However, they would probably be astounded to know that, according to the House of Commons Select Committee on the Environment:

THE UK DISCHARGES MORE RADIOACTIVITY INTO THE SEA THAN ANY OTHER NATION . . . SELLAFIELD IS THE LARGEST RECORDED SOURCE OF RADIOAC-TIVE DISCHARGE IN THE WORLD. THE ANXIETY AND CONTROVERSY WHICH THIS AROUSES IN THE UK IS WELL KNOWN. IT ALSO CREATES ANXIETY IN OTHER NATIONS. WE FOUND, FOR EXAMPLE, THAT THE SWEDES COULD IDENTIFY RADIOACTIVE TRACES IN FISH OFF THEIR COAST BEING LARGELY ATTRIBUTABLE TO SELLAFIELD, GREATER EVEN THAN THE CONTAMINATION FROM ADJACENT SWEDISH NUCLEAR POWER STATIONS. SIMILAR EXPERI-ENCES WERE REPORTED TO US BY THE ISLE OF MAN GOVERNMENT. THAT THE UK, WITH A COMPARATIVELY SMALL NUCLEAR INDUSTRY, SHOULD BE SO DRAMATICALLY OUT OF STEP IS A CAUSE FOR CONCERN.[15]

This once proud nation has become the world's nuclear dustbin. A number of countries, including Germany and Japan, terrified of their own radioactive wastes, pay Britain to take these distasteful burdens off their hands.

Since it was acquired by the Ministry of Supply in 1947 for the construction of two air-cooled nuclear reactors, Sellafield has had almost 300 accidents, including a core fire in 1957 that was, until Three Mile Island, the most serious accident to occur in a nuclear plant. Enormous amounts of radioactive waste material are routinely pumped from it into the Irish Sea through a pipeline $1^1/_2$ miles long, or vented through smokestacks into the air. Plutonium from Sellafield has been found in Ireland, Iceland, Sweden, Denmark and Belgium. In the village nearest the plant, one child in 60 dies of cancer, and comparable rates have been found in other villages in the region. However, no one is prevented from fishing in the area, although fish caught there are 5000 times more radioactive than those caught in the North Sea. The government has issued no warnings about the hazards of living or holidaying in this part of Cumbria, or of growing or marketing food in this region known to be polluted by radioactive wind and rain. [16]

Rather than attempt to reduce the amount of radioactive pollution emanating from Sellafield, the British government seems hellbent on increasing it. Under construction since the 1980s, the thermal oxide reprocessing plant – THORP – at Sellafield finally received the go-ahead from the government in December 1993 to take in most of the world's nuclear waste for reprocessing. As long ago as 1986, the House of Commons Select Committee was dubious about its financial viability; today, there is little doubt that THORP will be an economic disaster.

But it will also be the cause of thousands of deaths. According to the International Commission on Radiological Protection, there are 0.05 deaths per man-Sievert (m-Sv; the unit of a collective dose of radiation received by all members of a population), or one death per 20 m-Sv. The UK's National Radiological Protection Board has estimated that THORP will annually add 4100 m-Sv to the environment from increased discharges into the sea and air; these 4100 m-Sv equal 205 deaths a year, and if the plant runs for at least ten years (which it is expected to do), that means that there will be an additional 2050 radiation-caused deaths from THORP, not counting any that might result from accidents. [17]

TICKING CHEMICAL TIME BOMBS

Human debris clogs not only our skies but also our water. Rivers, once able to cleanse themselves with their powerful currents, are becoming overwhelmed with our refuse; bottles, cans, paper, plastic and other rubbish litter their banks. Lakes are suffocating under the advance of detergents; bubbles froth at their edges, and algae, feeding on the phosphates in the detergents, spread across their expanse, sucking oxygen from the water and depriving the lakes of life. Even the oceans, previously thought to be limitless dumping grounds for all of humankind's detritus, are finally rejecting the endless stream of wastes, spewing hypodermic needles and oil-covered wildlife on to their beaches. These are the obvious signs of modern society's destruction of the environment's natural balance, and should be of concern to every one of us.

However, what we should really fear is, again, what we cannot see.

Too often we drink tap water without realizing its potential hazards. After all, if it comes from a tap, it must be pure, mustn't it? In the United States 50 years ago, that may have been true, but it is no longer, and what is happening there reflects the problems now faced by most developing countries.

Tap water originates either from surface water, such as streams, lakes and rivers, which, in England and Wales, accounts for about two thirds of drinking water, or from groundwater coming from vast underground networks called aquifers. Between its point of origin and its final destination, the water we drink may be assaulted by a wide array of chemicals and outright poisons from a number of sources.

Toxic waste dumps provide what American industry believes to be the best final resting place for the 263 million tonnes (290 million tons) of hazardous chemical wastes produced by the United States every year. However, the EPA admits that there is no way to prevent even the most carefully constructed injection well, pond, lagoon or landfill from leaking and eventually contaminating water supplies far below ground. Of the approximately 300,000 toxic waste sites across the US today, 1000 are on the EPA's national priority list for clean-up, and it is predicted that an additional 9000 will soon join them. The estimated cost for cleaning up these 10,000 sites has already been put at hundreds of billions of dollars, yet it is only a matter of time before leaks occur at every toxic waste dump.

Landfills are another graveyard for hazardous substances such as cleaning fluids, home and garden pesticides and heavy metals. No measures whatsoever are taken to prevent the toxic residues of these wastes from slowly leaking into groundwater supplies, although, in the UK, waste disposal companies try to collect and treat them, but with little success. Today the US has a total of 360,000 active landfills and an equal or even greater number of closed dumps. At present, almost 40,000 of the sites are believed to be contaminating groundwater; the cost of cleaning them up is about the same as for toxic waste dumps.

With the explosive growth of the car industry in the 1950s and 1960s came the need for petrol and other petroleum products. More than 2.5 million storage tanks containing these substances were buried in the US, and today the EPA estimates that perhaps 35 per cent of them are leaking into water supplies. One gallon of leaked petrol per day is enough to contaminate groundwater for hundreds or even thousands of years.

Taking all these sources of toxic pollution together, there is approximately one ticking chemical bomb per square mile in the United States. And these are not the only potential hazards to drinking water.

PESTICIDES, SEWAGE AND ACID RAIN

Pesticide use nearly tripled in the United States between 1965 and 1985, and in 1990, 28,000 tonnes (30,850 tons) of pesticides and herbicides were used in the UK alone. At some point, much of the pesticides and herbicides sprayed on to plants will be washed off on to the ground, where they will make their way to the groundwater supplies. The extent of American contamination is unknown – no state bothers to monitor pesticide run-off. But a report on London's drinking water found that no supplies were completely free of herbicide residues. The pesticides simazine and atrazine, used by local authorities and British Rail to control weeds, were finally banned in August 1993 because they were so often found in tap water.

Sewage, both human and animal, poses additional problems. Waste treatment plants in many cities only partially treat sewage before discharging it into rivers and lakes and into the sea. A few places don't even bother to do this, but simply run long pipes into waterways, discharging wastes in their natural states. In Britain, surfers have banded together to protest against the pollution of beaches in this way.

Not only must human wastes be considered but also animal wastes from farms and large meat production centres. Tons of manure are produced, all of which has to be moved, stored and spread on fields as fertilizers – without allowing it into the water supply. Yet some of it does get in, and with it comes nitrates, used in chemical fertilizers. In 1991, 3 per cent of water samples taken in England and Wales exceeded the limit set by the government, mainly in southern, eastern and central England. Reboiling nitrate-laden water increases the concentration of the pollutant.

High levels of nitrates can lead to a very rare condition in bottle-fed babies called methaemoglobinaemia, or 'blue baby syndrome', which reduces the flow of oxygen to the brain and other tissues. The last confirmed case in Britain was in 1972, and most cases have been associated with water from private wells that was also contaminated with bacteria. The body converts nitrates into nitrites, which have been shown to cause cancer in animals. There is also a theoretical link between nitrates and stomach cancer in people.

The old saying 'What goes up must come down' certainly holds true for the polluting gases sulphur dioxide and nitrogen oxide. Produced by industry, they are transported for many miles on wind currents, then return to Earth in the form of acid rain. The toxins leach into groundwater or run off into lakes and rivers, stifling life as they go. This form of water pollution has affected much of the eastern United States, as well as northern Britain, Western Germany and much of Scandinavia. A majority of the European pollution originates in Britain, but thus far, the government has failed to admit its responsibility, despite international protests.

HOW LOW IS SAFE?

Despite the growing number of hazards to drinking water, many officials still insist that it is pure and unadulterated. Although the enormous increase in sales of bottled water indicates that the public is becoming aware of the risks, too many people still believe the official line and simply assume that, because they are hooked up to a public water supply, the government will protect them from water contamination. This is not true. Although regulations require routine monitoring and treatment of water supplies, and that water must meet minimum quality standards, this does nothing to guarantee the purity of tapwater.

The number of contaminants monitored – 30 are required in the US by EPA regulations – is small in comparison to the number of toxins that may actually be in the water. Testing is the only way to determine contamination since many toxic chemicals cannot be seen or tasted. In the United States, more than 2000 toxic chemicals have been found in drinking water since 1974, nearly 200 of which are either known or suspected causes of cancer, cell mutations, nervous system disorders and birth defects. [18] In addition, an estimated 1900 to 2100 water contaminants have never been tested for toxicity to humans.

Even if potentially harmful contaminants are discovered – and violation of standards due to lax enforcement occurs far more often than it should – many pollutants cannot be removed using current treatment methods. So, rather than cause a public panic, officials report nothing. Or they may report contamination but then claim that the level is too low to be hazardous. But how can a low level of a contaminant be considered safe for human consumption if it has never been tested? In the UK and the rest of the European Community, some standards – e. g. those for pesticides – are not based on scientific evidence of health risks, but on the lowest limit that could be detected at the time the EC Drinking Water Directive 1980 was drawn up.

Contaminants in drinking water may go undetected or unreported to the public for months or even years. A prime example of this has happened in Phoenix, Arizona, where the contamination of a large proportion of the area's water supply by trichlorethylene (TCE), an industrial solvent, was brought to light by the *New Times*, a local newspaper. [19] The culprit, Motorola, is an $11 billion multinational electronics manufacturing company and the state's largest employer, with several plants in the Phoenix region. From the 1950s to the 1970s, it legally dumped thousands of gallons of chemicals into unlined lagoons and dry wells and even down the drain, but as early as 1966, the company knew that this could have serious consequences. Yet no investigations were carried out, and the public was not warned by the local news media or by state and federal regulators, and certainly not by Motorola itself.

Today, nearly 40 years later, present and past employees of the company, and others who have lived for years next to the two plants with the worst pollution records, are afflicted with leukaemias as well as diseases of the kidney and liver and the immune and central nervous systems. Legal battles over who is responsible for the damage and the clean-up are just beginning, and Motorola has already spent nearly $30 million (£20 million) on trying to remove the chemical from the ground-water supply.

However, groundwater that is polluted cannot cleanse itself as, say, rivers can; the pollutants can remain in it for decades or longer. The National Rivers Authority in Britain, responsible for protecting ground-water, says prevention is not only better than cure – in some cases, there is no cure. This, according to some American scientists, is the situation in Phoenix: it may take the aquifers up to 1000 years to be purged of the TCE naturally, and at present, no other way of getting rid of the chemical is known.

This is only a single example of what is happening all over the world. It is estimated that, if water pollution continues at current rates, as much as one quarter of the world's freshwater supply could be unsafe for human consumption by the end of the 1990s.[20] What sort of future will our children have?

DELIBERATE POLLUTANTS?

So far we have looked at pollutants that have somehow unintentionally leaked into drinking water. However, as if these weren't bad enough, water treatment plants routinely add their own supply of chemicals in the name of good health.

Fluoride has attracted controversy ever since it was first added to water supplies in the 1950s. Some scientists maintain that it builds strong teeth and bones, yet studies have revealed that the same decrease in tooth decay rates have been shown in children living in areas with fluoridated water and in those who don't.[21] Other health experts point to the link between fluoride and mottled teeth, bone and joint deterioration, bone cancer and damaged immune systems, as well as Alzheimer's disease, migraines, brain tumours and various other neuropsychiatric disorders. Long-term effects of fluoride ingestion may also include headaches, ringing in the ears, depression, confusion, drowsiness, visual disturbances, severe fatigue and loss of memory.[22]

In the United States, 6500 Maryland residents suffered such neurological symptoms when an 'overdose' of fluoride was accidentally dumped into their water system in 1979. Fluoride is a toxic substance. It serves no nutritional need, is not compatible with normal body functions and can interfere with proper enzyme functioning. If countries such as

France, Germany, Austria, Belgium, Denmark, Greece, Holland, Italy, Luxembourg, Norway, Spain and Sweden have banned the adding of fluoride to public water supplies, why is it still being added in the United States and in parts of the United Kingdom?

While it still is, make sure that you don't give yourself an 'overdose'. Find out from your water company whether your water is already fluoridated (as it is in Birmingham and elsewhere) or already contains a relatively high level of natural fluoride (as it does in, say, Hartlepool). If either of these is true for your area, avoid using fluoride toothpaste and certainly don't give your children fluoride tablets or drops.

The addition of chlorine to water supplies stems from the very real fear of waterborne diseases such as typhoid, cholera and diphtheria, which once were responsible for the deaths of hundreds of thousands of people. Chlorination of water does reduce the risk of infectious diseases, but also causes a whole gamut of new contaminants called trihalo-methanes (THMs), created when chlorine reacts with organic matter such as particles of rotted leaves or insects. Chloroform, one of the four major THMs, is suspected of causing bladder cancer.

The best way to rid water of chlorine is to install an activated carbon filter. Alternatives include boiling water for two or three minutes, then cooling it for drinking, or letting it stand overnight before using it.

GREENER PASTURES?

Developed societies produce mountains of refuse every day. For example, every American generates more than 2 kg (5 lb) of solid rubbish daily, or nearly one ton a year. But there and elsewhere in the West, this vast accumulation goes unnoticed because of our reliance on a system we all take for granted – rubbish collection.

While we bicker among ourselves about whose turn it is to take out the trash, officials in heavily populated areas are quietly tearing their hair out trying to find somewhere to put it all. In the United States within the next ten years, four states – Florida, Massachusetts, New Hampshire and New Jersey – will close virtually all of their currently active landfill sites. [23] Some large cities already transport their refuse across state lines and pay smaller communities to deal with it. This is a growing issue across North America, and the problem is even greater in smaller, yet more overcrowded countries such as Britain and Japan. What do you do with your rubbish if no one comes to collect it?

The potato peelings, cat litter, used tissues, empty containers, day-old newspapers and other things we casually dump into bin liners and take to the front of our homes for collection are fast becoming a threat to health. From landfill sites – whether active or closed – seep toxic wastes that soak through the ground to poison water supplies. Once a site has been closed, it remains practically useless for anything else. The inevitable nooks and crannies formed by squashed, discarded objects make a fantastic underground maze for insect and rodent colonies. Decaying garbage also produces a tremendous amount of gases, some of which are toxic and some of which are flammable, giving rise to the danger of explosions and fires. If rubbish is incinerated instead, poisonous chemicals are emitted into the air, and the ash that remains becomes just another hazardous waste to be sent on its way to another overloaded waste site. Even rubbish dumped at sea comes back to haunt us in the form of filthy beaches and poisoned seafood.

Ancient societies could simply move on to greener pastures and leave their rubbish behind, but our backs are against the wall. Not only do we have no place to go, but the wastes that our civilization is leaving in its wake will not disintegrate and return to the earth as the ancients' did, but will remain to pollute the soil and air for hundreds of years.

The normal waste products of the average household are bad enough, but yet again, it is what we don't see or know about that may be far more deadly – and it may just land up in our own backyards. Just as city officials are facing a shortage of landfill sites for household rubbish, large industrial companies are facing a shortage of dumping sites for their toxic by-products. Hauliers of hazardous wastes may be transporting their poisonous loads past your door every day in unmarked lorries or trains. You may not be aware that this is happening until an accident occurs and the truth hits the headlines. Hauliers have even been known to let wastes slowly drain out across the countryside or dump their loads on to the roadside, on waste ground or into rivers in the middle of the night.

INDOOR POLLUTION

Too often we think of our 'environment' as a place far removed from us – say, a national park where we go to view forests and dales and moorland and breathe in the good, clean air. Yet we know now that industry's chemicals have touched every part of this 'environment'. But our offices, living rooms and even the interiors of our cars are all part of our own personal environments, and industry's pollution of our world begins right here in the great indoors – in our homes, our workplaces, wherever we are.

While outdoor pollution is dispersed to some extent by wind and rain, chemicals used indoors remain relatively concentrated and, as a result, are potentially more hazardous. A study by the US Consumer Product Safety Commission revealed the presence of as many as 150 different chemicals indoors compared to ten or less outside.[24] The Total Exposure Assessment Methodology Studies, carried out by the EPA in the United States over a period of ten years, revealed that typical indoor levels of some toxic pollutants can be up to 20 times higher than those outdoors. [25] These indoor levels would be considered illegal if they were to occur out of doors, yet we spend 80 to 90 per cent of our time breathing this chemical-laden air. According to Lance A. Wallace, an environmental scientist at the EPA, these findings 'are so at odds with conventional wisdom . . . that most people have not yet grasped their importance.'

Unfortunately for a woman I know, it took years for her to grasp that importance, to realize that it was actually her personal environment that was slowly poisoning her. Margaret now believes that her illnesses began when she was four or five years old and became progressively worse as she grew older.

As a child, she suffered from irregular heart palpitations and aches and pains in her arms, legs and stomach. As an adolescent, she was routinely troubled by sore throats, severe acne and headaches. Depression followed her throughout her life. When she was in her late 20s, symptom upon symptom slowly began to appear until she was almost completely debilitated. Her feet hurt and arthritic-like pains struck different parts of her body at various times. She began to develop varicose veins, and when she didn't have diarrhoea, she suffered from constipation, which led to haemorrhoids. Her sense of taste almost vanished, and after meals, she suffered from stomach pains and 'wind' and felt sick, ravenous or sleepy. Menstrual periods, times of crippling agony, left her exhausted for several days afterwards. Tension stiffened her body and kept her awake at night, and sore throats came and went frequently for no apparent reason. She began to experience facial pain, loss of memory, weight problems and near total exhaustion round the clock.

It was at this point that, overwhelmed by her multitude of ailments, Margaret began to lose hope, and she seriously contemplated suicide. Then she met a friend of a friend who was suffering in the same way, and she began to realize that she was not simply a headcase, but someone who was very ill with very real problems. Gradually, with the help of her friend, it dawned on her that it was her surroundings that were making her sick, and she began to eliminate those items from her home that caused her such severe physical reactions.

It is only now, after several years of 'clean' living, that Margaret can lead a somewhat normal life. She must still monitor her surroundings, taking care to avoid certain products, places and chemicals, but she improves daily. Her case is an extreme example of how an indoor environment can affect a person; millions of people may be affected in minor ways by the same chemicals that made Margaret suffer so drastically.

According to the Board of Environmental Studies and Toxicology of the US National Research Council, approximately 15 per cent of Americans – or more than 30 million people – are adversely affected by chemicals found in the home, in offices and elsewhere indoors.[26] There are many symptoms of chemical toxicity, varying in severity according to each individual's sensitivity to a particular substance. These symptoms include: headaches, joint pain, fatigue, dizziness, behaviour changes, mood swings, insomnia, memory loss, constipation, abdominal pains, nervousness, confusion, depression, loss of sex drive, skin rashes, coughing, wheezing, nausea.

Because chemical toxicity isn't yet widely recognized and, in many cases, symptoms are so widespread, many people just accept them as a part of daily life. Rather than eliminating the cause(s) of their suffering, they continue to live in misery. But this may have far worse effects than might be imagined. It is now believed that people who have low-level, repeated contact with certain common household chemicals may gradually develop subtle brain and nerve impairments. Chemical toxicity may affect to different degrees anyone of any age, but in the elderly, the unborn, young children and people with prior respiratory and/or cardiac problems, it can cause severe problems – and sometimes it can be fatal.

The good news is that, unlike outdoor pollution, the air quality in our homes is well within our control. Freedom from chemical sensitivities will, for many, require only minor changes in lifestyle, although for the extremely sensitive, monumental alterations may be necessary. However, before any steps towards better health are taken, it is crucial to understand our potential enemies.

POISONOUS VAPOURS

Indoor air contamination is usually associated with the vapours and particulates produced from a variety of man-made sources. Indeed, some of the most lethally polluted air may be the result of using everyday household items. Gases from cleaning supplies, appliances and pesticides and smoke from cigarettes combine with 'biologicals' and radon (*see later*) to form an invisibly toxic but breathable soup.

It begins when we roll up our sleeves and prepare to do battle with the dust and dirt in our homes. We proudly open our war chests of 'harmless' furniture and floor polishes, window cleaners, bleaches, oven and drain cleaners, ammonia and other cleaning supplies. While the labels of virtually every container are plastered with dire warnings to the consumer about the results of drinking the chemicals within, most say nothing about the effects that the vapours might have on our bodies. The list of ingredients won't be of much help, even if we knew anything about the chemicals: because of 'commercial confidentiality', the law does not require a complete list.[27]

The most dangerous ingredients in these products are organic chemicals that are used for their ability to dissolve other substances and evaporate quickly. Immediate symptoms on exposure to them can include eye and respiratory tract irritation, nausea, headaches, dizziness, visual disorders and memory impairment. Long-term effects include kidney and liver damage and cancer.

Although most people realize that a chemical caustic enough to clean an oven must be harmful to the human body, many are unaware that even such everyday items as hairspray, air fresheners, antiperspirants, nail varnish, perfumes, moth balls and dry-cleaning fumes on clothes can cause toxic reactions. Methylene chloride, a substance that has a high risk of causing cancer, can be found in many of these items. Perchloro-ethylene (PCE), a common dry-cleaning solvent, has also been linked with cancer. Nothing that has been manufactured or treated chemically is immune from producing toxic vapours.

Despite our tremendous reliance on the products we consider everyday household items, there are alternatives. Borax, vinegar, corn-flour, baking soda, lemon juice and plain hot water, in various combina-tions, provide a startling array of natural cleaning products, ranging from window cleaners to scouring powders, spot removers to furniture pol-ishes. If concocting your own cleaners is too much of a hassle, make sure you treat the chemical substances in your home with care. Throw away partially empty containers and old and unnecessary chemicals; buy limited quantities of the chemicals to begin with; and reduce your exposure to all their vapours.

Other pollutants we are even less likely to consider dangerous, but which may be far more serious to our health, are combustion by-products. The gaseous contaminants and particulates emitted by wood stoves, fireplaces, candles, paraffin heaters and lamps and gas ap-pliances, as well as those that leak into homes from attached garages, all contribute to poor indoor air quality.

The major pollutants produced by these sources are nitrogen dioxide, carbon monoxide, sulphur dioxide and particulates (i.e. smoke). Low levels of these vapours in a home can cause fatigue in healthy people, and episodes of increased chest pain in those with heart disease. Higher levels can cause chronic bronchitis and other respiratory infections, headaches, eye, nose and throat irritation, dizziness, nausea, weakness and confusion. Extremely high levels may even result in unconsciousness and death. Long-term exposure to low levels of these gases and particu-lates may lead to emphysema and cancer.

Another danger inherent in combustion by-products is that they can reach unhealthy levels within a home and overwhelm those living there before anyone is aware of the problem. It is estimated that carbon monoxide (CO) – a colourless, odourless, tasteless gas – is responsible for half the fatal poisonings in the United States each year. In Britain, CO from faulty gas appliances kills 50 people annually. Yet pollution from combustion appliances should not be a serious problem if they are properly installed, vented and maintained.

SECOND-HAND SMOKING

It has been proved that smoking is hazardous to your health. But smokers seem unimpressed by the fact that hundreds of thousands of people die every year from smoking-related diseases – for instance, in any five-year period, more Americans die from smoking than died in all the wars that the US has ever fought. The fact that the incidence of lung cancer has increased dramatically since the 1930s apparently means nothing either.

Although tar and nicotine are the first harmful substances that come to mind when one thinks of cigarettes, pipes and cigars, tobacco smoke contains an additional 1500 to 3000 chemicals, including carbon monoxide, hydrogen cyanide and benzene.[28] Tobacco itself may carry pesticide residues from when it was growing, combustion particles from the curing process, and flavourings and sweeteners that companies add to improve its taste – all of which are inhaled when the tobacco is smoked.

It is well known that smoking causes lung cancer. Additional health problems include heart and circulatory system disease, chronic bronchitis, emphysema, anaemia, chromosome deterioration, bone marrow damage, leukaemia and other cancers throughout the body. Pregnant smokers are more likely to give birth to premature, underweight or stillborn babies.

Considering the multitude of ways that smoking can affect the body detrimentally, it is amazing that anyone smokes at all any more, especially since smokers are not the only ones affected. According to the collective results of more than 20 studies in Britain, non-smokers living with smokers are 10–30 per cent more likely to develop lung cancer than those living with non-smokers.[29] The EPA has stated that passive smoking (also called second-hand or involuntary smoking) causes between 500 and 5000 deaths annually in the US alone. The findings of the US National Council for Clean Indoor Air are even more shocking: they reckon that passive smoking is responsible for 46,000 deaths in the United States every year.[30]

Passive smokers are prey to these sometimes fatal illnesses because, unbelievably, the sidestream smoke they inhale is more dangerous than the smoke that smokers themselves are breathing into their lungs. It may take an adult passive smoker some time to become a statistic, but household tobacco smoke affects children far more quickly. A possible link has been made between sudden infant death syndrome (SIDS) – i.e.

cot death – and parents who smoke. Studies have shown that the children of smokers are more likely to: develop bronchitis and pneumonia in their first years; be, on average, 1 cm (about $1/2$ in) shorter than their friends at primary school age; lag, at age 11, up to six months behind their classmates in reading, maths and other subjects; and have a high incidence of dying from leukaemia, both earlier and later in life. Research in Sweden, reported in the *British Journal of Industrial Medicine* in July 1991, also showed a link between exposure to tobacco smoke as a child and the development of 'sick building syndrome', which we will come to shortly.

It is unlikely that any one of us would open a gas oven to heat our homes – we know that it would be too dangerous. Yet many smokers never consider the dangerous pollution they add to their homes by smoking, or the bodily harm they are doing to themselves and, more importantly, to their loved ones.

A FATAL GAME OF GOLF

None of the products we bring into our homes is as lethal as pesticides. The suffix *-cide* is derived from the Latin word meaning 'to kill', and that is exactly what pesticides were created to do, whether the object of this lethal ability be insects (insecticides), rats and mice (rodenticides), mites (miticides), weeds (herbicides), germs (germicides) or moulds (fungicides). Despite the warnings of potential danger that they bear, these products are frequently used far too casually, with little thought of the consequences.

An estimated nine out of ten American households use pesticides. In a frantic search to control the 'undesirables', Americans spend $630 million (£420 million) a year on over-the-counter pesticides and an additional $2.5 billion (£1.7 billion) for professional exterminators.[31] Although these products are recognized as killing agents, tons of them are being sprayed and powdered in the very spaces in which we live and work. The chilling truth is that, while experts may know that an insecticide will kill a particular bug, little is known about how it will affect a human being. The World Health Organization states that, every year, about 3 million people suffer acute, severe poisoning with pesticides, and the Pesticides Trust in Britain reckons that some 20,000 of these individuals will die – primarily those involved in the manufacture of these substances or their use in agriculture. But it is difficult not to fear the effects of pesticides even in the relatively low amounts used in the home.

Immediate symptoms of pesticide poisoning are eye, nose and throat irritation, blurred vision, twitching, loss of coordination, mental confusion, digestion disturbances, weakness, dizziness, headaches, palpitations and fatigue. Long-term effects may include depression, memory loss, anxiety, paranoia, central nervous system disorders, liver and kidney ailments and possibly even Parkinson's disease. The phrase 'long-term effects' does not only refer to everyday use of a pesticide over a period of years. These chemicals are more insidious than that. Such effects can be caused by the accumulation of these substances in body fat, or their continuing presence in areas where they have been used. Some pesticides have been known to contaminate a space for as long as 20 years!

One of the most horrendous examples of just how lethal pesticides can be involved a healthy US Air Force pilot in Arlington, Virginia, who decided to play golf on a course that had recently been sprayed with a fungicide. Shortly after he teed off, he began suffering flu-like symptoms, headache, a rash and a high fever. By the next day, his body was covered with severe blisters. Two weeks later, he was in a coma. Before the end of the third week, most of his skin had peeled off. He eventually died of kidney failure and pneumonia.[32] If this could happen in the open air, just imagine what could happen when pesticides are used indoors.

Fortunately, there are natural ways to avoid the need for pesticides in the home. The most simple of these is to keep your home clean, store food in closed containers and empty rubbish bins regularly. Plug any holes and cracks that pests might use to enter your house or flat. If you have to resort to commercial chemicals, use them strictly according to the manufacturers' directions and make sure that where you use them is well ventilated. Only employ well-known, reputable pest control companies.

SICK HOMES

Substances that have managed to seep their way into a home or have been deliberately introduced are not the only causes of toxic reactions. The building itself and its furnishings might also be at the root of chemical sensitivities. So many people are now affected by the construction of their homes – and workplaces – that illnesses caused by them are collectively known as 'sick building syndrome'.

Over the past few decades, the use of chemicals in the production of construction materials has increased over five-fold, perhaps to the benefit of the building industry but not to the health of the buildings' inhabitants. Once they are part of a structure, these materials emit vapours, some of which can be extremely toxic even to the hardiest of individuals.

To make matters worse, the energy crunch of the 1970s created the concept of the sealed building. While this may promote energy efficiency, such a structure does not 'breathe'. Instead, vapours from cleaning products, dust, smoke, pollen, gases such as radon (*see later*) and chemicals emitted from construction materials all become trapped inside and may rise to toxic levels. It would not be entirely wrong to say that, in tightly sealing our homes and workplaces against outdoor elements, we have actually created our own personal gas chambers.

Biological contaminants, or 'biologicals', may accumulate, too, and cause a variety of symptoms similar to those due to chemical exposure. Common household dust – carrying the faeces of house dust mites, mould spores, pollen, animal and human dander, bacteria and viruses, fabric and insect particles as well as chemical residues – can produce all the symptoms of allergies, including itchy urticaria (nettle rash), sneezing, watery eyes, coughing, shortness of breathe, wheezing, dizziness, lethargy, headaches and digestion problems. More serious respiratory conditions such as asthma, hypersensitivity, pneumonitis and allergic rhinitis (nose inflammation) may develop if a person is exposed to high levels of biologicals. Children, elderly people and those with allergies, lung diseases and other breathing problems are particularly susceptible.

The growth in biologicals in the home is usually in direct proportion to the humidity maintained inside. House dust mites, whose faeces contain a powerful and very common allergen, tend to be most prolific at 70 per cent humidity, so it is advisable to maintain a relative humidity of 30–50 per cent in winter and 40–60 per cent in summer to minimize their numbers. To prevent breeding grounds for mould and mildew, appliances containing standing water, such as vaporizers, humidifiers, air conditioners and refrigerators, should be emptied and cleaned regularly. Water-damaged materials, such as carpets, rugs or furniture, should be cleaned and dried thoroughly or replaced.

While hoovering may appear to be the most logical way to control dust, many machines without adequate filters simply fling dust and particles into the air. To remove biologicals from floor coverings properly, a central vacuum-cleaning system, a water-based vacuum or one specially designed for people with allergies should be used. Also, vent all exhaust fans used in kitchens and bathrooms, including clothes driers, to the outdoors. Perhaps the most important thing to remember is simply to keep your home clean.

ASBESTOS AND LEAD

Asbestos, a fibrous mineral once used extensively in building materials, is one of the most deadly indoor pollutants. Although considered the perfect construction material in the early decades of this century, by the early 1930s it was officially recognized by the British government to be an extreme health hazard. Its use in buildings and appliances is now prohibited, but it can still be found in older structures – around hot water and steam pipes, as boiler wraps, in vinyl flooring, ducts and furnaces, decorative wall and ceiling coatings, insulation, roofing, textured paints, fireproof board, acoustic ceiling tiles, door gaskets, appliances such as ovens and toasters, vehicle brake linings and even children's toys.[33]

Unlike other indoor pollutants, asbestos does not emit any noxious gases. However, when it becomes loose, is damaged or decays, microscopic mineral fibres escape into the air. These tiny, sharp particles are inhaled and lodge in people's lungs, where they do not dissolve but can cause asbestosis, a lung disease that is usually fatal, as well as cancer of the stomach and of the membrane surrounding the lungs (mesothelioma). Asbestos exposure produces no immediate symptoms, and it can take 15–30 years for asbestosis or cancer to develop. There is a cure for neither.

If you find asbestos in your home, *do not touch it.* Contact your local environmental health officer immediately. You will have to arrange to have it either removed, encapsulated or sealed off. It is vital to understand that, if you go the removal route, it must be done by professionals. Although this may be expensive, experts consider it the only permanent solution. Don't be surprised if the workers brought in to do the job arrive dressed as if about to enter a toxic waste dump – asbestos has the potential to be that lethal.

Lead is another health threat posed by many older homes. In Britain, it most commonly leaches into the water supply through old pipes and water tanks (this use of lead was banned in 1976). Lead-based solder on copper pipes (banned in 1989) may also contribute to lead levels. If you are worried about your water, take a sample – retrieved first thing in the morning, after the water has been standing overnight, when the lead level will be at its greatest – to your local environmental health officer for testing.

Lead is also frequently found in paints used on houses before the 1950s. Lead compounds were added to both interior and exterior paints to make them shinier, to fix colours and to make them last longer. It was not until 1976 that the US Consumer Product Safety Commission lowered the amount of lead allowed in house paint and, then, in 1978, banned it completely. Other developed countries soon followed suit.

Another, rather unexpected source of lead exposure is lead crystal. The British medical journal, the *Lancet*, reported in January 1991 that the lead level in port kept in a lead crystal decanter for four months rose from 89 to 5331 micrograms/litre – more than 100 times the permitted level in water. Brandy decanted for five years contained a staggering 21,530 micrograms/litre.

Lead ingestion may produce a variety of severe side-effects, including brain damage, stunted growth, hearing loss, and blood and kidney diseases. Even at low levels, it is toxic to many organs of the body, and can cause high blood pressure in adults. At high levels, it can be fatal.

Lead is particularly dangerous to children because their tissues absorb the substance more easily, and their low body weight ensures that even low concentrations are more damaging. Children are also more likely to play in areas contaminated by lead and then put their fingers or lead-contaminated objects into their mouths. Delays in physical and mental development, lower intelligence, shortened attention spans and increased behavioural problems have all been attributed to lead exposure.

Just as with asbestos, it may be best to leave the removal of lead to the professionals. Lead paint can flake into microscopic particles or very fine dust, making it an insidious enemy; its removal requires protective clothing, an extremely good ventilation system and thorough cleaning of the area when finished. You may be able to receive a council grant to help with the cost of replacing lead pipes and tanks.

The easiest way to reduce exposure to lead in tapwater is to allow the water to run for a few minutes before using it. Also, if you have a lead immersion heater, never use hot water from the tap for drinking or cooking: heat increases the corrosion of lead, making the water in the tank more highly contaminated than cold water coming in from the mains.

FUMES FROM WALLS AND FURNITURE

Another problematic material used in the construction and insulation of many homes is formaldehyde, a chemical most people associate with biology lab specimens. Formaldehyde fumes are produced particularly by particle board and plywood, but are also emitted by chip board, gypsum board, laminated lumber, vinyl imitation wood panels, plaster, stucco, wallpaper, paint, concrete and glues and adhesives. Many of these products can be found in the subflooring, work surfaces, cupboards and panelling of homes, but even upholstery and curtains can emit this toxic vapour. Perhaps the most common source for the fumes is urea formaldehyde cavity wall insulation. Although the amount of formaldehyde emitted slowly diminishes over time, it may take several years before the fumes are at a level low enough to be harmless. The Building Research Establishment in the UK recommends not draught-proofing for 12 months after installing urea formaldehyde insulation.

Even at very low levels, formaldehyde may cause minor eye, nose and throat irritation, shortness of breath, headaches, nausea and lethargy. Low concentrations may also aggravate coughs, sore throats, colds asthma, and may even induce vomiting and diarrhoea. Higher levels may cause other symptoms such as gastrointestinal disturbances, dizziness, insomnia, depression, fatigue, menstrual and other gynaecological problems, feelings of chest constriction, muscle and joint pains, blood clots, phlebitis (vein inflammation) and heart irregularities. Extended periods of exposure are now believed to be a possible cause of cancer.

There are a number of ways of reducing levels of formaldehyde in the home. Removing the source may be the most effective method but will probably be the most expensive if the culprit is subflooring or insulation. Treating subflooring or walls with a sealant will prevent at least a proportion of the fumes from escaping. An unusual but reportedly effective way to reduce formaldehyde vapours is to install houseplants that absorb the gas – philodendrons and spider plants are particularly good at this.

Of course, simple ventilation will reduce formaldehyde levels, although you have to be careful that, during the cold months, you aren't also heating the great outdoors; heat-recovery ventilators may help. It is also important to control the indoor temperature and humidity of a home as many construction materials emit more fumes in warm, humid environments. Finally, don't buy furniture containing materials that will emit formaldehyde. There's no point in making the problem even worse than it already is.

You may be able to avoid buying furniture containing formaldehyde, but it is almost impossible to avoid plastics. Products made from this oil-based material come in every size and shape imaginable. Plastics have many names; acetate, acrylic, polyester, polyurethane, polystyrene, polyvinyl chloride, nylon, vinyl are just a few. Unfortunately, many plastics, especially soft ones, emit invisible toxic vapours, particularly in warm areas with high humidity. While emissions from hard plastics gradually decrease, softer varieties can emit vapours indefinitely, causing fatigue, headaches and upset stomachs in those who breathe in the fumes.

Plastic emissions within a home may come from such construction materials as vinyl sheet flooring, but they usually originate from plastic furniture, appliances with plastic parts and items such as plastic lamp shades, shower curtains, table cloths and mattress covers. If you find that you or those who live with you are experiencing any inexplicable symptoms, and you cannot find another cause, try removing the plastic objects around you.

THE RADIOACTIVE HOME

Radon, a naturally occurring indoor contaminant, has received much publicity in recent years. A heavy, colourless, odourless, nonflammable gas, it is produced from the breakdown of uranium in the ground. The highest concentrations of radon are generally found in rocky places. In the United Kingdom, the areas most affected are Cornwall and Devon, although pockets of high levels had been found throughout the country. The only way to find out if it is present in your home is by the use of radon detectors.

While harmless out of doors, radon can seep into homes, become trapped and build up to hazardous levels. It breaks down into decay products known as 'radon daughters' or 'progeny', which can bombard the body, especially the lungs, and cause lung cancer. The National Radiological Protection Board (NRPB) estimates that at least 100,000 homes (out of 21 million in Britain as a whole) are badly affected, and that radon is responsible for about 2500 deaths from lung cancer every year.

There are a number of ways in which radon can enter a home. While it is easy to imagine this pollutant silently creeping around a house trying to find a way in, it is more probable that, because atmospheric pressure is usually lower inside than out, the building itself is actually sucking in the gas. Foundation cracks, floor drains, floor and wall joints, cellar windows and even concrete walls and floors provide the openings that radon needs to seep in. Modern double-glazed, draught-proofed, insulated dwellings make very effective radon traps.

If you are worried about radon, contact the NRPB and ask them to carry out a survey for you. Two detectors will be delivered, one for the living room and one for an occupied bedroom; they will take readings for about three months. If your radon levels are high, you should take steps to keep the gas out. If you have suspended floors (i.e. with airbricks around the base of the building), you will have to make them relatively airtight by covering them with sheet plastic and installing a fan system to draw the radon outside. Concrete floors need to have all cracks and breaks sealed with a special plastic; then a small hole must be dug under the house, where the radon will collect and then be transported outside with a fan system.

Since July 1988, all new homes in the worst affected parts of Devon and Cornwall have had to be radon-proofed, and this may be extended to other parts of the country. If you are protecting an older house, you can apply to your local council for a means-tested grant to help with the cost.

HAZARDOUS NOISE

The amount and variety of toxic pollutants that can affect the air and water in the average home is frightening, especially when many of these substances are either invisible to the naked eye or perceived as harmless. However, two more forms of indoor pollution have recently been discovered to be health hazards and are slowly gaining the attention they deserve.

Sit quietly and listen for a while. Then list all the noises you take for granted every day: traffic roaring by, aeroplanes soaring overhead, garden gates clanging shut, doors slamming, kids crying, telephones ringing, dogs barking – even your refrigerator hums. And to think that, normally, you would never give a second thought to any of these sounds.

Noise is an irritant that many of us have learned to tune out mentally. To our ancestors, sounds signalled danger, and their senses were attuned to react accordingly. But today some people have grown so accustomed to our generally noisy world that peace and quiet have actually become irritants. Such individuals have televisions and radios blaring the entire day and cannot function without some type of audible distraction in the background.

Noise levels become dangerous when they reach 80–85 decibels – the volume of an electric razor. Continuous exposure to sounds as loud or louder than this will cause damage to hearing. It is not damaged immediately by most loud sounds; rather, deafness is a process that takes place over time, during which a person is subjected repeatedly to high levels of noise. Airports are probably the noisiest places to live near, but even appliances, such as vacuum cleaners and hair driers, children's toys and rooms with bad acoustics can play havoc with your hearing. Studies have shown that approximately 9 million Americans have incurred hearing loss due to noise pollution – nearly a third of all cases in that country.[34]

Doctors are becoming increasingly alarmed by the growing number of young people with hearing loss. Research at Keele University has shown that listening to loud music – either at discos or concerts or via stereos or Walkmans – can cause at least a degree of deafness. At the other end of the age scale, it is sad to think that we have become so hardened to noise pollution that we now consider hearing loss to be a normal part of growing old. It is *abnormal*. In research carried out on a tribe living in the Sudan under Stone Age conditions, scientists found virtually no deterioration in the hearing of older members.[35]

Noise not only affects our hearing but also our subconscious. As we strain to ignore or adapt to noise we cannot control, we develop a multitude of health problems. The most common of these is hypertension (sustained high blood pressure), which, in the United States alone, affects over 15 per cent of the adult population.[36] Our bodies jump to alertness when subjected to noise just as our ancestors' did; yet there is no need for flight, and so we subconsciously turn that 'flight energy' inwards. The result: a build-up of stress and tension. Recent studies have also correlated noise pollution with more serious illnesses such as heart disease, ulcers, asthma, colitis, antenatal complications and emotional problems. Some research even suggests that those who live near large airports are more likely to be hospitalized for psychiatric illness and have a higher suicide rate than those who live in quieter areas.[37]

CURRENT DANGER

The most potentially dangerous type of indoor pollution is relatively unknown. Only recently has it been recognized as possibly one of the most malignant threats of our modern age. What is this new hazard?

Environmental electricity, or electromagnetic radiation (EMR).

To understand fully how electricity may affect our bodies, it is important, first, to realize how intricately life itself is linked to the Earth's electromagnetic fields, its own natural energy. This pulsates not only through the Earth's core but also through every organism. The most obvious example of its power is its effects on the migratory patterns of birds, which are believed to be controlled by the seasonal changes in the Earth's electromagnetic fields. But this energy not only changes the outward behaviour of organisms; it can also alter the activity of their cells. It is at this level that man-made electricity begins to interfere with nature.

Since Thomas Edison invented the lightbulb in 1879, people have created a multitude of electrical inventions and have then produced them on a vast scale. In effect, what we have done is to create our own electromagnetic fields, at times counter to the Earth's natural ones. While some types of electricity are believed to be healing to the body, and form the basis for what is known as 'electromedicine', others are beginning to be seen as destructive.

The dangers of exposure to high levels of ionising radiation – e.g. gamma rays and X-rays – are well known. However, research has only recently revealed the possible hazards of extremely low frequency (ELF) and microwave radiation. This type causes the 'electropollution' that is generated in the home by the constant use of a wide variety of electrical appliances: lamps, televisions, stereo equipment, telephones, microwave ovens, computers, electric blankets, hair driers . . . the list goes on.

Microwave ovens work by bombarding food with electrical radiation – electrical waves – to increase the vibration of the water and other molecules that make up the food, generating heat in the process. Some researchers are afraid that ELF radiation from the appliances we so much take for granted today may be affecting us at a microscopic level in much the same way that microwave ovens cook food. This type of non-ionising radiation does not destroy cells, but it does shake them up. The danger involves the entire chemical make-up of the human body, for many vital functions depend on the natural electrical energy between cells.

While it is true that cancer has not been irrefutably linked to a person's exposure to household electricity, growing evidence has revealed that the small amounts of radiation we receive from appliances may be dangerous in other ways. For example, a study at the University of Colorado in 1984 showed that there was an above-normal rate of miscarriage among almost 1700 pregnant women who slept under electric blankets: three-quarters of the miscarriages occurred during the winter months when the blankets would have been used virtually every night.[38]

Electromagnetic radiation has been tentatively linked to depression and suicide, cataracts, reduced heart efficiency, leukaemia, sudden infant death syndrome (cot death), Alzheimer's disease, Parkinson's disease, autism in children and chronic fatigue syndrome. In addition, it may play a role in reducing the function of the immune system, increasing susceptibility to such infectious diseases as AIDS and herpes.[39]

By presenting information such as this, the intention is not to panic readers, simply to warn them of potential hazards. Particularly if you are pregnant, take precautions with home computers. Don't sit too close to the family television, avoid standing in front of microwave ovens when they are in operation, and remove any unnecessary electrical appliances from beds and bedsides.

THE OFFICE ENVIRONMENT

Although a great deal of our time is spent at home, the majority of us spend our waking hours at our places of work. Some occupations involve more exposure to dangerous substances than others. Radiologists are in continual contact with radiation. Decorators are exposed to harmful fumes. Farm workers use poisonous pesticides. Firefighters sometimes breathe in tremendous amounts of smoke and chemical vapours. Compared to these occupations, an office job may seem a safe haven . . . but it's not.

The average office setting may pose a variety of dangers to employees' health. Unfortunately most workers have much less control over their work environment than they do their homes, and often they are unwillingly exposed to substances that can do harm.

The British architect Thomas Saunders, an expert on indoor pollution, has explained how women could be affected more by office environments than men. Because most women – in their skirts and tops – are relatively less well covered than men, who usually wear jackets and/or long-sleeved shirts, they are more exposed to chemical contact. Women also tend to wear more synthetic materials, which create static and attract dust that may lead to adverse reactions. Immobile and/or repetitive jobs such as typing are usually done by women, and the physical positions required to perform this work may throw the body out of line, leading to stress and illness.

Women are also more likely to work in open-plan offices without access to daylight and surrounded by noise, confusion and chemicals from distant parts of the building, all of which they have no control over. A lack of control over one's environment can be physically and psychologically damaging, and may eventually lead to illness.

However, extensive exposure to certain indoor pollutants can affect anyone – male or female. Hazards that might be encountered include not only those found in homes, such as dust, tobacco smoke, carbon monoxide and asbestos, but also industrial chemicals, poor lighting, massive electromagnetic radiation from electrical equipment and high levels of noise. Every one of these may contribute to increased illness and absenteeism, diminished morale and, consequently, reduced productivity.

Like homes, most offices have their share of common-but-hazardous items. Paper copies fresh from a stencilling machine, carbon paper, typewriter correction fluid, typewriter ribbons, inks, felt-tipped pens, adhesives and the spray-on fixative used by graphic designers can all produce noxious vapours. Symptoms produced by these include headaches, dizziness, burning eyes, blurred vision, itching, sore throat, stuffy nose and lightheadedness. People who are especially sensitive to such substances may have even more severe reactions.

Office supplies are not the only sources of chemical vapours. Many machines employed in businesses use dangerous chemicals and emit harmful fumes. The ubiquitous photocopier is one such device. Because these machines give off vapours from the inks, dyes, powders and other chemicals they need to operate, they should be placed away from direct contact with employees. Lengthy exposure to such chemical fumes as trichlorethane can cause dizziness, headaches and even, eventually, liver damage; another chemical, trinitrofluorenone, may produce mutagenic effects. Methanol is a lung, eye and skin irritant, and is capable of affecting the central nervous system, as well as causing liver damage. Ammonia and ozone are other vapours emitted by office equipment.

Hidden from view but still present are the pesticides and cleaning fluids used by all building maintenance staff. The primary difference between those we use at home and those used in work environments is the strength – industrial products are usually much stronger than those bought over the counter. In fact, some disinfectants used commercially are not available to the public because of their strength and, hence, their toxicity. Vapours from these substances may linger in the air or be circulated through the ventilation system to different parts of a building, causing adverse reactions in people who are not directly involved in their use.

THE DARK SECRETS OF LIGHT

Most people wouldn't think that light could pose a 'hazard' in offices. Because of this, many employers overlook the effects that lighting can have on their workers, despite the fact that a number of experts now claim that good lighting is vital to our productive well-being. Recent studies are providing evidence that a lack of exposure to natural light can actually have detrimental effects on physical and mental health.

Natural sunlight contains the full spectrum of wavelengths – not only the visible light that we can see as the colours violet, blue, green, yellow, orange and red, but also the infra-red and ultraviolet waves that are invisible to the human eye. Although many experts believe that this natural light is essential to human health (for one thing, we create vitamin D from it), at work we are often shut away indoors and actually expose ourselves to light that may be unhealthy.

Incandescent bulbs provide light primarily from the red part of the spectrum; cool-white fluorescent strip lighting emphasizes only the yellow-green portion. Scientific researchers are finding more and more evidence that such artificial lighting produces negative effects on health. Common ailments linked to it include fatigue, depression, decreased performance, diminished immunity, reduced physical fitness and perhaps even impaired fertility. Too little sunlight may cause hyperactivity and changes in heart rate, blood pressure, electrical brainwave patterns, hormonal secretions and the body's natural cyclical rhythms, as well as vitamin D deficiency. These are all considered symptoms of what is called 'malillumination'. What the lack of vitamins and minerals is to malnutrition, the lack of full-spectrum light (i.e. sunlight) is to malillumination.

While artificial light may be harmful in general, certain types may produce particularly negative effects. Fluorescent lighting is believed to emit enough ultraviolet radiation to increase the risk of non-malignant skin tumours in some people. The flickering that occurs when it is on, although barely perceptible to the human eye, is perceived subconsciously and may cause irritability, headaches, eyestrain and fatigue, and may even trigger seizures in susceptible epileptics. High-pressure sodium vapour lamps can also cause eyestrain, headaches, nausea and irritability.

COMPANY CACOPHONY

Noise affects us in the workplace perhaps more than in our homes, chiefly because we often have no control over the sources of this pollution. Typewriters and computers, building heating and cooling systems, copying machines and simple conversation together produce a cacophony that makes it hard for anyone to concentrate.

To counteract the natural noisiness of most work environments, and to provide some privacy among employees, many large offices pipe in what is called 'white noise' – a type of humming static that is meant to cover up the multitude of other sounds. White noise is not hazardous in itself, but it does become just another sound in the jumble already present.

What *is* hazardous is a workplace's total sound energy – that is, its level and duration – entering the ears on a daily basis. Imperceptibly, you may begin to strain to make yourself heard or to hear others over the noise surrounding you. This can lead to stress, and when the stress builds, illness and absenteeism results.

COMPUTER STRAIN AND PAIN

It seems that the more technologically advanced our world becomes, the more we depend on the computer. Even the smallest business has one, and most large companies have literally hundreds, if not thousands. Advances in computer technology have proceeded at such an enormous pace that, until fairly recently, no thought was taken as to how human beings interacted with the machines themselves or how they might affect us. It was only when the users of computer keyboards and video display units (VDUs) began to suffer a host of symptoms that the business and computer worlds began to take notice of the very real hazards of this technology.

Working at a computer can be affected by the layout of the work-station – that is, the height of the desk and chair, whether you have to turn your head to see the screen, whether the keyboard can be moved and so on – and by the radiation emanating from the VDU. This is about the same as from a television, the difference being that employees sit much closer to computers than to their TVs at home. In addition, many people do not take breaks while working on computers, and computerized work tends to be more highly pressurized than the same work was in the days of manual or even electric typewriters.

Common problems that occur after working at computers for long periods include back and neck aches, stiff shoulders, eyestrain, arm pains, numbness and fatigue, and skin irritation and rashes. In those with photo-sensitive epilepsy, seizures might be triggered. Eye problems are also frequently experienced: VDUs will often exaggerate certain pre-existing conditions that the user was previously able to compensate for without difficulty. Colour-perception changes may also occur, and cata-racts are statistically more likely.

Perhaps the most serious condition experienced by computer users is repetitive strain injury (RSI). In the past, typists using old-fashioned typewriters would tire easily and take breaks. Those now using compu-ters do not expend as much energy so do not become obviously fatigued in the same way; however, the small, constant, repetitive movements of fingers, wrists and forearms creates strain that, in severe cases, can lead to agonizing pain and total incapacity. RSI is not limited to computer users: some manual workers – for example, chicken pluckers – have also succumbed to the condition, and have won compensation cases in court. Recently, however, RSI-affected computer users have received a set-back. In a case in the High Court in London brought by a sub-editor formerly with the Reuters news agency, and supported by the National

Union of Journalists, the judge denied the existence of RSI as a medical condition.

While His Honour may believe this, the European Community certainly does not. It issued a Directive that, in Britain, resulted in the Health and Safety (Display Screen Equipment) Regulations 1992, which came into force on 1 January 1993. These apply to 'all employed and self-employed workers who habitually use VDUs as a significant part of their normal work'. To comply, employers must:

- analyse employees' workstations and assess and reduce the risks.
- ensure that workstations meet minimum requirements.
- plan work so there are breaks or changes of activity.
- on request, arrange eye and eyesight tests, and provide spectacles if special ones are needed.
- provide health and safety training and information.[40]

In addition to the above known problems connected with computer use, there is also a substantial amount of anecdotal evidence – and a number of conflicting studies – implicating radiation from VDUs in a rise in miscarriages and birth defects.

'COMPUTER VIRUS'

With such an increasing number of extreme reactions to electrical appliances and other machines, it was only a matter of time before these illnesses were collectively labelled. 'Electromagnetic-hypersensitivity syndrome' (EHS) might aptly be defined as 'an allergic reaction to electromagnetic fields'.

Ann was a typical victim of EHS. For many years, she had worked as a computer supervisor for a large company, and during that time had suffered no major medical problems. Then one day she was asked to try out a new make of computer that the company was considering buying. It appeared to be the perfect machine: fast, powerful and easy to use.

On the first day, Ann enjoyed working with it, although that evening she went home with a slight headache. An aspirin took care of that. The next day, after she had used the new computer for less than an hour, the headache returned. She took another aspirin and decided she must be 'coming down with something'. However, soon after going back to working with the machine, she became nauseous and dizzy, and this time aspirin had absolutely no effect.

Ann went to the company doctor and was told that she had a slight fever and that, yes indeed, she appeared to be coming down with flu. After a couple of days off, she returned to work, thankful that she felt fine and was obviously recovered. But minutes after she turned on the computer, the nausea, dizziness and headache came back. She continued to work but soon began to experience severe fatigue, an inability to concentrate and difficulty with her vision. She struggled on, but when the symptoms became too much, she had to give up. She again went to see the company doctor, and this time mentioned that she thought perhaps something was wrong with the new computer. Back at home, she saw that her face and the exposed parts of her neck and chest were noticeably reddened.

She took a few weeks of sick leave. On returning to work, she went immediately to see the company doctor. This time she wanted a witness to her healthy condition before she began to use the new computer. She was told that, while she had been away, the manufacturer had checked her machine and had found it to be operating normally and not producing a harmful electromagnetic field.

Consoled by this news – but still wary – Ann returned to her office. She opened the door and immediately felt as if she had 'walked into a blasting furnace'. The entire room had been equipped with the new machines! She was able to remain in there for only a few minutes before she became extremely ill and was forced to leave. This time the company doctor suggested that perhaps she had some emotional or personal problems, and that it might be a good idea if she sought counselling for them. Ann refused to return to her office and, instead, left for home.

Soon, though, she noticed that her television and stereo produced the same symptoms as the new computer. Slowly, over the next few weeks, her conditioned worsened, until even using the telephone made her ill. She also developed what appeared to be allergic reactions to the vapours of such things as laundry bleach and perfume, and then even sunlight.

When her skin rash reappeared, Ann consulted a dermatologist. For the first time, she was not treated as if she had lost her mind. The doctor had seen cases like hers before, and suggested that an allergic reaction to electromagnetic radiation, such as that produced by the new computer, might be the culprit. He recommended a holiday in a very rural area to see whether the absence of electrical appliances and machines would cure her symptoms. Other patients of his had sometimes been able to return to a normal life after removing all electromagnetic fields from their environment for a time.

Ann took his advice and her symptoms did disappear. Unfortunately, when she returned to the city, her allergies returned, too. She never went back to her old job. She moved to the country and, today, is no longer plagued by her 'computer virus'.[41]

What Ann experienced is typical of what happens to many EHS sufferers: the abrupt onset of symptoms on exposure to a novel electromagnetic field, which slowly expands to include other electrical devices that wouldn't normally cause such reactions. While those with this syndrome may never progress beyond mild symptoms, others may develop severe neurological responses such as confusion, depression, decreased memory, sleep disturbances and even convulsions and grossly abnormal behaviour.

Although computers may be the most publicly emphasized source of radiation in an office, the effect of all electrical equipment on employees must be considered. Typewriters, fax machines, photocopiers, telephone systems and calculators, not to mention desk lighting, all produce ELF radiation, which can be added to that already produced in the home. In the end, most of us are bombarded with electrical waves of some kind 24 hours a day.

VENTING DISEASE

We have seen how industrial chemicals, lighting, noise, computers and radiation from electrical equipment can affect the majority of indoor workplaces to some extent. There is yet another form of indoor pollution that has recently caught the attention of employers. It is the by-product of what may actually be considered a 'building malfunction' as it is caused by the structure itself and results in illness among the occupants. Symptoms and diseases that have been traced back to commercial buildings – and, as we have seen, to houses and flats – are now grouped into two categories: sick building syndrome and building-related illnesses.

Sick-building syndrome (SBS) reveals itself as a collection of complaints including sinus congestion, eye, nose and throat irritation, coughing, wheezing, headaches, fatigue, dizziness, nausea, dry and/or itchy skin and rashes, difficulty in concentrating and sensitivity to odours. Often there is no clearly identifiable cause, and symptoms diminish or disappear after workers leave the building. A World Health Organization committee has estimated that up to 30 per cent of all new and remodelled buildings may have indoor air quality problems that could lead to SBS. But, in fact, almost every building, regardless of age or condition, may cause its occupants some discomfort at one time or another.

Building-related illnesses (BRI) are far more serious. They are usually associated with clinically defined diseases such as asthma, dermatitis, Legionnaire's disease, tuberculosis, influenza, measles, chicken pox, rubella (German measles) and hypersensitivity pneumonitis, some of which can be fatal. Although a distinction is made between SBS and BRI, SBS may, in fact, prove to be the initial stages of a BRI and, if left unchecked, may progress to one or more of these distinguishable diseases.

Most experts agree that SBS and BRI result not from a single phenomenon within a building but from a combination of factors. According to the US Environmental Protection Agency, the three major reasons for poor indoor air quality in office buildings are the presence of air pollution sources (discussed above), poorly designed, maintained and/or operated ventilation systems, and uses of the building that were unanticipated or poorly planned for when it was designed or renovated.

To begin with, design trends from the 1960s to the 1980s, as well as the energy crunch of the 1970s, affected not only residences but also commercial buildings. The move towards sleek glass and steel structures and the promotion of energy efficiency resulted in tightly sealed buildings with unopenable windows. Consequently pollutants have been able to build up inside. Dust, radon, vapours from cleaning solutions, particulates and gases from combustion sources, tobacco smoke, pesticides, asbestos fibres, formaldehyde – the whole gamut can become trapped within an office, only to be inhaled by employees.

Heating, ventilation and air conditioning (HVAC) systems were originally intended to prevent this from happening. These large mechanical systems should not only heat and cool a building but also draw in and circulate outdoor air, purifying it of contaminants in the process. However, several factors may restrict this equipment in its performance of these intended functions.

If the architectural and engineering phases of a building's design are not carried out with the structure's eventual indoor air quality in mind, it is highly likely that it will end up with inadequate ventilation. Improperly located vents may bring in air that has been contaminated with car and lorry exhausts, boiler emissions and fumes from skips, or they may carry air already vented from toilets, photocopy and supply rooms or building maintenance areas. Even if circulated air is purified, vents may have been placed in such a way that the fresh air does not actually reach the 'breathing zone' of the occupants.

Poor maintenance can compound these problems. HVAC systems may actually become a source of indoor pollution. Maintenance procedures are often lax or non-existent, or they may work against the HVAC systems' intended use. Vents may not be cleaned on a regular basis, and filters may not be changed or, if they are, various inappropriate replacements may be used to save costs.

Biological contaminants can multiply in cooling towers, humidifiers, dehumidifiers and air conditioners and on the inside surfaces of ventilation ducts. Another poor maintenance practice is the shutting down of a building's entire HVAC system during unoccupied periods. As a result, humidity soars, often to above 70 per cent, providing the perfect setting for the growth of mould and bacteria, which, once the building is reoccupied and the HVAC system is turned on, are blown into the office air. BRI are caused by this lack of maintenance.

The importance of proper maintenance of ventilations systems cannot be stressed enough. In 1984, the US National Institute of Occupational Safety and Health inspected over 400 'sick' buildings and found that almost half of the complaints could be attributed to inadequate ventilation.[42]

Cleaning and maintenance staff may also be slow to clean and dry or replace ceiling tiles, carpets, curtains, upholstered furniture and other items with porous surfaces that have become wet or soiled. Contamination of these surfaces also leads to the growth of biologicals if not properly treated.

The EPA's final reason for poor indoor air quality was the use of a building for which it was not intended. Pollutants can be circulated from portions of a building used for specialized purposes, such as restaurants, print shops and dry cleaners, into other areas in the same building. Exhaust fumes from vehicles, including carbon monoxide, can be drawn from underground carparks through stairwells and lift shafts. Those responsible for the renovation of a building, such as the remodelling of a warehouse into offices, may neglect to provide adequate ventilation for the new use.

Today, the public is becoming increasingly aware of the hazards posed by chemicals both indoors and outside. Débâcle after disaster after accident have gradually made their way on to the pages of our newspapers and on to our television screens, and this has led to the banning or restriction of such chemicals as DDT, Kepone, dioxin, PCBs, vinyl chloride, Chlordane and Alar. Employers are beginning to feel the full impact of SBS and BRI, largely due to the absenteeism of their employees each year – 500,000 work days are lost in the US alone.[43] Interior designers and architects are coming to realize that the buildings and interiors they design must provide healthy living and working spaces. In the United States, this has been hammered home by the number of recent court cases in which occupants made ill by buildings have successfully sued.

CHEMICAL HOLOCAUST

Perhaps the most horrifying of all is the sickness we are beginning to see around us every day; the family members we are losing to the diseases that medical technology, advanced as it is, has no way of curing; the new diseases that are cropping up each year; the known diseases that are now slowly changing and defying the knowledge of medical experts; the increasing number and different types of cancers. The question is: Where will it all end? Are we fast approaching a chemical holocaust, as some experts fear? Have we lost control of our own technology?

AIDS is often considered this century's medical crisis, but a few professionals now believe that AIDS is only one of many straws that will eventually break the proverbial camel's back. Some doctors predict that the most serious health problem in the 1990s and beyond will be the rise of immunological disorders, such as hypersensitivity and auto-immune diseases, conditions involving chronic inflammation, and increasingly virulent viruses. [44]

Despite mounting evidence from the scientific community that the massive amounts of chemicals we are exposed to every day are destroying the very fabric of our lives, governments, corporations and many conventional doctors still stubbornly refuse to acknowledge the existence of such widespread chemical toxicity. In turn, it is difficult for the public to comprehend that these 'institutions' – for years considered the pillars of society – are actually quite unconcerned about their health.

For too long, the average citizen has viewed a government seal of approval on a product or substance as the last word in safety. This is utter foolishness. How can society, in all honesty, place its health in the hands of an institution that has loosed such chemicals as DDT and dioxins on the public – and then palmed off any risks as 'insignificant'? In many cases, governments are unaware of the problem, have no control over it or simply don't care.

Corporations are often even more at fault. Most are aware of the types of complications that may arise from the chemicals they use in their products, yet they also know that they can escape restrictions and liability for these problems. There are many reasons for this sanguine attitude. First, linking a disease to a particular chemical is difficult as there are so many poorly understood diseases and so many poorly understood chemicals. Second, decades may pass between the initial exposure to a chemical and the development of the first detectable signs of an illness, by which time it is almost impossible to determine the cause. Third, whereas a chemical by itself may not cause harm, it can combine with others within the human body and together cause disease. The way chemicals react with other chemicals in this way is imperfectly understood. Fourth, chemicals may imperceptibly damage one of a person's body systems, such as the immune system, and this may lead to future secondary illnesses. Such diseases, however, are very hard to trace back to a particular chemical. Given these difficulties, it is no wonder that companies have been given virtual free rein over what they place on the market for public consumption.

Our last resort, the medical community, should be our protectors, yet they aren't. Orthodox doctors are trained to appreciate the results of drugs and state-of-the-art technology – all created to cure or treat diseases at a detectable (if not fully advanced) stage. Little is done to prepare most in the medical field to detect the earliest signs of the chemical poisoning that may later lead to disease, and even less is taught regarding the prevention of chemical toxicity.

However, the stiff resistance of government, corporations and orthodox medicine to the reality of chemical toxicity and the illness it brings to its victims is slowly being undermined by the sheer numbers of people being affected by chemicals in our environment. Gradually, larger and larger portions of the political, business and medical worlds are being forced to confront modern society's greatest threat: the chemical invasion.

Our bodies have taken thousands of years to evolve. While some speculate that they have not evolved enough to detect the chemicals that surround us in our environment, others disagree. Dr Kaye Kilburn of the University of Southern California School of Medicine suggests that, because the human nervous system is so highly evolved, its sensitivity to the environment is actually its undoing.[45] Whereas many dysfunctions of the human body may be attributed to anxiety, tension and ageing – that is, to psychological causes – it should always be remembered that they could be signs and symptoms of the body's reaction to chemical exposure.

The great majority of medical professionals are ignorant of the side-effects of chemical exposure and are not detecting the warning signs in their patients. The tragic plights of people who are so hypersensitive to chemicals that they become debilitated are well documented. Some of these individuals, afflicted by chemicals to the point that they are unable to work or find safe housing, become 'environmental refugees', forced to live nomadic lives in stripped-down caravans or old cars, vans, tents or sheds, isolated from society and without many of the basic necessities of life. Other victims are children, forced to live in 'glass cages' because of their bodily reactions to chemicals and so deprived of normal childhoods. Still others are people we encounter every day, who live half-lives, struggling with their symptoms. And there are those who, in the end, are completely overwhelmed by their illnesses and commit suicide.[46]

But there is hope. A growing group of doctors insist that the multitude of problems that people are experiencing today are not psychological, but in fact are the very real symptoms of our attempt to co-exist with chemicals. This relatively new field of research is called environmental medicine.

CHALLENGES

Dr Theron Randolph, considered the father of environmental medicine, was one of the first to document cases of people who were sensitive to exposure to chemicals in outdoor and indoor environments.[47] In his book, *Human Ecology and Susceptibility to the Chemical Environment*, he describes a medical condition that, over the years, has received several names, including environmental illness, ecological illness, 20th-century disease, total allergy syndrome and multiple chemical sensitivities. Today, 'chemical sensitivities' or 'environmentally triggered illnesses' (EI) are the terms most widely accepted, and are used to label ailments linked to synthetic chemicals and fibres, electromagnetic radiation and many other by-products of 20th-century life.

Leading the effort in EI diagnosis and treatment in the United States is the American Academy of Environmental Medicine (AAEM), known between 1965 and 1985 as the Society of Clinical Ecology. Today the AAEM has over 500 members, including medical and osteopathic physicians (many of whom also belong to the American Medical Association), other health professionals and scientists from many disciplines. Sister organizations can be found in many other countries, including Canada, Germany, Australia, New Zealand, China, Japan and Britain, where the British Society for Allergy and Environmental Medicine has been in operation for some years.

Environmental medicine is based on the fact that the human body and all its organs and systems are sensitive to the environment and may be adversely affected by exposure to the variety of harmful substances that we inevitably come into contact with from day to day. While the classical scientific model dictates that medicine should treat body parts as separate entities, environmental medicine treats the body as an organic whole, with the function of each part inseparably intertwined with and influenced by the complex interaction of every other organ and system.[48]

Environmental medicine is founded on the concept of homoeostasis, first described in the late 19th century by the French scientist Claude Bernard. This is the body's natural inborn drive to maintain the stability of its organic functions, even when faced with varying and unpredictable exposures to external and/or internal environmental stressors. These stressors include not only the potential hazards outlined earlier, but also foods, nutritional excesses or deficiencies, vibration, and changes in temperature and barometric pressure. Physical problems occur when the body can no longer adapt to these stressors and maintain homoeostasis.

EI are actually very complex to diagnose. People plagued with generalized feelings of illness, such as constant fatigue or headaches, often pass the symptoms off as the signs of an oncoming cold or bout of flu, or they acknowledge the problem but simply accept it as part of daily life. It isn't until one particular stressor suddenly overloads the body, throwing it into disorder and serious illness, that these individuals become concerned. Rooting out the cause of this ill health becomes more difficult because this time has elapsed.

Sometimes hypersensitivity to certain substances produces chronic symptoms – that is, those that surface after exposure to small doses of a toxin over a long period. A physician must again backtrack to find the initial poison. To complicate matters further, some EI produce recurrent or fluctuating reactions, or even seasonal variations in reactions. Symptoms may also involve more than one organ or system of the body.

Using past patient cases to determine the cause of another individual's problems can be misleading, as different substances can produce different reactions in different people. The amount of a substance that will produce an effect may also differ between individuals.

If a patient is suffering acute symptoms, this usually means that the reactions are a result of exposure to large doses of a toxin over a short period. The environmental physician will advise the patient to avoid the suspect substance for a time; then he or she will be brought back into contact with it and his or her bodily reactions will be measured.

Variations of this test are used throughout environmental medicine, especially for food sensitivities. For instance, in the *single food elimination/ challenge diet*, the one food that is believed to be causing problems is removed from a patient's diet. After four to seven days, the food is reintroduced and the person's physical reactions monitored. In the *multiple food elimination/challenge diet*, several foods are removed from the diet, then slowly reintroduced over a period of time. As for the *total elimination/ challenge diet*, also called 'diagnostic fasting', the patient eats nothing for several days and then foods are gradually reintroduced one by one.

There are other diets that can be followed. The *rare food diet* involves patients eating only what are termed 'rare foods', such as giraffe steaks; 'normal' foods are reintroduced slowly and the patient's physical reactions are watched closely. The *cave man diet* allows people to eat only very simple foods such as nuts, some grains, fruits and vegetables. This regime is very high in fibre and may also be used to detoxify the body. Finally, the *rotary diversified elimination diet* eliminates all food to which a person is allergic, and then, over a period of time, ensures that he or she eats foods from different food groups, never repeating the same foods on successive days. This is done to prevent the person from developing allergies to common foods such as wheat and eggs.

These elimination/challenge tests can be useful in pinpointing a stressor but are normally very time consuming. A less lengthy test is the *provocation/neutralization test*, also known as the 'maximum-tolerated intradermal dose test'. This introduces a possible stressor, such as car exhaust, to a person's system either through injection or drops placed under the tongue, where they will be readily absorbed. Reactions to the substance are measured. Slowly the strength of the stressor is reduced until, after many 'provocations', the diluted stressor neutralizes the person's reactions to the contaminant.

Other tests involving the skin are employed. The *intradermal serial dilution endpoint titration test* also requires the injection of a stressor.

This time, though, the skin's reaction to the contaminant is monitored rather than that of the body as a whole. If the skin at the point of the injection puffs up and/or reddens, the dose is reduced until the skin no longer reacts; the neutralizing dose has been determined. The *epidermal patch test* is a similar technique but relies on the skin's reaction to a substance placed on it rather than injected into it.

As in orthodox medicine, blood and other bodily fluids are tested by environmental medical doctors, and sometimes certain traditional drugs are used to alleviate symptoms. This often goes hand in hand with detoxification of the body through exercise and heat (e.g. saunas), and nutritional supplementation is the norm. However, educating patients about their specific problems and how to avoid contaminants is considered among the most important factors leading to health.

The techniques outlined so far can be carried out at an out-patient clinic. But for a person with a severe or complex case – the 'environmental refugee' – more drastic measures may be necessary. In these instances, a patient might be admitted to a specialized *environmental control unit* (ECU), where all environmental and dietary exposures are carefully controlled. After a five-day fast, the patient begins challenge tests; he or she will also be assessed psychologically and will be given counselling and advice on stress management.[49]

HOPE FOR THE FUTURE?

Although the evidence produced by monitoring patients treated by these methods strongly supports the ideology behind environmental medicine, traditionally trained doctors and allergists continue to belittle their medical colleagues who choose to practise in this field. Allergists are particularly vehement in their assertions that chemical sensitivity is a myth, that people cannot be 'allergic' to chemicals.

However, according to Dr Gary Oberg, past president of the AAEM and still head of continuing medical education for the society, the root of the disagreement between the two fields of medicine is merely one of definition. Allergists believe that only biological contaminants affect certain parts of the body – e.g. the respiratory system – to produce allergies. Doctors practising environmental medicine believe that not only biological contaminants but a whole host of other pollutants, including chemicals, can and do affect the entire body. Training orthodox doctors in environmental medicine would, says Dr Oberg, combine the best of both worlds. In addition, because it stresses prevention, environmental medicine would lead to infinitely healthier patients in the long run and would also drastically reduce the present high cost of medicine.

Despite the heated debates that continue to rage between professionals in environmental and orthodox medicine, the majority of today's medical community still does not endorse preventive medicine. At the same time, their patients are becoming increasingly disillusioned with current techniques used to diagnose and treat illness, as well as with the attitudes of government and corporations towards chemicals and how they affect people.

Support groups for those with chemical sensitivities are forming. The most prominent one in the United States is the Human Environmental Action League (HEAL) with nearly 200 active or developing chapters around the country and approximately 10,000 members. In the UK, as well as general environmental organizations – Friends of the Earth, Greenpeace, the British Ecological Society – there are a growing number of self-help/support groups for individual conditions with an environmental element, ranging from arthritis, migraine and childhood hyperactivity to eczema, schizophrenia and seasonal affective disorder.

Once health food shops were the only places where you could buy organic, chemical-free products. This is no longer the case. Mail-order businesses and other outlets for personal 'no-tox', 'low-tox' household items are springing up. These places offer everything from no-tox cleaning products to completely natural cosmetics and naturally produced bed linens. The relatively few architects who build only healthy homes with no-tox or low-tox materials are now in high demand, and in their wake have sprung up various companies to supply their needs. These produce no-tox and low-tox substitutes for insulation, paint, finishes and other previously unhealthy materials.

Although 'sick building syndrome' is a relatively new issue in both the United States and Britain, the same is not true of Germany. The *Baubiologie* movement – '*Baubiologie*' means 'architectural biology' – has been in existence for some time, and many of its adherents offer answers to the 20th-century problems of sick buildings.

Perhaps the most critical change occurring in the public's fight against chemicals is the increase in legal action taken against the various sectors of society that contaminate people with their products. Especially in the US, recognition of EI is advancing daily as more and more people successfully fight and win court cases against the companies that have made them ill through the negligent use of chemicals.

Where will the present massive production of chemicals ultimately lead? That's anyone's guess. However, it is becoming increasingly apparent that it is not (as the creators of these products so desperately want us to believe) leading us towards the improved lives we have been consistently promised.

CHAPTER FOUR

THE QUEST FOR OPTIMAL HEALTH

Today, it is an art just to be yourself. So many people are sheep. It is easy to conform to popular rules, regardless of whether they are sensible and not to think for yourself. I am astonished to find that so many of my friends read the same books, listen to the same music and wear practically the same fashions, although they are very different individuals. But the bestseller lists, the pop charts and popular magazines dictate such preferences.

Blind acceptance, it seems, has been a law of human nature throughout history. This is especially true of health treatments and medical procedures, which we have been expected to agree to without question. However, this sort of depersonalization can produce detrimental results when it comes to our physical and mental well-being.

Our health is technically defined as: a condition of physical, mental and social well-being with the absence of disease and other abnormal conditions. It is not a static condition; constant change and adaptation to stress results in homoeostasis.[1] When our health is in jeopardy, we are primarily treated with allopathic medicine – that is, modern medicine as we know it. An allopathic physician is one who treats disease and injuries with active interventions, as medical and surgical treatment, intended to bring about effects opposite to those produced by the disease or injury. The great majority of practising physicians in Western societies are allopathic.[2]

If this method of treatment were continuously successful, it would not be considered an issue for debate. However, it is now known that our present medical system is able to help only about 10 per cent of those who seek its services; in addition, 8–9 per cent of people who seek allopathic treatment are harmed by it. Therefore, statistically speaking, the benefits of our current medical system are insignificant.

This is not to say that a success rate of 10 per cent should be dismissed. If I were in a car accident, I would want to be rushed to the nearest modern-equipped accident and emergency department. If I broke a bone, needed artery bypass surgery or a liver transplant or wished to have a mole removed, I would insist on the services of a skilled allopathic doctor. This type of medical service is, for most part, crisis care, and calls for talented physicians and scientists.

But what about our health concerns the other 90 per cent of the time? Should they not be addressed with an equal amount of concern, dedication and respect? Should the professionals who can deal with them be cast aside, diminished as insignificant, ignored, ridiculed and attacked solely to preserve the status quo? Any mildly reasonable individual would come to the conclusion that, when it comes to our overall well-being, there is perhaps room for a variety of health-care disciplines and providers within society. Yet, the powers-that-be are vehemently opposed to such reasoning.

'NATURE CURES'

It wasn't so long ago that medical treatment comprised a number of techniques. They all had one thing in common, though – all incorporated 'nature' in their philosophies and respected the body and mind as a whole. 'Nature cures, not the physician,' wrote Hippocrates, the father of medicine. In fact, the word 'physician' is derived from the Greek word *physis*, which means 'nature'. But in the 19th century science overpowered nature, allopathy emerged and we soon became depersonalized body parts that were mechanically and chemically dealt with once disease set in or an injury was inflicted. Allopathic medicine served its purpose, but it completely disregarded prevention while ignoring our right to optimal health. This is not to say that, at the turn of the century, stupidity mercilessly struck the medical community or that the authorities' tunnel vision forcefully led them down a single, limited path. Instead, a newly established economic power structure saw an enormous opportunity to further enrich itself by creating a health monopoly.

In the United States, for instance, homoeopathy was strong enough in the early 1900s to rival allopathic medicine, but eventually it lost ground to the rising strength of the pharmaceutical industry. Further nails were driven into its coffin when the Rockefeller-funded American Medical

Association (AMA) commissioned the Carnegie Foundation to make an evaluation of the nation's medical schools, which led, among other things, to the closing of all homoeopathic medical schools and hospitals.[3] Today, more than 80 years later, the United States has the dubious honour of being the only nation on the planet where illness is a 'for profit' industry, with no incentive for keeping people well.

In Britain, too, the main ideal of the National Health Service – health care free at the point of delivery – is being undermined. The Conservative government's backing of private medical insurance (and, thus, private medicine), its insistence on bringing the rules of the marketplace into health care and its establishment of hospital trusts and fundholding GPs has led to a two-tier system of haves and have-nots, with the health of British patients of increasingly less importance.

However, allopathic medicine, with its emphasis on crisis management, appears at last to be pricing itself out of the market. In 1990, Dr Louis Sullivan, the US Secretary of Health and Human Services under President Bush, admitted that good health has been permitted to exist as a benefit for only those who can afford it and has not been made available to every citizen. He urged that Americans, once again, begin to take responsibility for their own well-being, and implored the medical establishment to reintroduce preventive care. After all, many of the leading causes of death for people between the ages of 25 and 65 are preventable.[4]

The entire Western world has sacrificed an astonishing number of its people to heart disease, cancer, injury, stroke, HIV infection, alcoholism and drug abuse – all avoidable to a large extent. In the US injury alone now costs well over $100 billion (£66.7 billion) annually, cancer over $70 billion (£46.7 billion) and cardiovascular diseases more than $135 billion (£90 billion).[5] If such expenditure yielded fruitful results, it might be considered justifiable, but the money spent usually does not produce cures, and the treatment often causes pain and other side-effects as disturbing as the disease itself. With an annual health bill of $1.5 trillion facing the US by the year 2000, according to government estimates, personal health management, medical self-care and alternatives to high-tech, high-cost medicine are now urgent priorities.

Whether you are paying for medical treatment directly, through insurance premiums or through taxes, it is an expensive proposition financially, not to mention the real cost in human suffering. Sophisticated technology for the diagnosis and treatment of disease has outstripped society's ability to pay for it. What is even more disturbing is that we have been forced to accept this 'preventable' burden.

Every society has within its power the ability to save lives lost prematurely and needlessly. But the health of a people should be measured by different criteria than simply death rates. Illness prevention, avoidance of unnecessary suffering, an improved quality of life and a quest for optimal health are gains that should benefit all people.

Many people have decided on their own that allopathy is not the last word in medical care. They have come to the conclusion that conventional medicine represents only one philosophy of health care and not always the best one. Allopathy's heavy reliance on invasive surgical procedures, antibiotics and other powerful biochemicals implies that you can only be helped at the very last stage of an illness. So little is done to prevent you from getting to that point. How often have you been told by a doctor to 'keep an eye' on a certain condition, only to watch yourself deteriorate into a worse state? I know a man who 'kept an eye' on his infected toe, while consuming a barrel of antibiotics and painkillers – until his leg was eventually amputated.

THE ROCKY ROAD TO OPTIMAL HEALTH

With alternative and complementary therapies, you get to practise 'empowerment' where your optimal health is concerned, in ways you probably never have before. You soon learn that your body is your own responsibility. Even the greatest doctors cannot heal you. They can only minimize obstacles and help you to strengthen your body's own healing process, of which you are the sole possessor. As someone once said, the purpose of the doctor is to humour the patient while nature does the healing.

At present, only a slender minority of us come anywhere near optimal health. The rest linger in health limbo awaiting a crisis to erupt. Although optimal health is readily at our disposal, many people limp along, never feeling fully charged with positive and productive energy. This may be due to the fact that it can take a while for symptoms to surface, but although you may be asymptomatic, that does not mean that all is well. It has become evident that the fatal diseases of our era begin many years before they are detectable. By the time symptoms actually appear, the chances of reversing the disease are slim indeed. Let's take the case of the late actor, Michael Landon. By the time his cancer was diagnosed, people could not believe how far the disease had progressed before it was detected. 'But that's the way it is with cancer,' most people in the medical community responded. It appears that we have an abundance of confidence in super medical technology until something happens to us and we realize what a rocky road it is that will lead us back to good health. There is obviously a vast difference between the absence of both recognizable and undetectable abnormalities and the state of optimal health.

The nature of chronic illness certainly makes obsolete the annual check-up, a peculiarly American ritual. The whole concept of the annual physical exam was introduced in the 1920s by the Metropolitan Life Insurance Company. Today, many experts believe it is a waste of time and money. The absence of symptoms does not equal good health. In fact, the clean bills of health that patients receive from their doctors upon completing a physical examination can be downright false. Many have gone to doctors with complaints and left their surgeries with a pat on the back and a prescription that does not cure the problem. Such was the case with my good friend, Anna. For nearly two years she visited a variety of doctors with various complaints, including a general lack of energy. Then, after yet another examination and being told she was fine, that she was just too stressed out over her job and family, a visible lump popped out of her neck while the patronizing physician was still speaking. A biopsy revealed lymph node cancer, and she barely survived six months of chemotherapy.

No, the physical exam cannot assure you of good health. Even the US government has stepped in lately to emphasize this. A few years ago, at the request of the government, a committee of physicians known as the United States Preventive Task Force reviewed all available evidence about preventing illness and concluded that it's pointless for all people to receive the same battery of tests routinely, regardless of their age, sex or symptoms.[6] According to the Task Force report, if prevention is to work, people must assume greater responsibility for their own health.

First of all, your body will most likely tell you when something has gone wrong, through symptoms such as pain, fever, nausea, fatigue and so on. Instead of suppressing these symptoms, this is a good time to find out what may be the underlying problem. Second, many clinical examinations and lab tests are not sensitive enough to detect chronic conditions at an early enough stage to be of help to you. Colon cancer, for instance, can grow for up to 15 years before most modern early-detection techniques can find the tiniest tumours.

A group of medical doctors recently concluded that 'for the asymptomatic [apparently healthy], non-pregnant adult of any age, no evidence supports the need for a complete physical examination as traditionally defined.'[7] They said that medical tests – including taking temperature, checking pulse and respiratory rates, testing reflexes and motor control and inspecting the thyroid, lymph nodes, lungs, liver, spleen, back, rectum and testicles – are of questionable or no value.

Others believe that the annual physical can actually be detrimental to those people who buy into its 'false reassurance' trap. If they believe that such a visit to their doctor will detect any abnormalities, which can then be cured, they will continue with such unhealthy lifestyle choices as eating a high-fat diet, not exercising and not learning how to manage physical, emotional and environmental stress.

FILLING THE GAP

Doctors, many of them being rational creatures at times, have not failed to take notice of the gap in the services they provide. The American Holistic Medical Association has announced that a good number of medical doctors are turning to holistic practices and adapting natural medicine to give their patients the best of both worlds. And not only in America. According to the *Jerusalem Post*, within the next five to ten years allopathy and many forms of complementary or holistic medicine will be well integrated in Israel.

Modern medicine has simply failed to keep many of its promises. A walk through any hospital is a disturbing reminder that allopathic medicine is virtually helpless in the face of enormous human suffering. Even common problems are at times beyond its reach. And there are orthodox medical professionals who claim that modern medicine has totally lost its way. It is difficult to view the widespread suffering and deaths caused by lethal yet preventable chronic diseases and think otherwise.

This realization was not lost on the British public. In the mid-1980s, reports suggested a growing use of various types of non-orthodox health care not generally available under the National Health Service. At about the same time, a report from the British Medical Association's board of science suggested that this might be a 'passing fashion'. By 1990, however, there was little to indicate that interest was waning. In fact, that the market for non-orthodox health care is 'buoyant' has been confirmed by a study by the University of Sheffield Medical School.[8] According to *Which?* magazine, many thousands of patients are seen every year by the approximately 50,000 holistic medical practitioners at work in the UK. Of these patients, two thirds are women and 36 per cent never consulted an orthodox physician. This trend naturally makes one ask: If an ounce of prevention is worth a pound of care, then why is that valuable ounce so rarely covered by insurance or the NHS?

Alternative and complementary therapies have always been a way of life among the more enlightened members of society. This has certainly been true of royalty and the upper classes throughout history and today, the Royal Family are keen to use holistic treatments as well as allopathic medicine. Although Prince Charles is the most prominent in this regard, the Queen Mother and the Queen have both been treated homoeopathically. The Duke of Gloucester is patron of the Homoeopathic Trust for Research and Education; Princess Diana and the Duchess of York engage in treatments ranging from acupuncture and colonic irrigation to zone therapy. The Prince of Wales has, in fact, become patron of the Marylebone Centre Trust, an NHS complementary medical general practice in London, while he openly encourages the use of alternative therapies to complement orthodox practices. Other converts include

Margaret Thatcher, Barbara Daly, Richard Branson, Sylvester Stallone, Paul McCartney, Richard Gere and Tom Cruise.

Those physicians who employ complementary therapies as well as modern-day medicine are primarily known as holistic doctors. They are attempting to go beyond the rigid parameters of what standard medical philosophy pontificates. Holistic medicine considers the complete person. It utilizes the body's vital energy, or life force, and its capacity for recovering with the aid of therapies that boost the immune system. Practitioners believe that an individual's well-being depends on both body and mind, and so they attempt to treat you as a whole person. Their holistic principles are based on the theory that the body has tremendous self-healing power and that this is accomplished by the body and mind together, not the 'healer'.

Although we have strayed far from nature, and we have traded in much common sense for sophisticated technology, we are slowly but surely re-emerging with the realization that our inner power is part of the healing process. The main purpose of any therapeutic discipline is to nurture the body's innate ability for healing. Thus, you have primary responsibility for your own good health. This doesn't imply that we stray totally from conventional care. Like other professionals, responsible holistic physicians have limits to what they can do. Cancer and congenital disorders are among the conditions that get referred to allopathic specialists. Complementary medicine is not aiming to replace our current system of health care; it is, as its name implies, seeking to complement it. It is filling in the gaps and helping patients in ways that modern medicine is unable or unwilling to address. The either/or approach is not at issue here. But one should first use the therapy that poses the least risk; conservative management of illness is preferable since the body usually heals best when interfered with least.

HOMOEOPATHY

Among the most popular alternative therapies is homoeopathy. In the United States, although there are only 5000 licensed homoeopaths (compared to 615,000 MDs) a recent poll suggests that 62 per cent of all Americans would accept such treatment, and of those who have already visited alternative physicians, 84 per cent say they would do so again.[9] Despite the lack of practitioners, one million Americans take homoeopathic medicine. In Europe, the practice of homoeopathy is far more widespread. In France, 30 per cent of the population have used homoeopathic remedies, and in Germany, 25 per cent of the physicians use them. In Britain, homoeopathy remains a part – albeit a small one – of the NHS, not least because of the Royal Family's enthusiasm for this form of alternative medicine at the time of the establishment of the health service in 1948. Even Mother Teresa has added homoeopathic services to the care she provides the destitute, because of their effectiveness and low cost. Still, homoeopathy lacks the full support afforded allopathic practitioners by the establishment.

Homoeopathy's progenitor was the German physician Samuel Hahnemann (1755–1843). Disillusioned by the medical practices of his day, such as blood-letting, leeching, purging and using toxic mercury remedies, he discovered the Law of Similars ('like cures like'), first introduced by Hippocrates. According to this theory, substances that cause symptoms similar to those caused by a disease can be used to cure that disease. Dr Hahnemann combined the Greek words for 'similar' and 'suffering' to name his new discipline: homoeopathy.

Homoeopathy developed long before the era of scientific medicine and still lacks the multitude of double-blind, randomized studies that are considered the hallmark of Western medicine. However, studies at the Glasgow Homoeopathic Hospital in the 1970s provided impressive results. Perhaps even more significantly, the benefits gained by animals given homoeopathic remedies seem to negate claims by orthodox practitioners that it is the placebo effect that makes human homoeopathic treatment so successful. But since the lion's share of medical studies are funded by drug companies, it may be a while before therapies such as homoeopathy, which stress prevention and offer cures to long-standing conditions, can be brought to the forefront.

Homoeopathy is most successful in dealing with chronic conditions such as allergies, recurrent infections, respiratory problems, skin disorders, digestion problems, reproductive difficulties, chronic fatigue, premenstrual disorders, headaches, immune system dysfunction and even emotional instability – areas of distress where modern medicine offers little or no relief. But most importantly, homoeopathy, like all other holistic approaches, zeroes in on prevention. A healthy lifestyle that includes proper nutrition, physical fitness, emotional balance, good environment and stress management are key factors. A homoeopath works within a system of medical care that emphasizes personal responsibility and fosters a cooperative relationship among all those involved. It encompasses all safe (and relatively inexpensive) modes of diagnosis and treatment while emphasizing the whole person – physical, emotional and spiritual.

At the time when Dr Hahnemann became disillusioned with allopathic medicine, the treatments available were ineffective and often lethal. Besides bleeding people sometimes to death and forcing vomiting, highly poisonous substances were prescribed as medicine. Now, as then, allopathic practitioners deal with the suppression of symptoms, while homoeopaths view them as the body's natural way of self-healing.

Orthodox health providers prescribe drugs to relieve symptoms and, when they disappear, presume the patient is cured. This is clearly not the case with homoeopaths (or other alternative and complementary medicine practitioners) who believe that symptoms are warning signs that the body's natural defence mechanism has weakened. From the homoeopathic viewpoint, drugs such as steroids and antibiotics may restore normal health in the short term, but they will not restore the person to a balanced state of well-being.

Although homoeopathic theory does not fit the drug model of medicine, homoeopathy's ability to help people has been repeatedly evaluated through rigorous scientific research. In a 1991 review of more than 100 clinical studies on homoeopathy published during the previous 30 years, 81 per cent showed that homoeopathic remedies had helped the patients treated.[10]

Homoeopathic medications are extremely diluted animal, plant or mineral extracts. These remedies consist of a minute dose of a substance that, in a healthy person, would produce symptoms similar to those of the disease. For instance, instead of suppressing a fever, a remedy may induce one (within a safe range) to further fight off an infection. Homoeopathic medicines are said to work by revving up the immune functions for overcoming the agents – i.e. viruses, bacteria, etc. – responsible for the ailment. However, the inherent paradox of how they actually work is probably the single most important reason for their lack of acceptance by modern science and medicine.

A decade ago, alternative practitioners appealed mainly to people who rejected mainstream medicine outright. But recently, affluent 20-something and 30-something professionals – health conscious and angered by what they perceive as conventional medicine's impersonal approach – are turning to what used to be traditional treatment.[11]

A Chicago-based allopathic doctor spoke of his frustration with the existing system. Dr Joel Sheppard said that many patients seem to be stuck in a revolving door with little hope of ever achieving health. 'We would work like crazy to save people's lives, and a couple of months later, they would be back with the same problem or something worse,' said Dr Sheppard. He blames our current medical approaches, believing they are merely stopgap measures, doing little to turn around the patient's deeper lifestyle and personal health problems.[12]

AYURVEDA

Some people, like Margaret Thatcher, have turned to an ancient medical practice known as ayurveda, which, like homoeopathy, concentrates on prevention rather than cure. It is based upon three concepts: (1) the recognition and evaluation of clinical signs and symptoms; (2) the acknowledgement that behaviour and environment influence health and disease; and (3) the belief that proper food and diet restore health. Physiological imbalances are treated through diet, herbal preparations and seasonal routines before they manifest themselves in illness.

Ayurveda is believed to be one of the oldest medical systems, dating back at least 5000 years. Its roots lie in ancient India and it still thrives outside Western societies to this day. The All-India Ayur-Veda Congress consists of 300,000 practitioners, while the 108 ayurvedic colleges in that country grant degrees on completion of a five-year programme. Ayurveda is also recognized by the World Health Organization as a leading form of preventive care. [13]

It is only very recently that ayurvedic medicine has made itself known to Western health consumers. Alarm over chronic diseases and modern medicine's inability to deal with them has led some people to this form of complementary medicine.

The Ayurvedic pharmacopeia includes thousands of plants and plant products, many of which function as therapeutic agents. The name 'ayurveda' is derived from two Sanskrit roots: *ayus*, which means 'life span', and *veda*, meaning the 'knowledge of science'. Ayurveda thus means the 'science of life'.

Ayurvedic diagnosis and treatment centres around the principles of biological individuality. It views emotional considerations as crucial to the development of the body's imbalances. A disorder of the immune mechanism is seen as a primary factor in the creation of disease.

According to ayurveda, three irreducible physiological principles known as 'doshas' regulate the different functions of mind and body. In Sanskrit, the three doshas are called *vata*, *pitta* and *kapha*. Everyone is endowed at birth with some value of all three, but in each person, the exact proportions vary and this determines the psychophysiological type. There are ten classic types, derived from combinations of the three doshas. [14]

Through palpation of the radial pulse, skilled ayurvedic physicians can diagnose conditions such as diabetes, neoplastic disease and asthma. Most importantly, such experts can spot imbalances at that crucial early stage, when there are no other clinical signs. Treatment then would prevent the further development of the disease.

The key factor in ayurveda is its emphasis on restoring balance to the doshas. This would prevent the onset of conditions that develop into chronic diseases. This is accomplished through the division of ayurvedic therapeutics into four areas: mind, body, behaviour and environment. Every patient is counselled and treated in all of these.

Mind over body has enormous clout in the practice of ayurveda. Whereas modern medicine considers the body a complex machine, ayurvedic philosophy views it as a physical expression of our higher consciousness. Thus, mental intervention in the treatment of illness is the hallmark of ayurvedic therapeutics. For instance, the practice of transcendental meditation (TM) is a commonly preferred discipline. While you are in a meditative state, metabolic changes actually bring you to restful alertness. Many studies have linked the use of TM and reduced illness, increased longevity and quality of life, and decreased anxiety, hypertension, cholesterol levels and substance abuse. [15]

But mind over body is most effective when the body is fully respected, and fuel for it plays a central role in ayurvedic medicine. Health is considered the normal human condition and results when the body remains in balance. This balance is achieved, in part, through proper diet, exercise, herbs and *panchakarma* – purification procedures that consist of medicated oil massages, herbalized heat treatments and elimination therapies. [16] The ayurvedic physician prescribes foods and therapies to balance the patient's *vata, pitta* and *kapha* as needed. Many patients are also encouraged to use specific herbs.

It is interesting to note that a select group of ayurvedic herbal compounds known as rasayanas are believed to increase resistance to disease and promote longevity. Two of these compounds, called Maharishi Anuit Kalah-4 and -5 (M-4, M-5), were studied at a number of American universities and other institutions. Both were found to reduce the incidence of chemically induced mammary carcinoma (breast cancer) in up to 88 per cent of experimental animals and caused up to 60 per cent of fully formed tumours in control animals to regress when they were subsequently given the herbal compounds. [17] Further, M-4 prevented experimental lung cancer in nearly 65 per cent of lab animals without any adverse side-effects. It is believed that M-4 and M-5 may contain powerful antioxidants. Both agents were proved to combat free radicals and reactive oxygen species, which are responsible for many chronic diseases, from cancer and heart disease to allergies.

Nevertheless, all the evidence in the world won't do you an ounce of good if you do not apply it. In preventive medicine, behaviour is the key to all success. According to a person's particular requirements, ayurveda strongly emphasizes daily and seasonal health routines. In fact, it has, for thousands of years, practised what modern medicine is just beginning to preach. Adequate rest, normal bowel function, proper food combining and timing and regular exercise are crucial factors in the attainment of optimal health.

Where the medical community has let us down, the US government has, uncharacteristically, stepped in, disseminating a mountain of evidence revealing the multiple health benefits of physical activity. Regular exercise has been proved to prevent and manage coronary heart disease, hypertension, diabetes mellitus, osteoporosis, obesity and mental health problems such as depression and anxiety.[18] Physical activity has also been associated with lower rates of colon cancer and stroke and may be linked to reduced back injury; in addition, physically active people, on average, outlive those who are sedentary. Increased physical activity can also help to maintain the functional independence of older people and generally enhance the quality of life for all.[19]

While you do all you can for yourself, the environment cannot be ignored. The well-being of an individual and the well-being of society are interrelated. The effects of living conditions, environmental pollution, food chemicalization, air quality, pure water and hygienic practices affect society as a whole and you as an individual.

Ayurvedic medicine considers your own psychophysiological type and assists you in dealing with various environmental conditions. Since everyone does not respond to all stimuli equally, learning how to best cope with your environment brings you closer to optimal health.

NATUROPATHY

In a quest for optimal health, some people have discovered naturopathy, a 19th-century European system that incorporates even older healing methods such as oriental medicine. It is a system of therapeutics based on natural foods, light, warmth, massage, fresh air, regular exercise and the avoidance of medications. Advocates believe that illness can be healed by the natural processes of the body.

In the last few years, naturopathy has once again received a good amount of attention. The practice declined in the 1940s and 1950s when pharmaceutical drugs and technological medicine took firm hold of the health community. At that time, the public bought into the 'magic bullet' theory and assumed that a particular pill would one day exist for every one of their ailments. But today, in the United States, even many insurance companies are encouraging their clients to seek naturopathic care, having found allopathic treatment far too costly.

Naturopathy, unlike other complementary medical disciplines, has a great deal in common with allopathy. Its roots are in conventional medical science. To qualify as a naturopath, standard pre-med courses are required, followed by two years of primary medical science and two years of clinical training in naturopathic therapeutics. The latter include clinical nutrition, counselling, medical herbalism, homoeopathy, natural child-birth, minor surgery, stress management and physiotherapy. In Britain, many naturopaths are also qualified osteopaths.

Naturopaths, like other complementary medical practitioners, view the patient as a 'whole' and not merely as a condition. Much emphasis is placed on discovering the root of an illness, and a patient's lifestyle may be adjusted to correct and/or prevent an ailment.

Naturopathic medicine has enjoyed great success in the treatment of both acute and chronic conditions. Unlike in allopathy, however, nutrition plays a central role in health maintenance: naturopaths study nutrition for at least 200 hours compared to the less than 20 *elective* hours offered to trainee orthodox doctors. Your naturopath may also be a trained homoeopath. Thus, by helping you to build up your immune system and improve your health habits, while at the same time not being ignorant of modern practices, he or she may provide you with the best of all worlds.

With its close association with modern medicine, one would think that naturopathy would receive its due recognition from the establishment. Yet, in the United States, naturopathy is licensed in only eight of its 50 states, and in the United Kingdom, naturopaths (while free to practise) are few and far between outside the major urban centres.

One of the world's leading naturopaths is Dr Jan DeVries, who has a long history of treating the Royal Family. His clinic in Scotland sees more than 3000 people each week.

Dr DeVries agrees with the holistic physicians that we humans must think more about nature and obey its laws. He blames many modern practices for the deterioration of our health. 'Civilized foods are mostly prepackaged,' he said in an interview in 1990. 'Nothing is better for us than fresh foods and fresh juices. The modern [ailments] such as candida and Epstein-Barr [the virus responsible for glandular fever] have all come from a weakened immune system. People flock to doctors, but the immune system is seldom treated. Problems of virus infections will fall away if the immune system is treated in a natural way.'[20]

Naturopathy is finding its way again. Of the 2000 naturopaths now practising in the United States, half of them emerged from medical school in the last decade. They realize that by allocating greater responsibility for well-being to their patients, questioning drug over-reliance and focusing on people's lifestyle decisions, preventive care will soon change the face of modern medicine.

HERBALISM

This form of medicine is the oldest healing art in the world. It utilizes herbs to tackle illness directly. A herbalist combines natural remedies to balance the body's essential life force, which the Chinese have called *qi* (pronounced 'chee'). Herbs can be administered internally or externally, in the form of tinctures, extracts, distillations, pills, ointments or plasters, prepared from whole herbs or roots without the elimination of a single element.

Before the technological and pharmaceutical revolution, Western medicine was primarily herbal medicine. To this day, the symbol of pharmacy is the mortar and pestle, which pharmacists used to grind medicinal herbs. The history of this form of medicine can be traced back through the civilizations of Rome, Greece, Assyria and Babylon to Sumerian times and even beyond. A cuneiform tablet from the library of Assurbanipal, King of Assyria (668–c.626 BC), at Nineveh (Iraq), and now in the British Museum, ends with a note saying that it was copied from a tablet that had been written in the second year of the reign of Enlilbani, King of Isan (c.2201–2177 BC). Thus, the Sumerian herbal was in existence in the second half of the third millennium BC.

With this astonishingly ancient pedigree, it is amusing that, nowadays, people seem to associate herbalism with New Age ideas. They can hardly take the credit for its existence. Many societies throughout the centuries have relied on some of the 750,000 species of flowering plants worldwide. In fact, 25 per cent of all allopathic prescription drugs today contain some active ingredients derived from plants. However, herbalists say, because they use the whole plant (or root) and not just the 'active ingredients', their treatments are far more gentle, with fewer side-effects, than pharmaceutical drugs.

Essentially, herbal preparations are prescribed to stimulate and support the body's own natural healing abilities. The immune system is a key target, and many herbs are used to reinforce it. They are also commonly prescribed to complement other treatments. For instance, naturopaths will regularly suggest tinctures, teas or poultices to help detoxify the body.

Herbalists have at their disposal compounds for a multitude of conditions. Throat infection, psoriasis, constipation and reproductive dysfunction are just a few problem areas that have benefited from the use of herbs. Some people opt for herbal remedy supplementation along with orthodox treatment.

It would appear that all the great natural healing arts only became despised or ignored in the 20th century. Herbalism, like others, was swept aside, unexamined and unexplored, accused of being unscientific superstition because it was antiquated and (God forbid) traditional. Such a verdict was accepted without any case for its defence being heard.

There remains a widespread misunderstanding of what herbalism really is. In reality, no tenable grounds for disagreement exist between traditional herbalists and modern scientists who are searching for measurable truth about substances. Both have – or should have – the same goal: to cure disease and to relieve suffering by any means that is safe and effective. Advocates of any one discipline should never assert that they alone know the cure for all diseases. The English King Henry III (1207–72) understood this when he enacted legislation to protect herbalists from prosecution by the Company of Physicians and Chirugeons.

Hippocrates wrote: 'We know the nature of medicaments and simples [respectively, herbs used medicinally and the medicines made from them] and make many preparations with them, some in one way and some in another. Some simples must be gathered early, some late, some we dry, some we crush.' He left a list of 400 'simples' employed by him and his forebears, and half that number are still in general use today.

Modern herbalism is based on theories and principles that centre around 'living medicine'. Since plants alone have the power of building up organic life from inorganic material, they form an active or living medicine. Herbalism works according to the law of nature, and herbs are the natural cures for human disease and ill health.

Non-poisonous herbs form the exclusive *materia medica* of herbalism. They have a dual function: they are food as well as medicines, and so build up general health at the same time that they cure any specific disease. It is believed that very small doses, if continued for a long time, are more effective than large quantities administered once. In this respect, herbalism owes something to homoeopathy but differs from it widely in theory and practice.

The first aim of all herbal treatment is to purify the bloodstream of any poisons and to create a normal functioning of the ductless glands (e. g. pituitary, thyroid). This is followed by attempts to make the various organs of the body work properly. Each herb has a specific sphere of influence within the human body, and by selecting the most suitable, the herbalist can treat any organ he or she desires.

However, herbal treatment, being particularly designed to deal with chronic complaints, is generally slow in effect. It is seldom possible to state how long a cure will take. It will vary according to your individual characteristics and those of any specific disease as it affects you, and months may pass before herbal treatment begins to show results. The cure of chronic conditions that have sometimes been developing since birth must inevitably be a lengthy business. The aim of herbs is not to rid the body of symptoms, but to cure the disease itself. Obviously, this takes longer than the quick suppression of symptoms, which leaves the disease intact. However, the slow process of herbal treatment effects more radical and complete cures than other more rapid methods.

In the 1990s, certain herbs will be making news as never before. Eighteen of the most prominent American herbalists have picked the top ten herbs that will dominate the market.[21]

- **Echinacea** is known to activate leukocytes, the crucial white blood cells that act as scavengers to free radicals. Additionally, it fights infections and speeds up wound healing.
- **Ginseng** is widely used to improve the functioning of the central

nervous system. It also soothes stomach upsets and can normalize blood pressure, control stress and, yes, even improve one's sex drive.
- **Ginkgo** has already made headlines as the 'smart herb'. It increases blood flow to the brain and stimulates mental alertness as well as overall cerebral well-being. It is also known to aid the body's vascular system, combat free radicals and, among other functions, act as a neuro-transmitter.
- **Garlic.** When it comes to this herb, your grandmother was not wrong. This is an anti-cancer, anti-ageing, antibacterial, antiviral agent and an immuno-stimulant. It successfully lowers cholesterol, and its revolu-tionary effects in the treatment of AIDS patients are receiving fame.
- **Chamomile** is another golden pick by the herbalists. Its function as a mild sedative and stomach relaxer is well appreciated.
- **Astragalus** is, say the herbalists, the most important herb for strengthening the immune system. It also acts as a blood tonic and helps to regulate fluid metabolism.
- **St John's wort** is known for its positive results in cases of trauma and burns. Recent studies suggest that it can also be quite useful in the treatment of AIDS, influenza, urinary tract infections and mild depression.
- **Dandelion** made the list for its high content of vitamin A, which acts as an antioxidant. The herb and root are ideal liver and kidney tonics.
- **Dong quai**'s most powerful asset may be its contribution to treating breast cancer. Studies are currently under way to substantiate this claim further.
- **Rosemary**'s aroma, says one herbalist, helps you feel clear-headed and calm. This herb can be used to tackle bad breath, high blood pressure, female problems, digestion disorders, poor circulation and, if you can imagine it, baldness.

Last year alone, Americans spent nearly $1 billion (£667 million) on herbal remedies, and the demand for this medical practice has yet to peak. Herbalists are content to base their case for herbalism on the fact that plants do have curative powers against human disease – the thou-sands of cases thus cured are more than enough evidence to back this claim. However, both the US and UK governments choose to ignore this. In the US, proposed Food and Drug Administration (FDA) regulations would restrict the sale of medicinal herbs unless they have gone through clinical trials, which would cost close to $400 million (£267 million) for each herb. The FDA says this would eliminate 'phoney' herbal products; herbalists point to the preface of the FDA's *Dietary Supplement Task Force Final Report* (May 1992), which states that one reason for these restrictions would be to keep the American pharmaceutical industry viable. There have also been calls for the same sort of regulation of herbal products in the UK.

ACUPUNCTURE

The Prince and Princess of Wales have made acupuncture (as well as homoeopathy, naturopathy and aromatherapy) accepted and respected in their native Britain. Although the US Food and Drug Administration considers this 4500-year-old Chinese medical practice experimental, about 240,000 treatments are administered every week in the United States. Chronic pain is readily tackled with the use of fine needles to stimulate nerve impulses to redirect channels of energy found beneath the skin. Thus, by balancing the body's energy levels, good health is restored.

One of the reasons why our culture may be uncomfortable about acupuncture is that it doesn't function the way we are conditioned to think. Western medicine is based on physical principles while acupuncture deals with 'energy' that cannot be seen or handled in our traditional medical manner. The Chinese claim that all our bodily functions, emotions and thoughts are the end result of a sophisticated interplay of subtle, internal energies. An acupuncturist would say that, before you come down with hepatitis or glandular fever, you first experience an energy imbalance. Therefore, his or her mission is to balance your level of energy to prevent an adverse condition or to cure the illness.

While treating your illness, acupuncturists rely on the complex circuitry in the body, which consists of about 50 meridians and hundreds of acupoints. Meridians are related to primary organs, while acupoints are areas of access to them. Qi, the vital energy or life force, is thought to flow through the meridians and strengthen the organs to maximise their functions. Illness may occur when the flow of qi is blocked or hyperactive.

Besides acupuncture, oriental medicine balances qi using a number of other methods including the burning of medicinal herbs over acupoints (moxibustion), precise body massage according to meridian theory (shiatsu), and the use of Chinese herbs. Many holistic practices may be self-prescribed and treated, but this is not recommended with acupuncture. The subtle bodily energies it deals with are powerful, and mishaps in stimulation can be dangerous.

In recent times, acupuncture has been used successfully to treat drug abusers, female infertility problems, insomnia, chronic fatigue, respiratory and digestion disorders. Other ailments that respond well include degenerative arthritis, muscle spasms, back, shoulder and neck pain, tendinitis, tennis elbow, arm, wrist and hand pain, as well as hip, thigh, knee and ankle problems. Acupuncture is especially efficacious with sports injuries, since it rapidly speeds up circulation to injured areas and decreases inflammation. Other conditions that benefit from acupuncture are migraine and tension headaches, facial pain, constipation and irritable bowel syndrome. Great degrees of improvement through the use of acupuncture have also been noted in the treatment of immune system problems.

Last year I visited a drug rehabilitation centre in Dallas, Texas. There I met James, who had opted for rehabilitation over prison for his drug problems. He had great difficulty dealing with symptoms of withdrawal, which, he said, included overwhelming anxiety, nervousness, irritability, headaches, occasional nausea and, not least, a constant craving for cocaine. Out of desperation, he chose acupuncture treatment and soon began to experience an ease and relaxation that, he said, he had not known in a decade.

Addictive disorders such as drug abuse, smoking and alcoholism respond well to acupuncture because it blocks withdrawal symptoms. After a month of three sessions a week, James began to make new plans for his future. Today, he is halfway through earning a degree in engineering, has remarried and is living near Houston. He credits acupuncture and the other complementary therapies he used later for his new 'life of normalcy'.

Others have experienced similar results. In 1990, for example, the *Lancet* reported on studies that assessed patients who had been treated with acupuncture techniques for alcohol dependence. The results indicated that, compared to a control group, members of the treatment group were admitted less frequently to detoxification centres and expressed a diminished need for alcohol after acupuncture was performed. [22]

About 200 drug treatment programmes in the United States rely on acupuncture to ward off the side-effects of drug withdrawal. They don't consider such treatment a cure, but it allows the person to have reduced cravings so that counselling becomes more effective in assisting behaviour modification.

Acupuncture has reportedly been used in private American clinics since the early 1980s as a treatment to relieve stress and improve the quality of life for carriers of HIV. Now it is being studied at the University of Miami School of Medicine. This pilot study, which began in June 1991 and which receives absolutely no outside funding (participants have to foot part of the bill themselves), is the first of its kind at a leading university to take a critical, scientific look at the treatment's efficacy. Early results are promising: patients, who are given acupuncture in combination with Chinese herbal supplements, report easier sleep and increased energy. If the final results live up to their promise, perhaps researchers won't meet as much resistance in obtaining funding to conduct a randomized, clinical trial. [23]

Dr Matthew Lee, acting chairman of the department of rehabilitation at the Rusk Institute in New York City, uses acupuncture to treat
chronic head, neck, jaw and facial pain. He told *American Health Magazine* that 60 to 70 per cent of his patients respond within eight sessions. 'I
use acupuncture to break the cycle of pain, which then allows me to get
the patient to exercise and participate in standard pain management,' Dr
Lee said.[24]

Many believe that acupuncture should be the first line of attack for
chronic pain since it is far safer and often more effective than drugs. Dr
Bruce Pomeranz, a physiologist at the University of Toronto, says, 'We
may never prove all the mechanisms of acupuncture, but aspirin was used
for years before anyone knew how it worked.'[25] Acupuncture is increasingly available at NHS pain relief clinics in Britain, such as the Pain
Relief Centre at Walton Hospital in Liverpool.

If you are considering acupuncture, rest assured that there are no
known toxic, allergic or other harmful side-effects. The risk of infection is
eliminated through the use of sterile needles and antiseptic techniques.
However, to produce successful results, it is crucial that the acupuncturist has adequate training and clinical experience in anatomy and medical
and physical disorders. It is also important that he or she is a member of a
recognized society, such as (in Britain) the Council for Acupuncture,
which trains acupuncturists, vets their credentials and maintains a code of
practice.

CHIROPRACTIC AND OSTEOPATHY

'Oh, my aching back!' is spoken by eight out of ten of us sooner or later.
The odd thing is that medical science can do little more than prescribe
painkillers or muscle relaxants for this common condition. If these drugs
helped, most people would be satisfied.

It is reported that Americans, for instance, spend $60 billion
annually on back treatments, yet very little is known about how to treat
this ailment effectively. One can't help but come to the conclusion that the
mystery illness of our time is not cancer or cardiovascular disease or
AIDS, but back pain!

Lately, however, a good deal of attention has been given to both
chiropractic and osteopathy for their success in back pain alleviation. In
fact, these two 'manipulative therapies' have become the first choice for
potential relief from musculoskeletal complaints such as back pains, aches
and strains, whiplash injuries, arthritic conditions, bursitis and restriction
of movement.

According to chiropractic, the state of a person's health is determined, in general, by the condition of his or her nervous system. In most
cases, treatment provided by chiropractors involves the mechanical

manipulation of the spinal column, although some practitioners employ X-rays for diagnosis and use physiotherapy and diet. Chiropractic does not involve drugs or surgery. The theory behind osteopathy is similar, the differences in practice being that osteopaths place less reliance on X-rays for diagnosis, and they use more leverage and less direct thrust in their spinal manipulations.

A chiropractor is awarded the degree of Doctor of Chiropractic (DC) after completing at least two years of premedical studies followed by four years of training at an approved chiropractic school. Registered osteopaths in Britain have completed a four-year full-time course of training. Recently, legislation has been proposed that would make it against the law for non-registered osteopaths to practise – giving the profession the same status as orthodox medical doctors.

Chiropractors and osteopaths believe that, by keeping all the joints in your spine properly moving, they can prevent interference with your nervous system and thus allow your body's life force to express itself through your nerves. As people become more attuned with their bodies, the benefits of these manipulative therapies are soon realized. Such is the case with many athletes, dancers and performers. The US Olympic team employs the services of chiropractors at all Olympic games, and the Soviet Sports Committee also included a Western-trained chiropractor at all Olympic events.

Five per cent of Americans visit one of the 45,000 chiropractors at least once a year, at a total cost of $2.4 billion (£1.6 billion).[26] Results in the *British Medical Journal* may encourage the British public to seek such help for back pain as well. The *BMJ* reported the outcome of a three-year study, during which researchers at the prestigious Epidemiology and Medical Care Unit of the Medical Research Council in Harrow, Middlesex, studied more than 700 patients with muscle- or skeletal-related lower back pain, in 11 different towns and cities in England. The study concluded that, among people with severe and chronic pain, those being treated with chiropractic had a 13 per cent higher rate of improvement than those receiving hospital outpatient care.[27] Citing the economic benefits of relief from pain and disability – eliminating an estimated 290,000 sick days annually – the researchers recommended that the National Health Service consider offering chiropractic.

Previous studies had usually shown that the results produced by chiropractic treatment lasted for only a matter of hours after each session. This one demonstrated that the 378 patients receiving chiropractic care tended to have better results after six months than the 339 treated in medical clinics.[28]

A group of doctors at the University of Limburg in the Netherlands reviewed 35 clinical trials comparing chiropractic techniques of spinal manipulation and mobilization with other treatments, such as drugs, massage, physical therapy and exercises. They, too, acknowledged that manipulation can help relieve certain kinds of neck and back pain.[29]

Although chiropractic and osteopathy – both of American origin – were not formally introduced until the late 19th century, anthropologists have found evidence that the ancient Egyptians, Hindus, Chinese, Assyrians and Babylonians used hand manipulative techniques very much like the procedures applied today. But today's chiropractor, in particular, is going beyond the traditional hands-on spinal manipulation. Innovative and high-tech equipment for diagnosis and treatment, such as the dermathermograph to measure spinal heat and complex X-ray machines, as well as sophisticated mind/body models and theories, all promise to revolutionize the therapy.

MASSAGE THERAPY

Somewhere between Hippocrates and the Industrial Revolution, we lost all track of massage. So when the French discovered oriental massage it was news to the Europeans. However, it was a Swede, not a Frenchman, who popularized massage all over again in the early 19th century – hence, the term 'Swedish massage' for the basic body rubdown.

The practice of massage is a universal concept of healing. Those of us who are regular recipients know that we could not get through life without it. The manipulation of the body's soft tissues, through stroking, rubbing, kneading and tapping, increases circulation, improves muscle tone and relaxes the body and mind.

Besides simply making you feel wonderful, massage has many other therapeutic effects. It dilates the blood vessels which improves the circulation and relieves congestion throughout the body. It acts as a cleanser by stimulating lymph circulation and speeding up the elimination of wastes and toxic debris. Massage is famous for relieving tension and relaxing muscle spasms, but many are not aware that, by manipulating general circulation, it also increases nutrition of the tissues and stimulates the immune system.

But for most of us, the simple function of massage is to allow our minds to relax from their frantic activity. Tense muscles are frequently the result of psychological tension and pent-up emotions. Hence, a proper massage has a deeply relaxing effect which brings you to a place of physical and emotional well-being by increasing your energy level. Tension blocks energy; massage restores its balance to a normal, natural state. If fatigue is the first sign of ill health, then massage may be your first choice of action for relief. There are many forms of massage therapy, and here we will consider a few. Through experimentation, you will discover what works best for you.

Shiatsu, which means 'finger pressure' in Japanese, is the oldest documented form of physical therapy, dating back to the Yellow Emperor's dynasty (500 BC). It was introduced by Buddhist monks and, to this day, is believed to be the most flexible therapy. Marilyn Monroe thought so, among many others.

In shiatsu, the palms and thumbs apply pressure to the skin at places that often correspond to acupoints. Those who wish to get rid of a headache, for example, press their thumbs on a series of pressure points along the skull and the back of the neck.

Shiatsu is very effective for the ordinary aches and pains that result from bodily stress. Some believe this is because hard pressure exerted over the painful area causes extra blood flow there, which brings about relief. The blood functions as a natural purifier of the body, delivering antibodies and oxygen to the troubled area and taking away waste products, including carbon dioxide.

Others claim that shiatsu possibly acts like acupuncture, stimulating certain meridians and helping the body to heal itself. Then there are those who think that, when pressure is put on the head, this causes the release of natural substances known as endorphins, which are the body's own painkillers.

An altogether different form of massage is preferred by some people. What used to be known as 'structural integration' is now called **rolfing**, in honour of Dr Ida Rolf, who introduced this system of body education and physical energy. Rolfing is based on a set of principles concerning human structure. First of all, most people are believed to be significantly out of alignment with gravity. Further, we function better when we are lined up with the Earth's gravitational field. And our bodies are so adjustable that their alignment can be brought into harmony with gravity at any time during a lifetime.

Dr Rolf has said that the gospel of rolfing is: when the body gets working appropriately, the force of gravity can flow through; then the body spontaneously heals itself. Rolfing rebalances the body by bringing the head, shoulders, chest, pelvis and legs into proper vertical alignment. It is possibly the most complex of massage therapies, and generally is applied in ten sessions – each serving as a continuation of the last session and a progression to the next. The sessions are designed to uncover a structural ease and kinetic balance that is unique to each individual. The aim is to help you discover the most efficient way of using your body, given its limitations, liabilities and virtues.

Those who want a full body effect but not a full body massage may resort to **reflexology**. After a long day of frantic activity, a killer aerobics class or a long journey, I know of no better way to breathe life back into my body than some serious pressure applied to the soles of my feet. When a pair of hands covered in warm lotion begin kneading, prying at the toes, loosening each foot's 26 bones, 56 ligaments and 38 muscles, all accumulated stress simply seems to melt away. As a thumb methodically probes along the sole, between the toes, digging in painfully at points, the whole body begins to relax.

Of course, reflexology is far more complicated than what many of us simply consider to be a glorious foot rub. Although the Indians and Chinese have practised it for about 5000 years, it is believed that, at some point, this therapy gave way to acupuncture and began to play a minor role. But about the time that literature about reflexology began to appear in Europe, the great Florentine sculptor Benvenuto Cellini (1500–71) and others were already using strong pressure on their fingers and toes successfully to relieve pain elsewhere in their bodies. The relationship between reflex points and the internal organs of the body is thus used in the treatment of disease.

Body tensions are believed to manifest themselves in the hands and feet, thereby blocking energy. Through reflexology, the foot is manipulated in order to release energy, thus allowing the body to heal itself. Whole-body reactions are possible since there is a point on the foot that corresponds to every point on the body.

After shiatsu, rolfing and reflexology, to the lay person **aromatherapy** sounds like a luxurious beauty treatment rather than a therapy for optimal health. Of all the holistic practices, aromatherapy – treating the body and mind with essential oils of flowers and herbs – is just about the most popular.

The effects of aromatherapy preparations are achieved through the sense of smell, through absorption by the skin or both. Some are strong anti-microbial agents, about as effective as antibiotics. Others are used for psychotherapeutic purposes, ridding the mind and body of depression, insomnia or pre-menstrual syndrome (PMS). Essential oils are known to improve tissue regeneration, aid the sufferers of osteoporosis and arthritis, as well as speed up the healing of broken bones. Different essential oils have different effects on the mind and body. Lavender, marjoram and chamomile are soothing and stress-reducing. Rose, clary, sage and bergamot are used to lift the spirits, while sage and spearmint deliver alertness. Geranium, cypress and lemon are great physical invigorators, while ylang-ylang and sandalwood promise sexual arousal.

These effects have not been overlooked by certain corporations and informed individuals. They apply essential oils to their offices, board rooms, aeroplanes, cars or bedrooms, to achieve particular desired effects.

In Britain, there are two types of aromatherapy. 'Aesthetic aromatherapy' is carried out in a superficial way at beauty clinics and health farms, to induce a generalized feeling of well-being. 'Holistic aromatherapy' is, on the other hand, primarily therapeutic, carried out by well trained people to treat specific disorders. Holistic aromatherapists will ask clients for a medical history, and if a person has, say, serious heart disease, his or her GP will be informed before any treatment is started.

In Germany and France, health insurance covers spa and holistic clinic visits, which may include aromatherapy treatment. In the United States, the FDA does not recognize aromatherapy. The pressure on the American public not to accept this type of holistic treatment is so great that I cannot even buy peppermint oil at the Body Shop! It is against the law.

Most of us have an underdeveloped sense of smell. Bringing this sense to its peak capacity could open up a whole new pleasant and healing way of life for us. There are some 400,000 different scents on Earth; yet, we rely on a mere fraction for our occasional use.

The 1990s and beyond will see a drastic rise in degenerative diseases, exacerbated by continuous alterations in lifestyle and the deterioration of the environment. As an increasing number of illnesses result from the way we live, alternatives to our present health care system will become a necessity, not a choice.

CHAPTER FIVE

THE
VITAMIN
REVOLUTION

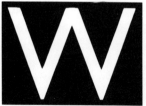hen the Dallas Cowboys enter the football field, they know that the best defence is a good offence. However, when it comes to nutritional and environmental assaults on your body and mind, just the opposite is true – good defence is the best offence. Therefore, we must act now to ward off the all-too-often devastating afflictions that modern-age living brings upon us.

In the 1990s, the term 'prevention' possesses a promise and a power as never before in the health field. In an era of chronic conditions where modern medicine has very little authority, nutritional science is on the threshold of tremendous new developments.

Nutrients, as we all know by now, are the source of life. In ancient Greece Hippocrates resorted to liver as a cure for night blindness, not knowing it was an excellent source of vitamin A. Centuries ago it was discovered that certain foods could cure or prevent such devastating diseases as pellagra, beriberi and scurvy. In the 20th century we discovered and isolated substances in food that provided cures to such serious ailments. Today much is known about the preventive and curative powers of vitamins and minerals. From colds to cancer, they have been identified as indispensable to our basic well-being and for our optimal health.

However, minerals and most vitamins cannot be produced in the body and need to be constantly resupplied as they are used up and eliminated. In addition, it is being increasingly recognized that the intake of these nutrients can be varied in such a way as to produce a significant improvement in general health and a decrease in the incidence and severity of disease.

Among the unconverted, however, are most allopathic doctors. Decades of public health policies provided by government – not to mention the influence of the pharmaceutical companies – have left these physicians thinking that we get every single nutrient we require, and in the right amounts, from our daily diets. But there are those who assert that, since the skills of these doctors are primarily used for the repair of faulty arteries, the setting of broken bones and the provision of chemotherapy to cancer victims, perhaps prevention is not their forte. Many people are no more likely to ask their doctors about nutrition and preventive care than they are to ask them to repair their cars or television sets – it simply isn't taught in medical school.

But as consistent evidence mounts from prestigious universities and other institutions around the world, that nutrients play a much more complex role in assuring vitality and optimal health than was previously thought, an increasing number of scientists and medical authorities are beginning to realize and admit that orthodox medical views on vitamins and minerals have been severely limited. After decades of treating nutritional supplements as marginally more useful than snake oil, mainstream medical experts are at last recognizing their unprecedented value. Vitamins, often in doses much higher than those usually recommended, may protect against a host of ills ranging from birth defects and cataracts to heart disease and cancer. Even more provocative are glimmerings that vitamins can stave off the normal ravages of ageing.[1]

In 1937 Azent Gyorgyi wrote that 'Vitamins, if properly understood and applied, will help us to reduce human suffering to an extent which the most fantastic mind would fail to imagine.' Only now, 50 years later, we are beginning to grasp the idea.

HEALTHY OR DISEASE-FREE?

Since the 1970s population studies from around the world have shown a consistent link between diet and health. It was discovered that people whose diet consisted mainly of fruits and vegetables had the lowest rates of heart disease and cancer. This new evidence led scientists to examine many individual nutrients, studying vitamins and minerals to determine what role they play regarding our health.

Their findings have been extraordinary. It has been determined that most people are not getting the vitamins they need, even if their diets are considered to be healthy ones. Most government-sanctioned recommendations for vitamin and mineral intake are based on the amounts of nutrients required to prevent serious deficiency diseases. However, this way of thinking is going the way of the dinosaur and the dodo. For instance, researchers have concluded that consuming vitamins C and E and beta carotene (a precursor of vitamin A) in amounts considerably higher than government recommendations can provide protection against chronic and often life-threatening illnesses, in addition to boosting the immune system and, to an extent, warding off ageing. As scientists have been made aware of the increasing significance between diet and health, they have inevitably declared that what is adequate and what is optimal requires more focused definition and consideration. In other words, do we wish to be truly healthy or merely disease-free?

'The field is currently undergoing a paradigm shift,' says Catherine Wateki, director of the food and nutrition board at the Institute of Medicine of the US National Academy of Sciences. 'We are now entering a second wave of vitamin research,' says Jeffrey Blumberg, associate director of the Human Nutrition Research Center on Aging at Tufts University in Boston, Massachusetts. 'The first wave was the discovery of vitamins and their role in combating nutritional deficiencies such as rickets and beriberi. That occurred in the first half of the century. Now we're on the second wave. You don't need to take vitamin C to prevent scurvy in this country today. But you could need it for optimal health and the prevention of some chronic diseases.'[2]

Recently, the prestigious New York Academy of Sciences held a conference for researchers to share their findings on the value of vitamins. 'The fact that it was held at all indicates a major shift in scientific opinion regarding the role of vitamins in disease prevention,' commented C. E. Butterworth Jnr, MD, professor of nutrition sciences at the University of Alabama at Birmingham.

As low as government standards are for optimal health, the majority of us don't even come close to meeting them. Less than one in ten of us eat five daily servings of fruit and vegetables, for example, thus keeping ourselves quite malnourished. Today, individual nutritional programmes can be designed to build up, balance or detoxify the body. Although supplements cannot replace a good diet, they are often necessary to help us deal with the extra physiological burdens that are placed on us. In the 1990s, as the result of excessive pollution, food chemicalization and stress, it has become crucial for us to guard ourselves by all available means.

Proper nutrition with supplementation is the best and most conven-ient defence. Since vitamins are food substances that are part of living things, an optimum quantity should, in most cases, keep us thriving. They are utilized in our bodies as co-enzymes, catalysts for physiological responses by the body to all sorts of stress. Vitamins regulate the body processes; hence, when you become inadequately nourished, the body/mind machine begins to break down. It may be years before the ill-effects of this malnutrition make themselves evident, but by then the condition may have caused extensive damage and may not be reversible.

THE 'TWINKIE DEFENSE'

Not only does our physical well-being depend on our nutrition, but according to recent findings, it also plays an amazing role in mental health. A great deal of criminal and antisocial behaviour may be related to nutrient deficiencies. These findings have not been lost on criminal lawyers. When a San Francisco mayor and his assistant were shot, the man accused of their murder pleaded the 'Twinkie Defense': temporary insanity as a result of hypoglycaemia (low blood sugar) from eating an excessive amount of cream-filled sponge cakes called Twinkies. Following a series of gruesome murders in Oceanside, California, court-appointed psychologists determined that, due to malnutrition during his early years, the accused was permanently and irremediably unfit for society. When an elderly man with no history of psychiatric ailments shot his wife and grandson, his physician determined that the cause was a prescription medication that had seriously altered the balance of calcium in his body.[3]

Today, you would be hard pressed to find a nutritional expert who did not believe that inadequate supplies of vitamins and minerals in the body can cause mental damage. Many mental conditions can be traced to the absence of specific vital nutrients.[4] Nutrition can prevent, treat or at least improve unpredictable swings in emotions, depression, Alzheimer's disease and other types of senility, confused behaviour, lethargy and a host of other common mental problems.[5] It is believed that even a slight deficiency has the ability to affect mental function dangerously, even if physical symptoms are not evident. The drugs used to treat mental disturbances tend to work against this law of nature, by altering the way in which nutrients function in the body. This leads to further deterioration.

Although nutrition and mental health are known to be closely associated, medical science is barely beginning to explain this process. For instance, severe mental depression and psychosis can be brought about by nutritional deficiency, but two decades have passed since the *Journal of the American Medical Association* began to publish articles that explained the connection. One of these stated that mental changes resulting from vitamin B_{12} deficiency are among the least publicized aspects of this condition. The milder symptoms may be a slight mood disturbance or mental slowness with difficulty in concentrating and remembering. However, the symptoms may be much more severe, with violent maniacal behaviour, severe agitation, stuporous depression, paranoia or the presence of overt visual and auditory hallucination. These mental status findings make it difficult to distinguish this condition from schizophrenia.

We have heard and read a great deal in the media recently about the battles of the famous with bulimia and anorexia, and the air has been full of accusations of outrageous behaviour. But anyone who is even remotely familiar with the ill-effects of such eating disorders will not be surprised, since the roots of such behaviour are biochemical. Depression is probably the leading outcome of malnourished individuals and is marked by distressing characteristics: low self-esteem, anxiety, agitation, social withdrawal, feelings of guilt, insomnia, impaired short-term memory, loss of appetite, weight loss, lack of energy, fatigue, pessimism and crying spells. Depressed people also have a tendency to exaggerate their problems and to emphasize their inability to deal with their environment. Dwelling on imminent doom and steeped in pervasive gloom, the individual can become wrapped in a morbidness that simulates the depersonalization of dementia.[6]

Thiamin, riboflavin, folic acid and vitamin B_6 all have important roles to play in the metabolism of neuro-transmitters involved in emotional disorders. These nutrients may be important in the cause and treatment of some types of depression, particularly those occurring later in life.[7] Long-term malnutrition can bring about the onset of further brain failure. The human brain comprises only 3–4 per cent of the whole body's weight, but the chemical burning which takes place there may be 25 per cent of the total; hence, the brain's fuel requirements are much higher than those of other organs. In addition, brain cells are not able to divide and rebuild on their own; they can only be replaced by carbohydrates, certain amino acids, vitamins and minerals. If your diet is inadequate in any one of the brain's nutritional requirements, its biochemistry will be altered and problems will follow. Even though the brain generally experiences a deficiency last, after the rest of the body has been seriously depleted of nutrients, all too often the nervous system is affected seriously – at times, irreversibly.

THE B-COMPLEX VITAMINS:
PLUSES AND MINUSES

VITAMIN B_{12} This nutrient is essential for DNA (genetic material) synthesis and red blood cell development. Prolonged deficiency results in pernicious anaemia, neurological deficits and gastrointestinal dysfunction. Vitamin B_{12} is only available from animal foods, including eggs and dairy products. These are avoided by strict vegetarians, and thus these individuals are considered to be at risk of deficiency of this nutrient.[8]

Although vitamin B_{12} deficiency is a common disorder, it often goes undiagnosed. Early signs may go unnoticed because the symptoms are often too general. Fatigue, for example, is probably the first manifestation, but it's also the No. 1 general medical complaint. Impotence, poor appetite, memory loss and inability to concentrate are other frequently missed signs, but they can also be caused by other things. Memory loss, for example, has been linked with heavy metals in the brain, herpes infections, alcohol abuse and vitamin B_1 deficiency. But in the context of a health-promoting diet and lifestyle, it is most prudent to consider the possibility of vitamin B_{12} deficiency.[9] There are several causes of deficiency. One is inadequate intake from the diet, and another is malabsorption, which may be diagnosed with the Schilling test. This procedure involves administering radioactive doses of vitamin B_{12} and measuring the 24-hour urinary output of radioactive material. The test gives false-positive results in up to 14 per cent of patients, particularly those with kidney disorders, but it is often able to distinguish between two types of malabsorption leading to vitamin B_{12} deficiency: classic malabsorption and pernicious anaemia. Malabsorption may be the result of various intestinal disorders such as internal strictures, diverticula, blind loops, fistulas and achlorhydria (lack of hydrochloric acid in the stomach). It can also be a side-effect of certain drugs such as Questran (cholestyramine), colchicine and oral contraceptives.[10]

A lack of vitamin B_{12} can cause even more harm than already mentioned, and deficiency is thought to be far wider spread than was initially suspected. For instance, various types of anaemia (an abnormal decrease in red blood cells) are a frequent occurrence in people with rheumatoid arthritis, a disorder characterized by inflammation of the joints, swelling, stiffness and pain. As well as vitamin B_{12} deficiency anaemia, they may experience anaemia resulting from deficiencies of other essential elements such as iron or folic acid.[11] Animal studies have shown that a lack of vitamin B_{12} decreases the ability of the body to produce antibodies, thus crippling the immune system.

Multiple sclerosis is thought by many researchers to result from a viral infection, perhaps one that occurred many years prior to the actual onset of symptoms. Few have considered the theory that the disease might be a complication of vitamin deficiency. In nine out of ten multiple sclerosis sufferers, blood abnormalities are present that are likely to be the result of a vitamin B_{12} deficiency. This is normally uncommon among healthy individuals under the age of 40, suggesting that the observation of this deficiency in patients with multiple sclerosis (which usually begins to show symptoms between the ages of 20 and 40) may be more than a matter of chance. A review of the medical literature has revealed that, in certain studies of multiple sclerosis, abnormally low levels of vitamin B_{12}

in both the blood and the cerebrospinal fluid have been found.[12]

The *British Medical Journal* has reported a case of misdiagnosis of leukaemia when a vitamin B_{12} deficiency was the real problem. This individual's symptoms included weight loss, anorexia, tiredness, shortness of breath, nosebleed, jaundice, tachycardia (abnormal increased heart rate) and low concentrations and physical abnormalities of the white blood cells. Examination of a bone marrow sample showed large immature white cells, and a diagnosis of acute leukaemia was made. However, the results of blood chemistry testing showed low levels of vitamin B_{12} and after the administration of this nutrient, an immediate improvement in the patient's white blood cells occurred. Two weeks after this treatment, only a few immature cells could be seen in the bone marrow.[13]

Another article in the *British Medical Journal* stated that vitamin B_{12} deficiency can cause psychological symptoms which may vary in severity from mild disorders of mood, mental slowness and memory defect to severe psychosis. A report in the *Lancet* concluded that screenings for vitamin B_{12} deficiency should be routine among psychiatric patients. However, a prolonged deficiency of this vitamin can cause such extensive damage to the nerve sheaths that the illness may become irreversible.

Besides depression and other mental disorders, vitamin B_{12} deficiency may also cause headaches, faulty memory, imbalance of posture, nausea, numbness and double vision.

THIAMIN (VITAMIN B_1) Major food sources of thiamin include brewer's yeast, wheat germ, whole grains, soybeans, pumpernickel bread, milk, peanuts, pecans, cashews, orange and grapefruit juice. As mentioned earlier, a diet high in empty calories (i.e. junk food) has been linked to neurotic behaviour. Many people suffering from thiamin deficiency report pains in the chest and abdomen, sleep disturbances, aggressiveness, hostility, fevers, digestive tract complaints and chronic fatigue. When given thiamin supplements, most sufferers notice marked improvement or lose their symptoms completely.[14]

In an experimental study reported in the *American Journal of Clinical Nutrition*, five out of nine normal volunteers placed on a thiamin-deficient diet developed depression and irritability. In severe thiamin-deficiency, psychiatric disturbances such as delirium tremens, impaired gait, mental confusion, hallucinations, fatigue and ocular degeneration ensue. Alcoholics are especially vulnerable to this type of deficiency.

Researchers have also connected thiamin deficiency to anaemia, anxiety, Crohn's disease, diabetes mellitus, glaucoma, multiple sclerosis, neuralgia and Parkinson's disease. In animal studies, thiamin deficiency has been shown to impair the immune system.[15]

Thiamin deficiencies have also been linked with malignant tumours of the blood. A case was reported in the journal *Cancer* of a patient with acute myeloid leukaemia complicated by severe right-sided congestive heart failure, who responded to treatment with thiamin. The report suggested that clinicians should be alert to this often undiagnosed, potentially fatal but easily treatable deficiency in non-alcoholic patients with fast-growing haematologic cancers.[16]

Vitamin B_1 deficiency has been further linked with heart ailments. Congestive heart failure is the inability of the heart to pump blood efficiently, resulting in the accumulation of fluid in the rest of the body. This condition is also characterized by weakness, breathlessness and abdominal discomfort. Diuretics – agents that increase the elimination of fluid – are the drugs of choice for treating congestive heart failure. However, long-term treatment with diuretics such as frusemide may cause various side-effects, such as thiamin deficiency due to loss in the urine. This can be successfully treated with thiamin supplements.[17]

A wide range of health problems may be produced by a deficiency of B vitamins. The *Lancet* reported an interesting occurrence among Southeast Asian and Japanese men who immigrated to the United States – they dropped dead. It turned out that this group are at high risk of a peculiar form of sudden death. The typical victim is a man around 33 years old without indications of heart disease, who dies suddenly in his sleep. It has been determined that this is associated with a simple deficiency of thiamin.[18]

In 1988, according to the *New York Times*, three hospital patients receiving intravenous feeding died because the intravenous solution was deficient in thiamin. Such a deficiency can, said the report, develop within a week with feedings that are 70 per cent glucose.

FOLIC ACID (FOLATE)   One of the most common deficiencies in Western societies is of another of the B vitamins, folic acid. It is important in reproduction because it is needed for the synthesis of DNA (deoxyribonucleic acid), the genetic material found in every cell.

It is recommended that everyone – all ages, both sexes and all radical groups – take more folic acid, but women and black people are especially at risk of deficiency. Studies indicate that smokers, those taking oral contraceptives and anticonvulsant medications, and those drinking alcohol are also at high risk.[19] If the right foods are chosen, meeting the body's needs for this nutrient is not difficult or expensive. The best sources are cooked dried beans, green leafy vegetables, orange juice, liver, yeast and whole grains.[20] Signs of folate deficiency include cracked lips and corners of the mouth, anaemia, gastrointestinal disorders (such as malabsorption) and infertility.[21] When the body is deficient in folic acid, a person may, in extreme cases, experience mental confusion, irritability, weakness, lack of energy, forgetfulness, debilitating diarrhoea, insomnia and anaemia.[22]

An extremely positive piece of evidence showing the importance of vitamins has demonstrated the role of folic acid in preventing neural tube defects in babies, such as spina bifida. In the *Medical Journal of Australia*, a leading article from the University of Otago, New Zealand, reported on a major multi-centre study of folic acid supplementation and these congenital defects. This showed that taking 4 mg/day of folic acid before conception and in early pregnancy substantially reduces the risk of recurrence of neural tube defects in women who were at high risk because they have already had an affected child.[23]

Such findings have caused even die-hard sceptics to reconsider their positions. 'I was in front of the band of nay-sayers,' admitted Dr Godfrey Oakley, director of the birth defects and development disabilities division at the Centers for Disease Control in Atlanta, Georgia. 'But I changed my mind when I saw that folic acid can prevent certain birth defects.'

As well as preventing neural tube defects, some findings have suggested that folic acid may protect against cervical and lung cancer.[24] All these developments have sparked off a surge in research into this nutrient.

Folic acid deficiency can sometimes be misdiagnosed. The *British Medical Journal* reported the case of a woman patient who had an upper respiratory tract infection, inflammation of the stomach and tongue, diarrhoea and excess 'wind'. She also had abnormally long and heavy menstrual periods and spontaneous bruising and bleeding, was feverish and had toxic confusion. Blood samples showed abnormal white blood cells, including immature ones. A bone marrow specimen revealed abnormalities which suggested promyelocytic leukaemia. However, concentrations of folic acid in the patient's blood were found to be very low, and it was concluded that, as a result of this deficiency she had developed megaloblastic anaemia (in which the fewer than normal red blood cells are overly large and primitive). After treatment with this B vitamin, her blood and bone marrow cells became normal. The researchers concluded that severe vitamin B_{12} deficiency and severe folic acid deficiency can cause abnormalities in the blood cells and in the precursor cells of the bone marrow.[25]

NICOTINIC ACID (VITAMIN B_3) We now come to nicotinic acid (vitamin B_3), also known as niacin, niacinamide and nicotinamide. In the body, it is responsible for releasing energy from carbohydrates, protein and fat in food. Major food sources of this vitamin include brewer's yeast, tuna, peanuts, whole grains, chicken, swordfish, liver, beef, almonds, lamb, oysters and salmon. A lack of nicotinic acid is related to alcoholism, hardening of the arteries, diabetes mellitus, difficult menstruation, gout, muscle abnormalities, multiple sclerosis, neuralgia, schizophrenia and tardive dyskinesia.[26]

A severe shortage of nicotinic acid can lead to pellagra. The symptoms of this serious deficiency illness include mental aberration, hallucinations, depression, irritability, anxiety attacks, confusion, dermatitis, debilitating diarrhoea, vomiting and emaciation. However, sufferers have been almost miraculously cured within 48 hours after the administration of the principal missing nutrient.

The interaction of nicotinic acid with zinc metabolism in alcohol abusers is of particular concern. Chronic alcoholism is often associated with decreased consumption of protein and with vitamin deficiencies. Pellagra, which usually results from a diet based on maize or sorghum, can also surface in chronic alcoholism. Research has shown that, in alcoholics, the metabolic pathways involved in the metabolism of nicotinic acid are affected, and that these problems may be related to underlying deficiencies of B-complex vitamins. Similarly alcoholism is known to be associated with chronic depression of zinc levels, which can trigger difficulties with several enzyme transport systems. These data point to the fact that alcoholism can include a zinc deficiency which can, in turn, cause deficiencies of other nutrients, particularly nicotinic acid.[27]

B-complex vitamins, omega-3 fish oils, vitamin C and zinc all help to alleviate skin disorders from acne to eczema and psoriasis. These problems are exacerbated by stress, birth control pills, environmental pollutants and ingredients in some commercial cosmetics. In *Orthomolecular Medicine for Physicians*, Abram Hoffer MD discusses the case of a 16-year-old boy who was depressed because of a severe case of acne. The patient was started on a sugar-free and milk-free diet, along with a daily dose of 3 g of nicotinic acid, 3 g of vitamin C, 250 mg of vitamin B_6 and 220 mg of zinc sulphate. One month later his face was better, and after three months, it was almost clear.[28]

VITAMIN B_6 (PYRIDOXINE)   The physiologically active form of vitamin B_6 (also known as pyridoxine) is involved in the metabolism of amino acids, nucleic acids, glycogen, porphyrins and lipids. Consequently, vitamin B_6 affects hormone modulation and the function of red blood cells, as well as the immune and nervous systems. This vitamin may also be involved in the development or treatment of various disorders such as heart disease, asthma and cancer. Inadequate dietary intake of vitamin B_6 is common in both the United States and Britain, particularly among elderly persons and pregnant and breastfeeding women.[29] Diets deficient in vitamin B_6 usually result in altered zinc metabolism, reduced copper absorption and altered iron states.[30]

The *Lancet* reported a study where 70 to 80 per cent of 630 women with premenstrual syndrome (PMS) obtained relief after taking 80–200 mg of vitamin B$_6$ daily. No nerve damage was reported and side-effects were minimal. However, it should be remembered that relatively high doses of vitamin B$_6$ can damage nerves – some unconfirmed reports suggest even doses as low as 100–200 mg a day can do this. Therefore you should never take more than 50 mg of the vitamin per day unless advised to do otherwise by your doctor.

Researchers at Kaiser Permanente Medical Center in Hayward, California have reported that vitamin B$_6$ is useful in treating diabetic neuropathies – the disturbed nerve function associated with diabetes. Vitamin B$_6$ therapy also resulted in a reduction in necessary insulin and oral medications.[31] Twelve severely depressed patients with coeliac disease (a malabsorption condition of the small intestine caused by an intolerance to the protein gluten in wheat, barley and rye) were given 80 mg of vitamin B$_6$ daily for six months. According to the *Scandinavian Journal of Gastroenterology*, all of them had been on a gluten-free diet for many years. After six months on the vitamin therapy, depression had improved significantly in all the patients.

RIBOFLAVIN (VITAMIN B$_2$)   This nutrient is essential for cell growth and to release energy from food. A deficiency in it has been closely associated with cataracts, the progressive, usually age-related degeneration of the lens of the eye, resulting in loss of lens transparency and blurred, distorted vision. Cataracts are responsible for more than 40 per cent of the cases of blindness in the world. Factors associated with the development or progression of cataracts include general predisposition, metabolic diseases, nutritional disorders, drug therapy, ionizing radiation (e.g. X-rays), exposure to damaging light (ultraviolet and infra-red) and increasing age. It is recommended that those with a genetic predisposition to age-related cataracts minimise the other risk factors throughout the full span of their lives, and that biological defences should be maintained by eating a balanced diet containing adequate riboflavin and other vitamins.[32]

VITAMIN K: BABIES AND BLOOD

Today, nutrition and vitamin supplementation is being used as never before both to prevent and to heal various damaging illnesses. For instance, one of the most serious health problems facing premature babies may be handled very simply by giving vitamin K to their mothers.

Vitamin K, isolated in the late 1930s, received its initial 'K' from its Danish discoverer Henrik Dam, who dubbed it the *Koagulationsvitamin* because of the role it plays in blood clotting. Deficiency in children and adults is very rare, since this nutrient is found in most vegetable foods and some is synthesized by 'good' bacteria in the intestines, from where it is absorbed into the bloodstream. However, newborn babies may suffer from a lack of vitamin K since their intestines are bacteria-free for the first few days, and milk is a poor source.

Intraventricular haemorrhage (IVH), or bleeding in the brain, happens in roughly 40 per cent of the babies born at 30 weeks or less (at least 10 weeks early). It can result in cerebral palsy and mental retardation. Doctors believe IVH occurs because the baby's blood vessels are too immature to stand the surges of the blood pressure that occurs following delivery, so they burst.[33]

Haemorrhagic disease of the newborn is a condition occurring in infants younger than six months, which is characterized by spontaneous bruising and/or bleeding; it includes IVH. The diagnosis is made when other causes of these symptoms, such as inherited disorders of coagulation or disseminated intravascular coagulation (in which small clots form throughout the body), have been eliminated. Haemorrhagic disease of the newborn remains an important problem in Britain. However, the risk of developing the disease is more than 13 times greater for babies given oral vitamin K than for those given intramuscular injections of it. Babies given no preventive vitamin K at all are 81.7 times more likely to develop the disease than those who receive the vitamin.[34]

NUTRIENT SUPERSTARS:
VITAMINS C AND E AND BETA-CAROTENE

The latest nutrient superstars are vitamins C and E and beta-carotene, a precursor of vitamin A. They are crucial because they are antioxidants, which guard the body from damage by unstable molecules called free radicals. We have been hearing a great deal about free radicals these days – many people think they are disobedient political renegades! But the free radicals we are talking about can do far more harm to society if given the opportunity.

We briefly looked at free radicals in the discussion about irradiated food in Chapter 2. These chemical substances alter or destroy healthy cells and are believed to be the primary sources of the leading killers of today – cancer and heart disease – while they contribute enormously to the development of other chronic conditions. These unstable molecules have part of their structure missing, and they try to replace the absent bits by taking them from other molecules. When this happens, a reaction or series of reactions take place that are like an explosion, and extensive harm can occur to cells. Free radicals destroy cell membranes, cause tissue damage and are believed to play a serious role in tissue degeneration. Cigarette smoke, carbon monoxide, environmental pollution and food chemicalization are among the major sources of oxidative stress – that is, the process of the release of free radicals.

Reports from the division of immunology of the University of Pretoria in South Africa reveal that activation of phagocytes – cells of the immune system that engulf and digest invading viruses and bacteria – is accompanied by a burst of cellular activity and increased consumption of oxygen, leading to the formation of oxidants (i.e. free radicals). These can suppress the immune system, cause cancer and inactivate an enzyme that is essential for healthy lung function.

We have, biologically, a built-in antioxidant mechanism, but it is of limited usefulness. The extra antioxidant support we require to combat modern-day living must be supplied from nutrients. 'Population studies have shown a clear association between diets high in antioxidant nutrients and protection against cancer and heart disease,' says Dr Marion Nestle, professor of nutrition at New York University.[35] Studies to determine exactly how this process takes place are currently under way. Fifty per cent of the work being undertaken today at the US National Cancer Institute chemo-prevention branch concerns antioxidants, and in 1992 the UK government funded a three-year research programme to gain a better understanding of the role of these protective nutrients.

All living cells require enormous quantities of energy to function, and since the processing of oxygen – oxidation – is the basic source of energy, it is the basic source of life. Without oxygen, our cells die in just a few minutes. However, at times, oxygen itself can be toxic and harmful. One of the most important findings in medicine has been the discovery of how this element functions at the molecular level, producing by-products (free radicals), and how living cells handle such by-products.

As we have seen, numerous external factors induce free radical formation in our bodies. Radiation, smoke, heat, alcohol and pollution by such gases as nitrogen dioxide, carbon monoxide and ozone are among the leading offenders. Bodily injuries are also known to release free radicals in your system. But even if you lived under perfect conditions, your body would naturally produce a certain amount of free radicals on its own: white blood cells produce them as weapons against infectious organisms such as viruses and bacteria. If genetic material is harmed by free radicals and isn't completely repaired, the damaged DNA is replicated in new cells.

However, living cells do possess the ability to fight back. Just as the body can fight infections, it has a way of controlling free radicals. This task is performed by the free radical fighters we know as antioxidants. Certain antioxidants are dietary nutrients, while some, such as enzymes and other compounds, are created by the cells themselves.

FIGHTING THE FREE RADICALS   Fortunately, we can exercise reasonable control over the external assaults that can lead to free radical formation. We can also eat diets rich in vitamins C, E and beta-carotene. Once these nutrients are absorbed by the body, vitamin C is present in blood and all other extracellular fluids, vitamin E and beta-carotene are in fats (lipids) in the blood and in fat deposits, and vitamin E is also found in cell membranes. These molecules are thus readily available to each cell.

It is easy to see why vitamin C is one of our first lines of defence. Researchers have discovered evidence that it may block the conversion of nitrates and nitrites into cancer-causing compounds. Inadequate levels of vitamin C in the body have been associated with various types of cancers, especially those of the stomach and oesophagus. However, this potent antioxidant cannot be stored by the body because it is water soluble and excess amounts are excreted in the urine. That is why a constant resupply is crucial.

Daily supplements of vitamins A, C and E have been shown to reduce cell abnormalities that can develop into bowel cancer. This finding was the result of a six-month preliminary study conducted at the University of Bologna in Italy, which was reported recently in the United States in the journal of the National Cancer Institute. People who had growths removed from their colons were given daily 30,000 IU* of vitamin A, 70 mg of vitamin E and 1000 mg of vitamin C. When the study ended, the specimens from the people on the vitamin regimen showed a significant reduction in abnormal cell growth not found in the tissues of people who had taken placebos (pills containing no vitamins or drugs). High doses of vitamins C and E are known to be safe, but the University of Bologna investigators expressed caution about the long-term safety of the relatively high doses of vitamin A used in their study. Investigators have reported toxic responses in people taking between 20,000 and 50,000 IU daily for several months.[36]

In an important new experiment, Dr Bruce Ames and his colleagues at the University of California at Berkeley showed that low levels of dietary vitamin C result in higher levels of free radical damage in human sperm and thus could increase the risk of birth defects.[37] Conversely, vitamin C supplementation has been shown to increase the chances of fertility in male smokers. The clumping of sperm (agglutination) can act as a deterrent to their ability to fertilize an egg. Researchers have noted that the higher the amount of vitamin C supplementation, the more remained in the blood serum and the higher the quality and viability of sperm.

Vitamins E and C, with their powers to combat free radicals, are

*IU = international units. 100 IU = 30 micrograms.

now being used to treat Parkinson's disease. This is characterized by tremor, muscular rigidity and weakness and abnormal gait, and usually begins in individuals over the age of 50 and progresses over time. In Parkinson's, there is a loss of certain neurons in the brain, leading to a reduction in the levels of dopamine, a neuro-transmitter. This process may also cause the oxidation of catecholamines (neuro-transmitters of which dopamine is one), resulting in the production of free radicals, which can cause further damage and destruction. Conventional therapy involves treatment with the drug levodopa to increase the amount of dopamine in the brain. Because antioxidants such as vitamins E and C can protect tissues from damage caused by free radicals, researchers have concluded that antioxidants may be beneficial in the treatment of early Parkinson's disease.

MULTIFACETED VITAMIN E   Although you may be in general good health now, if you are physically active an antioxidant shortage may already be taking place inside your body. Investigators at the Research Center on Ageing at Tufts University in Boston, Massachusetts have proposed that physically active individuals who consume oxygen at a rate 20 to 40 times higher than that found in resting subjects have higher dietary requirements for the antioxidant vitamin E to counteract an increase in the production of free radicals.[39] A number of studies have even suggested that vitamin E has a beneficial influence on physical performance and a protective action against exercise-induced muscle damage.

When vitamin E was discovered in the early part of this century, no one could imagine just what implications this nutrient would be found to have for our overall health and well-being. The most fascinating aspect of vitamin E's multifaceted action is its action as an immune system booster. It also seems to bolster cell membranes, strengthening their defences against pathogenic (disease-carrying) bacteria and viruses.

Patrick Quillen PhD told *Let's Live* magazine that 'long-term subclinical deficiencies of vitamin E probably surface as common diseases (such as heart disease, cancer, senility, allergies, cataracts and premature ageing) rather than a neat and concise vitamin deficiency disease.'

The No. 1 killer in the Western world today is heart disease, and one can't help but wonder to what extent deaths from this could have been prevented by nutritional means. As far back as the 1940s, two Canadian physicians, Evan and Wilfred Shute, made a correlation between heart disease and vitamin E. They were the first to note that the tremendous rise in cases of heart failure had occurred at the same time that wheat germ – naturally rich in vitamin E – was eliminated from flour through modern milling practices. They were also first to question the role of atherosclerosis and fat in the development of heart disease. The doctors' theory that vitamin E helped prevent heart attacks has since been proved in a number of cell and animal studies which demonstrated that vitamin E inhibits blood platelets from clumping and so are less likely to block arteries. Other studies showing vitamin E's effectiveness against free radicals have testified to its role in preventing the damage that often accompanies circulatory problems.[40]

As recently as 1993, researchers at the University of Toronto reported findings that showed that large doses of vitamin E administered daily during the two-week period before patients had coronary bypass surgery reduced the 'metabolic dysfunction' in the heart muscle that generally follows such surgery. The World Health Organization conducted their own studies and concluded that low levels of vitamin E in the blood are strongly associated with increased deaths from heart disease. In addition, Dr Terrence Yau stated at the 63rd scientific sessions of the American Heart Association that vitamin E 'is the only antioxidant to penetrate the lipid membrane around the heart muscle cell to reach the sites where free radicals do their damage.'

According to the *International Journal of Cancer*, adequate vitamin E intake is associated with a drastically decreased risk of cervical cancer. The taking of vitamin E and A supplements was additionally associated with a lowering in the risk of invasive cervical cancer. The Institute for Breast Disease of the New York Medical College reports that between 50 and 60 per cent of patients experiencing impaired immunity against their own breast tumours had an improved immune response after taking either vitamin. And when both were taken simultaneously, 80 per cent of the patients improved.

The *Nutrition and Cancer Journal* has linked low levels of vitamin E and lung cancer. A study of vitamins A, C and E in lung cancer sufferers showed that the patients had 'significantly lower mean serum levels of carotenoids (e.g. beta-carotene), vitamin E and total cholesterol than the control group. Vitamin E was lower in hospitalized patients with lung cancer than in other hospitalized patients, even after adjusting for total cholesterol levels.'

A VITAMIN FROM PIGMENT   That other super antioxidant, beta-carotene, is converted into vitamin A once consumed. It is usually found in dark green, yellow and orange vegetables and fruits. The red and yellow pigments that given their colour are known as carotenoids, of which beta-carotene is one. It is believed that their purpose in the plants themselves is to guard against solar radiation damage. In other words, these are free-radical scavengers in plants as well as in the body. At least 70 studies have found that people who don't eat enough fruits and vegetables have a higher risk of cancer, particularly lung cancer.[41]

Best known for its high concentration in carrots, vitamin A (also known as retinol) is necessary for reproduction, cell development and vision. A deficiency may result in biological changes that resemble precancerous conditions.

It certainly seems as if leading scientists at the National Research Council and the National Cancer Institute in the United States have been catching 'carrot fever'. Literally hundreds of scientific papers demonstrate that vitamin A has cancer-protective effect on animals, and epidemiological studies of smokers show that those with the lowest beta-carotene intake are at greatest risk for lung cancer.[42] Scientists believe beta-carotene helps prevent cancer by reducing cell damage caused by highly reactive oxygen ions, the free radicals, also known as singlet oxygen. One group of researchers has called beta-carotene 'the most efficient singlet oxygen [eliminator] thus far discovered'.[43]

Vitamin A helps fight infection. In animal studies, supplements of this nutrient have boosted immune system responsiveness.[44] In humans, vitamin A deficiency is associated with a higher incidence of infection, and high doses of the vitamin* markedly reduces immune-suppressive effects of surgical anaesthesia and cancer chemotherapy and radiation.[45] Also, vitamin A has been shown to speed wound healing in laboratory animals, which has special implications for a certain proportion of the human population. The incision wounds of diabetics recovering from surgery often heal very slowly; it is now believed that, just as supplemental vitamin A improves immune function in lab animals, it is especially useful in preventing wound infection and promoting wound healing in diabetic patients who have undergone surgery.[46]

Children are especially at risk of vitamin A deficiency. Measles, for instance, remains a devastating disease worldwide and no specific treatment is available. The illness depresses vitamin A levels, and vitamin A deficiency in young children with infectious disease is associated with increased mortality.[47] Studies suggest that vitamin A therapy may have a protective effect. According to the *New England Journal of Medicine*, vitamin A therapy significantly reduces the severity of the disease and the numbers of deaths in children with measles. Therefore, researchers stated, all children with severe measles should be routinely given vitamin A supplements, whether or not they are thought to have a nutritional deficiency.[48]

Children can be affected in other ways. Infection and malnutrition are the major contributors to childhood mortality in developing nations. A particularly devastating consequence of vitamin A deficiency is xer-

---

*See p. 140 for information on the dangers of high doses of vitamin A.

ophthalmia, which in its advanced stages results in blindness. It is less widely appreciated, says the *Lancet*, that there is a strong correlation between xerophthalmia and a high risk of infection, particularly of two of the most serious among children in the developing world: diarrhoea and pneumonia.[49]

RAISING HOPES: VITAMIN C   Other ways in which vitamin therapy can make an impact on modern health continue to be discovered at an astonishing rate. Vitamin C, for instance, is raising the hopes of scientists in a wide range of medical fields.

Researchers at the University of Texas Health Center at Houston have concluded that vitamin C can destroy some bacteria associated with diseases of the mouth and gums. It also helps protect cells against some viruses, including ones known to cause certain types of cancer, and even – in the laboratory – inhibits the growth of the HIV virus that can cause AIDS.[50]

Yet other studies proclaim that large doses of vitamin C may ease the side-effects of radiation therapy. It has also been shown to ward off the toxic effects of Adriamcin, a widely used anticancer drug, as well as the side-effects of interleukin 2, which is currently used in experimental cancer treatment.[51]

It has been known for decades that vitamin C protects against cardiovascular disease, but scientists were at a loss to explain why. Studies at Harvard University's School of Public Health have shown that it can prevent the buildup of 'bad' cholesterol, which can lead to coronary artery disease. However, Nobel prize winner Dr Linus Pauling has another, plausible explanation. A study conducted by Dr Matthias Rath at Hamburg University in Germany, and since repeated at the Linus Pauling Institute of Science and Medicine in Palo Alto, California, indicated that it is not low-density lipoprotein (LDL) cholesterol – the bad kind – that clogs arteries and causes heart attacks and strokes, but something called 'lipoprotein (a)'. Individuals have varying amounts of lipoprotein (a) in their blood; in fact, some people have 1000 times as much as others. The higher amount, the greater risk of a cardiovascular catastrophe, says Dr Pauling. Drs Rath and Pauling add that people with low levels of vitamin C may also have weakened blood vessels.[52]

Heart disease is the No. 1 killer in industrialized nations. In the United States it accounts for nearly 50 per cent of all deaths each year, and an additional 10 per cent of deaths are due to strokes. In other words, atherosclerosis (clogging of the arteries) and other types of arteriosclerosis (hardening of the arteries) are jointly responsible for 60 per cent of the US mortality rate. Heart disease begins in all of us during childhood and progresses at varying rates during adult life. However, it usually remains undiscovered until symptoms strike. These are the result of the gradual narrowing of arteries to the heart muscle or brain, reducing the blood supply until part of the tissue dies.

For years, however, we haven't been told the truth about the true causes of heart disease. The most famous study in the world, begun in 1948, involved the residents of Framingham, Massachusetts, and was conducted by the National Institutes of Health. Although it showed no significant correlation between dietary cholesterol intake and blood cholesterol levels, yet the myth that said there was such a connection grew out of that study – and then out of control. At least eight other clinical trials conducted in the United States, the United Kingdom and Scandinavia between 1965 and 1972 also showed that changing the amount of dietary cholesterol had no significant effect upon heart disease.[52]

Despite the fact that important studies conducted in more than 15 countries linked a high intake of sugar with heart disease, this received no media attention. And as far back as the 1940s, studies began to document links between vitamin C levels and arteriosclerosis, but this too prompted no interest in the media. Even as long ago as 1947, it was first suggested in an article in a medical journal that vitamin C should be used in the treatment of heart disease. By 1953, an intimate relationship between vitamin C, cholesterol synthesis and arteriosclerosis had been documented, and this was proved again in 1959, when it was shown that arteriosclerosis can be reversed with vitamin therapy.[53]

Vitamin C has been shown to modulate cholesterol metabolism by increasing the rate at which cholesterol is removed from the body by its conversion into bile acids and excretion via the intestines. The vitamin increases levels of HDL – high-density lipoprotein, the good kind of cholesterol – in the body and, through its laxative effect, accelerates the elimination of waste, thereby acting to decrease the reabsorption of bile acids and hence their reconversion to cholesterol.[54]

Researchers in the United States, the United Kingdom and throughout the rest of Europe have concluded that vitamin C can ward off heart disease. Deaths due to heart disease and stroke are remarkably low in southern Italy and Switzerland where vitamin C intake is plentiful. In Northern Ireland, the mortality rate for the same conditions fall somewhere in the middle of the global scale, and vitamin C consumption there is between adequate and marginally low. In Scotland, however, vitamin C levels are extremely low, and the death rate from heart disease is very high. Such consistent data are very difficult to ignore.

CANCER AND CATARACTS   Scientists around the world are reporting on the benefits of vitamin C in unprecedented volume. From

Gynaecologic Cancer Research at the Albert Einstein College of Medicine in Bronx, New York, comes evidence suggesting that women who show signs of cervical dysplasia (changes in the cells lining the cervix, which may have cancer implications) are also found to have vitamin C deficiency. Administration of supplements (1 g daily for six months) was effective in raising blood vitamin C levels, and the scientists' optimistic prognosis for recovery proved correct.

A lack of vitamin C has, like riboflavin deficiency, been linked with cataract formation. Eye fluids are normally rich in this vitamin (and other antioxidants), which may guard against sunlight-induced free radical formation in the eyes. From the department of epidemiology of the University of Western Ontario in Canada, biochemical evidence suggests that oxidative stress caused by a build-up of free radicals induces cataracts in the elderly. Vitamins C and E were administered to halt the process.[55] A recent study concluded that the cataract sufferers generally had lower serum levels of vitamins C and E or beta-carotene, but after they had taken vitamins C and E, a 50 per cent reduction in the risk of cataracts was noted.[56] Similar conclusions were made by scientists at the department of human nutrition and health in Basel, Switzerland.[57]

According to researchers at the Philadelphia College of Podiatric Medicine, vitamin C therapy may soon be a supplemental or alternative choice of treatment for rheumatoid arthritis sufferers. Researchers there found that taking vitamin C reduced both pain and arthritic swelling.[58]

The *Indian Journal of Medical Sciences* reports that vitamin C is able to destroy bacteria such as *Staphylococcus aureus* (which causes wound infection), *E. coli* (implicated in many intestinal illnesses), *Corynebacterium diphtheriae* (involved in diphtheria) and *Mycobacterium tuberculosis* (responsible for tuberculosis). Researchers claim that the vitamin possesses the power to neutralize, inactivate and render harmless a wide variety of bacterial toxins.[59]

From the University of Göteborg in Sweden, evidence suggests that a lack of vitamin C in your diet interferes with the body's absorption of iron. Thus, increasing the amount of vitamin C-rich foods eaten will allow maximum iron function in the body.

More than 90 epidemiological studies from the School of Public Health at the University of California, Berkeley show that vitamin C is a powerful anti-cancer agent. Cancers especially responsive to therapy with this vitamin, either to reduce them or prevent them altogether, include those of the oesophagus, oral cavity, stomach, pancreas, cervix, rectum and breast.[60]

Vitamin C is known to be a strong preventive against breast cancer. Women who have the highest intake of vitamin C from their diets have the lowest risk of breast cancer, and women who get the least vitamin C have the greatest risk.[61] In another study by Dr Pauling, high doses of vitamin C delayed the formation of breast tumours in mice bred to develop breast cancer. Tumours took 125 weeks to appear in the treated mice, compared to 83 weeks in the untreated ones.

A combination of vitamins C and B_{12} may have a unique cancer-fighting effect. That is the news from researchers at the Mercyhurst College Cancer Research Unit in Erie, Pennsylvania and the Roswell Park Memorial Institute in Buffalo, New York. In their experiments, 40 mice were injected with cancer cells, and 20 of them were also injected with special forms of vitamins C and B_{12}. Fifty per cent of the mice that received the vitamins were still alive and tumour-free after 60 days; all 20 of the untreated mice died within 19 days.

ASTONISHING DISCOVERIES   Even biochemists are amazed at the new ways that vitamin C can prevent and help to alleviate human suffering. One discovery that is particularly astonishing is that even minor vitamin C deficiencies, as are present in one third of a 'normal' population, can be extremely harmful. For instance, such an apparently minor lack of this nutrient may induce the depositing of cholesterol beneath the linings of arteries and lead to arteriosclerosis.[62]

One seems to come to the inevitable conclusion that, without an adequate intake of vitamin C, you couldn't get out of bed in the morning – or ever. The vitamin is crucial for breathing, heartbeat and a multitude of other body functions. It is a vital component of collagen – the white fibres of connective tissue that form the packaging material of the body, ranging from simple tissue to large artery walls and ligaments – and is the cellular glue connecting all these cells by electrical magnetism. Vitamin C also helps iron in the formation of red blood corpuscles, which bring oxygen to all the cells. The adrenal glands contain the highest quantity of vitamin C. Vitamin C is necessary for the body to produce carnitine, which is used in energy production.

If your body contains 4500 mg of vitamin C per gram of blood, you should have plenty of energy for each day's activities and for optimal health.[63]

Symptoms of a vitamin C deficiency are many, but loss of energy is among one of the first. In the United States, a lack of energy, or fatigue, is the seventh most common reason for visiting a doctor, accounting for more than 10 million visits annually and more than $300 million in medical costs. In a recent study of 18- to 34-year-old women, 40 per cent reported feeling tired most of the time.[64] Easy bruising and having difficulty coping with stress are also common symptoms of vitamin C deficiency, as are allergies to foods and medications, bleeding gums, cuts that won't heal, poor memory, mental depression, restlessness, bad

breath, frequent colds or flu, inability to adjust to hot or cold environments, elevated cholesterol and triglyceride levels, and stretch marks on
arms, legs and hips.

Advanced vitamin C deficiency can make itself evident through such
signs as drooping skin, thickened lips and many red lines in the whites of
the eyes. At times, women's menstrual bleeding becomes very scanty,
and premature menopause has been known to result from shortage of
vitamin C, as well as calcium, iron and vitamins B_{12} and D.

Key contributors to vitamin C deficiency include poor eating habits,
physical exhaustion, mineral deficiencies, excess acid and salt in the
body, insufficient exercise, extreme stress, severe illness, surgery, cuts
and bruises and certain medications. Some of these last, which may
destroy the vitamin C in your body for up to two months after you stop
taking them, include: aspirin, barbiturates, adrenaline, stilbestrol,
oestrogen, sulphonamides, aluminium chloride, antihistamines, thio-
uracils (e.g. propylthiouracil), thryoid extract and atropine.[65]

Much of the vitamin C you need can be obtained from fresh orange
and grapefruit juice, papaya, guava, kiwi fruit, Brussels sprouts, green
peppers, cantaloupe melons, asparagus, alfalfa and many bean sprouts,
watermelon, tomatoes, berries, broccoli, potatoes, bananas, raw cab-
bage, lemons, spinach and cherries. Fruits that were picked green and
not properly tree- or vine-ripened contain much less of the vitamin. Also,
as pointed out in an earlier chapter, the adulteration of food greatly affects
its vitamin value; thus, supplementation may be necessary. Since vitamin
C plays an important role in every single cell in your body, whether it be
an organ, gland or muscle, the slightest deficiency can and does wreak
havoc. It is also important to note that this single vitamin will not, on its
own, solve all the problems mentioned here, but works in conjunction
with all other essential vitamins, minerals, amino acids and enzymes,
while your body and mind further relies on pure water, sufficient rest,
exercise and a decent environment to achieve optimal health.

VITAMINS, HIV AND AIDS   Nutritional science is on the threshold of
tremendous new developments. Recently, 130 physicians and researchers from 46 countries converged on Washington, DC for a revolu-
tionary conference on the topic of vitamin C. Forty papers were
presented, 33 of which claimed that vitamin C can prevent cancer. Others
raised interest concerning vitamin C and AIDS.

There is one reason why such an important conference could be
conducted in Washington with US government sanction. The work of the
inexhaustible Dr Linus Pauling, two-time Nobel laureate, has finally
swayed world opinion and respect in his favour. Dr Pauling first became
interested in vitamin C when he discovered that most animals manufac-

ture vitamin C at a rate that, if scaled up to human body weight, would be the equivalent of about 10,000 mg daily. Human beings are unable to produce any vitamin C at all.

At the Washington conference, Dr Raxit Jariwalla of the Linus Pauling Institute turned attention to studies concerning vitamin C and the HIV virus that causes acquired immune deficiency syndrome (AIDS). These found that large amounts of vitamin C suppressed the HIV virus when the vitamin was placed in HIV-injected cell cultures. Dr Jariwalla said that the ability of vitamin C to suppress acute HIV infection and to inhibit viral replication in chronically infected cells indicates that the vitamin works at a stage in the HIV life cycle that is different from the stage that is targeted by the AIDS drugs AZT (zidovudine) and alpha-interferon. In contrast with AZT and some of the other drugs that produce very serious side-effects in some patients, he continued, vitamin C given orally is virtually harmless. About the only side-effect reported is mild diarrhoea, which indicates that the tissues are saturated with the vitamin for the time being.[66]

The idea that vitamin C can retard the growth of the HIV virus is quite extraordinary. AIDS patients who had taken high doses of the vitamin experienced a marked improvement in their condition. Vitamin C is also known to act against other viruses, including the Rous sarcoma virus, a member of the retrovirus family that also includes HIV. The effects of the vitamin were tested by Dr Jariwalla and his colleagues on two different lines of HIV-infected white blood cells known as T-lympho-cytes. In chronically infected cells, vitamin C helped to reduce by over 99 per cent the levels of transcriptase, an enzyme crucial to virus reproduc-tion. In freshly infected T-lymphocytes, vitamin C also blocked virus-induced cell fusion, a sign of early viral infection.[67]

Other researchers have reported on problems with vitamins B_6 and B_{12} in those who are HIV positive. Deficiencies in vitamin B_6 develop in individuals who are infected with the human immunodeficiency virus type 1 (HIV 1), at the third stage of HIV infection, as classified by the Centers for Disease Control in Atlanta, Georgia. This happens even if the intake of the vitamin is normal. Deficiencies of this nutrient, which have been shown to cause abnormal functioning of the immune system, were analysed in 44 homosexual men who had Stage III HIV infection. The degree of dysfunction was found to be related to the status of vitamin B_6 in the individual.[68]

It has also been noted that persons infected with HIV are especially likely to suffer a deficiency of vitamin B_{12}. Although this has been attributed to an abnormality of gastrointestinal function, the precise cause is not yet clear. A recent study has indicated that about 7 per cent of patients who are HIV positive but show no symptoms have vitamin B_{12}

deficiency, and the proportion rises to 15 per cent among those with symptomatic AIDS. The evidence suggests that vitamin B_{12} deficiency may be a common and treatable cause of neurologic defects in some HIV-infected patients.

Further, there are those who claim that poor nutrition can be the underlying cause of death in people with AIDS, and that it can hasten the physical deterioration of individuals with HIV infection. Dietician Marcy Fenton of the Los Angeles AIDS Project says that an aggressive, individually tailored nutritional programme is crucial to slowing infection, increasing the efficiency of medical treatment, and enriching quality of life. She claims that practitioners must be aware that good nutrition is not an 'alternative therapy'; it is a fundamental component of medical care.[69]

Scientists at the Sixth International Conference on AIDS agreed that nutrition should play a key role in AIDS treatment. Researchers from the New York Medical College at Valhalla reported that, although all of their test subjects had adequate caloric and protein intake, nearly 90 per cent had diets deficient in at least some vitamins and minerals. This indicates that malabsorption or altered metabolism may be a factor in HIV disease.

Stanford University researchers who studied patients on the drug AZT found that, in the first 12 months of treatment, all measurements of nutrients remained normal. However, after that, a decrease was noted in total protein consumption, and by 16 months, the patients in the study were found to have decreased body weight, body mass and body fat percentage. As a result of these findings, the researchers recommend nutritional intervention early in the course of HIV infection. Investigators at the University of Miami School of Medicine suggest that even marginal vitamin B_{12} deficiency in the context of HIV infection can contribute to impaired mental function.

Jean-Louis Vilde and his colleagues at the Bichat–Claude Bernard Hospital in Paris set out to determine whether the weight loss seen in otherwise clinically stable HIV-positive patients is due to increased energy expenditure when these people are at rest. Dr Vilde's team concluded that there are three mechanisms of malnutrition: a loss of appetite (which, he said, is extremely common in HIV-positive patients), malabsorption of nutrients, and high resting energy expenditure. Italian researchers at the University of Pavia also determined that antimicrobial and nutritional therapy including vitamins and minerals can restore and maintain weight and energy in AIDS patients, enhancing resistance to opportunistic gastrointestinal infections.

As preliminary and new as these data are concerning the nutritional implications of HIV and AIDS, results are already proving quite promising. For example, the hospital Germans Trias i Pujol in Barcelona reports that half of their AIDS patients respond to aggressive nutritional supplementation.[70]

BANNING SUPPLEMENTS?

With all the breakthroughs taking place in the field of nutritional research, and in view of all the life-sustaining properties that nutrients possess, it is truly dismaying that the US Food and Drug Administration (FDA) is once again attempting to ban supplements. If the FDA has its way, the dietary supplements that most of us require for optimal health and disease prevention will disappear from the shelves of American supermarkets and health food shops. The FDA has, instead, chosen to brand the findings of some of the world's most respected scientists and medical authorities as insignificant and downright negligent.[71]

The FDA has been diligently trying to have this ban on supplements enforced since the early 1970s. It took an Act of Congress (the 1973 Proxmire Bill) to prevent this. But the agency has stepped up its harassment of health food companies in recent times, and two Congressional bills, recently proposed, will (if passed) make matters significantly worse.

If public safety were an issue, such action might be condoned, but in 50 years of sales of vitamin supplements, there has never been a vitamin-caused fatality from self-administration reported in an adult or child in the United States. However, each of the following has been responsible for disability and death: peanuts, strawberries, rhubarb, undercooked pork, broad beans, chicken and shellfish.[72]

Where the United States leads, the United Kingdom usually follows. The citizens of England, Wales, Scotland and Northern Ireland may soon find that they, too, are unable to buy the vitamin supplements they need to achieve optimal health.

MINERAL VALUES

S taying well is fast becoming a global way of life, as opposed to continually attempting to cure ills. The fitness boom of the 1980s shed light on the dangers of sedentary living, and most people are now aware that vitamin C can help colds. But when it comes to minerals, they know little more than that calcium has something to do with their teeth and bones.

Scientists, however, have recently placed minerals right at the head of the queue. They are beginning to establish a connection between these nutrients and leading chronic diseases such as high blood pressure, cardiovascular disease and chronic pain, as well as cancer.

In the field of nutrition, the significance of minerals, especially trace elements, has not been adequately emphasized. Our diets not only consist of fats, protein, carbohydrates and vitamins, but also a multitude of minerals – more than 60 of them – which play crucial roles.

It is staggering to discover that in the United States 99 per cent of the population is deficient in minerals which usually results in some illness. [1] As stated previously, the chemicalization of soil and agricultural produce has altered the quality of our food. The mineral content of fruits and vegetables depends on the minerals in the soil in which they are grown. Since many of the fruits and vegetables we buy are grown in poor, mineral-depleted soils, we can no longer rely on them to obtain basic, life-sustaining nutrients. Similarly, the mineral content of animal products varies, depending on the feed that cattle, pigs, chickens and so on have been fed and the soil on which it was grown. Growing evidence indicates that we may be slowly starving to death without knowing it.

Millions of the body's cells die daily and must be replaced with new ones for us to remain healthy. Minerals permit this process to occur naturally, unless, of course, you did not consume a diet that contains adequate amounts of them. Minerals are the basic building blocks of all living things. Vitamins, amino acids, enzymes and the other complex substances the body needs to build new and healthy cells are all dependent on minerals, including minute amounts of difficult-to-obtain trace elements. Experts say that cell breakdown, which leads to degenerative diseases, is a direct result of the absence of these substances. [2]

So what exactly are minerals? Well, they are the basic inorganic elements of the Earth's crust. Carried into the soil, groundwater and sea by erosion, they are taken up by plants and consumed by animals and humans. These inorganic substances remain as ash when animal and plant tissue is burned, and are found in the tissues and fluids of all living things. Minerals are located in our bones, teeth, soft tissues, muscle, blood and nerve cells. About 4 per cent of human body weight consists of mineral matter. Minerals are a crucial part of every single body function and they are as necessary to us as oxygen. Your body cannot utilize many vitamins from food without the necessary minerals.

In other words, the minerals that are nutrients are absolutely essential to numerous vital processes in the body, from bone formation to the functioning of the heart and the digestive system. Many are needed for the activity of enzymes, proteins that serve as catalysts in the body's chemical reactions.

The minerals in food are indestructible – even if you burn your food to a cinder, it will retain all its original minerals. However, when food is boiled, some of its minerals are dissolved into the water and then discarded. Minerals are also often processed out of foods, such as when whole wheat grains are refined to make white flour. [3]

Of the 60 minerals so far found in the human body, medical researchers consider 22 to be essential. Seven of these – calcium, chloride, magnesium, phosphorous, potassium, sodium and sulphur – are known as macro-minerals (major nutrients) since the body requires a great deal of them. The remaining 15 minerals are found in tiny amounts and are, therefore, called trace elements or trace minerals. Our daily requirements of these are minuscule, generally in quantities of micrograms (one-millionth of a gram). You should not, however, discount the vital importance of these trace elements. For example, the iodine that comprises only 0.00004 per cent of your body is crucial to the 2 per cent that is calcium. The secret for optimal health is to maintain the proper mineral balance. Too much can be as harmful as not enough.

The United States government has established a Recommended Daily Allowance (RDA) for six major minerals: calcium, phosphorous, iron, magnesium, zinc and iodine. It has also established estimates of safe and adequate intakes for certain trace elements, including copper, manganese, fluorine, chromium, selenium and molybdenum.

In 1991, the UK government's Committee on Medical Aspects of Food Policy abandoned RDAs – which had previously been defined as 'the amounts sufficient, or more than sufficient, for the nutritional needs of practically all healthy persons in a population' – in favour of measurements that take into account the concentration of nutrients in the body, the absence of signs of deficiency and the balance of nutrients, among other things. They first came up with Dietary Reference Values (DRVs), which range from the lowest intakes that will meet the needs of some individuals, to the Reference Nutrient Intake (RNI), which is the point above which an intake of a particular nutrient will almost certainly be adequate. The Committee has established RNIs for 11 nutrients: calcium, phosphorous, magnesium, sodium, potassium, chloride, iron, zinc, copper, selenium, iodine. In addition, they have set 'safe intakes' for manganese, molybdenum, chromium and fluoride.[4]

So how do you know if you are mineral deficient? For starters, you may be missing that rosy glow on your cheeks, or your fingernails may break easily, or perhaps your teeth are cavity prone. Maybe your cuts and scrapes don't heal as quickly as they should or your hair has lost its lustre. But, most often, mineral deficiency or imbalance is what causes just about the most common medical complaint, accounting for excessive visits to doctor's surgeries – chronic fatigue. For our cells to produce the maximum quantity of energy, the body must have both the proper amounts of minerals and an adequate ratio of major minerals and trace elements.

Besides the problems already mentioned, a variety of illnesses as well as premature ageing are signs of mineral deficiency. But perhaps the most shocking mineral-deficiency symptom is sudden death. Several lines of evidence suggest that intakes of minerals may influence the risk of coronary disease, particularly sudden death from heart attack. Most research on this topic has focused on mineral intake from 'hard' versus 'soft' drinking water. However, a study conducted in Maradabad, India examined another major source of minerals – the diet.[5] It concluded that, among people predisposed to coronary disease, a diet rich in minerals can reduce the incidence of sudden cardiac death.

CALCIUM: A MULTI-DIMENSIONAL MINERAL

Although osteoporosis and premenstrual syndrome (PMS) have both been closely associated with a lack of calcium for some time now, the multi-dimensional role of this mineral is yet to be fully appreciated.

Many women have come to accept painful periods as a way of life, but such is clearly not a normal physiological condition. For instance, cramping pains with a period may be caused by mineral deficiencies such as low calcium and magnesium levels. Other common symptoms of PMS include: physical exhaustion, dizzy spells, difficulty with concentration, poor memory, irritability, depression, poor circulation, intolerance of the cold, weight gain, abdominal bloating, heavy periods, fluid retention, breast tenderness, tension, mood swings and headaches. In addition, there is often a loss of interest in sex, as well as joint stiffness, uncontrollable bingeing on food, constipation, diarrhoea, recurrent thrush infections, hot flushes, general debility, lack of stamina, and a very telling complaint of feeling 'like death' on awakening.[6] Yet these symptoms can act as a warning of low calcium levels. It is far better to spot this when period pains are a problem than to continue to suffer from a calcium shortage and fracture a hip in old age.

Osteoporosis is a crippling condition characterized by dramatic bone loss throughout the skeletal system, which results in honeycombed, fragile bones. Over two million people in the United Kingdom – 1 in 3 women and 1 in 20 men over the age of 60 – are afflicted with this illness, which results in 40 premature deaths each day.

Calcium is the leading mineral linked to osteoporosis, which is why Britain's National Osteoporosis Society recommends calcium intakes of 1500 mg/day in women over 45.[7] However, other major minerals, trace elements and nutrients contribute to healthy bones. The bones function as a warehouse where many vital minerals are stored for the body to utilize. In fact, your bones store 99 per cent of the body's calcium and 85 per cent of its phosphorus. Without phosphorus, your bones could not develop and mature properly; nor could the body control the calcium balance. The trace elements fluoride, copper, silicon and vanadiun and the amino acid leucine participate in calcium metabolism and bone mineralization. Researchers are currently testing osteoporosis treatments using fluoride and boron.[8]

Calcium's effects on the body can be far-reaching and, sometimes, dramatic, yet many people do not realize all that it does. Few are aware, for instance, that calcium protects the immune system from poisoning by heavy metals such as lead and cadmium (*see later in this chapter*), which pollute the environment. A number of studies show that we have an abundance of lead in our bodies, about 500 times greater than just a few generations ago. Cadmium adds to the burden as it enters our body via water pipes carrying 'soft' water or is inhaled in cigarette smoke and from air pollution.

Calcium has also been proved to prevent cancer of the colon and rectum. Additionally, along with magnesium and potassium, it has been shown to prevent high blood pressure: a calcium deficiency can cause overproduction of the hormones cortisone and aldosterone which, in turn, causes the kidneys to hold salt and water; the blood volume swells and results in high blood pressure. The mineral further helps by making blood clotting possible. Without adequate calcium, many seriously injured people would bleed to death.

Most recently, calcium has received wide recognition as a mineral that can lower blood cholesterol. Researchers fed large daily amounts of calcium (710 mg in foods and 2660 mg in supplements) to volunteers whose initial cholesterol levels were just under 250. Within four days, these levels dropped an average of 14 points. The researchers then lowered the prescribed calcium intake to 1600 mg per day for three weeks. Blood cholesterol dropped by as many as 48 points, often removing individuals from dangerous levels. Triglycerides plummeted by as many as 115 points. The higher the cholesterol and triglyceride levels initially, the more significant their drop. Researchers found that the sharpest declines occurred during the first week and held firm until the end of the study.[9] Studies similar to this have been successfully repeated by other scientists.

Calcium deficiency in the blood can cause a variety of other problems, including toxaemia of pregnancy, anxiety, hyperkinesis, otosclerosis and alcoholism.

Mild calcium deficiency is also noted for causing nerve sensitivity, paraesthesia ('pins & needles') muscle twitching, brittle nails, irritability, insomnia, confusion and depression. As a calcium deficiency becomes more serious, muscle cramps, heart palpitations, numbness, tingling and tetany (the sustained contraction of some muscles, causing severe pain) may all be a result. Some scientists have concluded that multiple sclerosis is an illness due to a lack of calcium and vitamin D consumption in puberty.

Health fanatics and professional athletes don't underestimate calcium. They know that it is particularly important to performance. Every time a weight-bearing exercise is done, for example, bone metabolism increases. That means calcium turnover – from the bones to the blood, and back again to the bones – is stepped up. Exercise is supposed to cause the bones to retain more calcium and grow in strength, but when dietary calcium is inadequate, the bones can break more easily.[10]

One can easily get the impression that a calcium deficiency is an older person's problem and not be concerned about it in early life. However, researchers at Ohio State University found that a staggeringly small percentage of girls met their daily required calcium levels. Since this puts most girls at risk of developing osteoporosis as they age, researchers recommended drastically increasing calcium intake for teenagers. Since so many avoid milk, cheese and green vegetables for fear of gaining weight or simply because they don't like them, calcium deficiency results. Researchers note that a shortage of calcium during the teens and 20s may severely limit a person's peak bone mass, the point at which the skeleton is at its sturdiest and healthiest. After the age of 30, one's ability to maintain the skeleton declines and bone mass is lost.[11] The bottom line, they concluded, is that some women may increase bone density by increasing both their calcium and vitamin D intake.

MAGNESIUM: THE ANTI-STRESS NUTRIENT

Magnesium and calcium are closely related. Some 25 g of magnesium is found in the body, of which 70 per cent is combined with calcium and phosphorus in the bone salt complex. It is only in the last few decades that the vital importance of this nutrient has surfaced. It is crucial to so many body systems, particularly when it comes to enzymes: some 300 require this mineral as a co-factor. It is also essential for basic physiological processes such as the functioning of DNA, the transmission of nerve impulses and the contraction of skeletal and heart muscle.[12]

Many who suffer from alcoholism, diabetic coma, thrombosis, leukaemia, epilepsy and eclampsia have been found to have inadequate levels of magnesium. This macro-mineral is involved in several hundred enzymatic reactions, most of which assist in the production of energy and cardiovascular function.

Often referred to as the 'anti-stress nutrient', it functions as a natural tranquillizer, for it relaxes skeletal muscles and the smooth muscles of blood vessels as well as of the gastrointestinal tract. Magnesium may ward off heart attacks since it can prevent coronary artery spasm. Spasms of the blood vessels lead to a restricted oxygen supply, resulting in pain, injury or even death of muscle tissue. For optimal health, magnesium needs to be balanced with adequate calcium, phosphorus, potassium and sodium chloride (i.e. salt).

It is not difficult to obtain magnesium from our diets. Vegetables are generally an excellent source, especially dark green ones. Seafood also contains sufficient amounts. Nuts, seeds and pulses are also high in magnesium, as are whole grains and brown rice. But one must consume these foods as close to their natural state as possible. Magnesium-poor soil will not produce magnesium-rich food, while processing will discard much of the goodness. About 85 per cent of magnesium is forfeited during flour milling, for instance. Soaking and boiling food also deprives it of its vitamin and mineral content; hence, the water you throw away may be healthier than the food you eat.

Magnesium deficiency is quite common although rarely checked by doctors. Those of us who indulge in processed or fast food are particularly at risk. The average persons ingests about 120 mg of magnesium daily, although the UK reference nutrient intake (RNI) for magnesium is 435 mg for men and 390 mg for women. However, most orthomolecular nutritionists claim that our daily requirement is around 600 mg. Sometimes magnesium absorption problems occur when a person has suffered an injury or undergone surgery, and sufferers of diabetes and liver disease may have difficulties, even though they may be consuming an adequate amount of the mineral. Others at risk are users of alcohol, caffeine, sugar, diuretics or birth control pills. Certain mineral-rich foods such as spinach and chard contain oxalic acid, and wholegrain cereals, nuts and pulses contain phytic acid, both of which form insoluble salts with magnesium, resulting in its elimination rather than absorption.

Some early warnings of a magnesium deficiency include fatigue, loss of appetite, irritability, insomnia and muscle tremors. Some people may suffer from these at the same time as psychological disorders such as decreased learning ability, confusion, poor memory, feelings of apprehension and/or apathy. In certain severe cases of deficiency, delirium and hallucinations may actually occur.

At the Einstein College of Medicine and Bronx Psychiatric Center in New York, doctors began thinking about how magnesium might relate to mental illness. 'One thing we knew,' explained Dr Daniel Kanofsky, 'was that some people who are not schizophrenic but who are markedly deficient in magnesium can display symptoms such as depression, agitation, even hallucinations. We and others also found that antipsychotic medications can drive down magnesium levels in patients.'[13] These researchers naturally asked if perhaps the patients who don't respond to drug therapy were actually showing mental symptoms resulting from magnesium deficiency. Yet others may experience cardiovascular problems such as a rapid heartbeat. High blood pressure, arterial spasm and even heart attacks have been caused by magnesium shortages.

PHOSPHORUS: GOOD NEWS FOR RUNNERS

The difficulty with phosphorus is not obtaining it from our diets, but keeping the proper ratio with calcium.

Second only to calcium, phosphorus is the most abundant mineral in the body, comprising about 1 per cent of body weight. Every single cell contains phosphorus, but 85 per cent of it is found in the bones and teeth, and a relatively large amount is contained in the red blood cells.

The RNI for phosphorus is the same as for calcium – 625 mg for both men and women. But since most people consume far too little calcium, the average phosphorus intake is usually much greater, around 1500 mg. To maintain biochemical homoeostasis, the phosphorus-to-calcium ratio needs to be 1:1. If it isn't, this leads to a decreased body storage of calcium. Hence, even if you take calcium supplements, you may still develop a calcium-deficiency problem, with calcium and phosphorus competing for absorption in the intestines. Those who eat a good deal of meat (most protein foods are high in phosphorus) and consume soft drinks regularly can drastically increase their phosphorus supply. Dairy foods have a much more balanced calcium-to-phosphorus ratio.

A low calcium-to-phosphorus ratio in the body increases the risk of hypertension and bowel cancer. A proper balance helps in reducing stress and problems relating to calcium metabolism such as arthritis. Cancer researchers have discovered that cancer cells have a tendency to lose phosphorus more rapidly than normal ones; therefore, phosphorus supplementation could evolve as a supportive cancer treatment.

Phosphorus is crucial to energy production. It supplies the phosphate in adenosine triphosphate (ATP), a high-energy molecule that is the most immediate source of energy for cell metabolism. Replication and repair of your body's cells and tissues also could not take place without this mineral. Additionally, the phosphate in ATP is essential in protein synthesis and in the creation of the nucleic acids in DNA and RNA – the genetic code.

The American College of Sports Medicine suggests that 'phosphate loading' may actually improve energy metabolism and make muscle cells more efficient during endurance exercise. This greater efficiency may result in faster running times.[14] The College's studies reveal that runners who load up on phosphorus show a 10 per cent increase in performance. Additionally, researchers discovered that the runners had higher blood levels of haemoglobin (which transports oxygen throughout the body). Although further research is required, experts think that phosphate may protect red blood cells in some way.

It is important to note, however, that improved performance is a short-term gain. Our bodies can adapt to high levels of phosphate after just a week and excrete any excess in the urine; therefore taking extra supplements will not continue to improve performance. In fact, it could be harmful: a high phosphorus level can lead to a low calcium level, which in turn can result in bone mineral loss (osteoporosis). When a phosphorus deficiency does occur, however, the results are generally quite alarming. Fatigue, irritability, loss of appetite, anxiety, joint stiffness, bone pain and, in children, decreased growth and inadequate bone and tooth development may take place. Although it is not recommended that the majority of people supplement their diets with phosphorus, it is absolutely essential to monitor closely the phosphorus-to-calcium ratio.

POTASSIUM: ABSOLUTELY ESSENTIAL

Supplementation is often required for the mineral potassium, however. Considered absolutely essential for optimal health, potassium is the major electrolyte in the fluid within the body's cells, where it helps to balance the composition of this fluid in relation to that outside the cell. It is also essential for the transmission of nerve impulses, the contraction of the muscles and for releasing energy from protein, fat and carbohydrates during metabolism. Muscular weakness, a malfunctioning neuromuscular system, slow reflexes, fatigue, depression and mental confusion can often result from even a minor potassium deficiency, which the body is able to store only in very small quantities. Other possible outcomes of such a deficiency include cardiac arrhythmia and arthritis.

The Food and Nutrition Board of the National Academy of Sciences in the US has estimated the minimum requirement for potassium for men and women over 18 years of age to be 2000 mg per day; in the UK, the RNI is 3200 mg/day. One third of the potassium in our diets comes from fruits and vegetables; white potatoes provide one third of that. Meat, poultry and fish supply a further 20 per cent. Leafy green vegetables such as spinach, parsley and red leaf lettuce, as well as broccoli, peas and tomatoes, are all excellent sources. Citrus fruits, bananas, apples, avocado pears and apricots are potassium rich, too, as are whole grains, seeds and nuts.

It is important to note that, while magnesium helps maintain the potassium in cells, the sodium/potassium balance must be as finely tuned as those of calcium/phosphorus and calcium/magnesium. It has been discovered that a high-sodium/low-potassium diet affects the volume of blood in the veins and arteries and generally increases blood pressure. Diuretics tend to intensify potassium loss, causing a host of additional ailments. Thus the natural course of action is to eat a healthy, potassium-rich diet and avoid salty, processed items. To retain potassium in food, it is also necessary to cook foods in a minimal amount of water and for the shortest possible time.

The body stores a greater amount of potassium than sodium – generally, 9 oz to 4 oz. The Western diet, however, which tends to include excessive amounts of processed and devitalized convenience foods, is loaded with salt. The body ends up conserving sodium while barely hanging on to a small amount of potassium. Fortunately, potassium has a very high absorption rate, but it's also one of the most soluble minerals. Thus, most potassium is lost in cooking and through excretion via perspiration and urine, as well as through vomiting and diarrhoea. Further loss takes place as a result of consuming alcohol, coffee, cola drinks, sugar and diuretic drugs.

Potassium is the mineral most commonly prescribed by doctors.

Since it is essential to cardiovascular and nerve functions and is eliminated during diuretic therapy for two very common conditions – oedema (excessive tissue fluid) and hypertension (sustained high blood pressure) – its replacement with supplementation is vital. This is also a necessary response to a high-sodium diet. Severe elevations or depletions of potassium will cause harm or even death. An overdose is generally unlikely, however, since the kidneys will eliminate the excess, but those with kidney disease may be at risk. But overconsumption is rarely an issue, since potassium deficiency is the rule of the day.

Researchers have discovered that a high intake of dietary potassium may reduce the risk of death by stroke by as much as 40 per cent. A 12-year study involving 589 men and women near San Diego, California was conducted by Di Kay-Tee Khaw, professor of clinical gerontology at Cambridge University. Her findings have been corroborated by animal studies at the University of Minnesota and at Cornell Medical College, New York.

Dr Khaw concluded that the protection offered by dietary potassium is consistent for both men and women, and it is independent of dietary fibre and other cardiovascular factors. Although data from her study and others have suggested that an increased potassium intake works equally well with both the elderly and the young, Dr Khaw believes that the mineral might be especially effective for the elderly, because these individuals are usually more susceptible to the effects of sodium, which would be regulated by the potassium intake.[15]

SODIUM: THE EVIL MINERAL?

Is sodium the evil mineral? Hardly. We simply consume too much of it due to eating processed foods and the liberal use of table salt (sodium chloride). Sodium functions in combination with potassium, resulting in a normal balance of fluids within cells and outside of them. These two minerals must be balanced in the body so the nerves can react properly to stimulation and the impulses can reach the muscles for muscular contraction. Although sodium supplementation is rarely necessary, a deficiency – as can occur in athletes after sweating in hot weather – certainly can result in nervous disorders, cramps and low blood pressure, and it can even make one prone to infections.

Some 60 per cent of your body's sodium is found in the fluids around the cells, and about 10 per cent is located inside the cells. The remaining 30 per cent is stored in the bones. The mineral functions as an electrolyte (like potassium and chloride). It is intimately related to the movement of water. Water follows sodium throughout your body; every cell in your body contains sodium.

In industrial societies, the average adult consumes about 6 g daily.

In fact, it is not unusual for some people to consume more than 12 g of salt a day! In earlier times, for thousands of years, people's natural diet consisted of less than 1 g of sodium per day, which made high blood pressure practically unheard of. Salt is 40 per cent sodium and 60 per cent chloride. So, about one teaspoon of salt contains some 2 g of sodium. It is no wonder then that high blood pressure is epidemic in Western society. It is interesting to note that people who don't have access to packaged or fast foods report little or no hypertension.

Today, it is difficult to get away from sodium. Nearly all foods contain it, especially in the form of sodium chloride, including seafood, poultry and beef, and vegetables such as celery, beetroot and carrots. However, this is not the case with most wholesome natural foods. When processed foods become our primary diet, optimal health, or health of any kind, is an unlikely result.

IRON: ROSY CHEEKS AND PINK TONGUES

A lack of iron is a common problem – in fact, it is the second most common nutrition problem in the United States, following hot on the heels of obesity.

Some 50 per cent of the mineral content of the Earth's crust is iron, and it is believed to have been the first mineral to find itself in living tissue. It is now found in every single cell in your body – nearly all of it in conjunction with protein. The haemoglobin molecule, which carries oxygen throughout the body, consists of 60 to 70 per cent iron. Hence, a shortage of iron results in decreased haemoglobin and thus less oxygen to the tissues. Iron is also found in the liver, spleen and bone marrow, which can be turned to in time of additional need of iron for haemoglobin production.

Anaemia is a frequent result of an iron-poor diet and is not detected nearly as often as it should be. You must be quite seriously deficient in iron before it shows up on any deficiency tests, which does not make for easy diagnosis. An added iron supply is especially essential during infancy, childhood, adolescence and pregnancy. In older people, deficiency results due to poor absorption and poor diet. Higher requirements are also necessary for women during their child-bearing years, since they must compensate for blood lost during periods; it is estimated that, even in affluent countries, at least 10 per cent of menstruating women suffer from iron deficiency.

Generally, when your body requires additional iron, absorption tends to improve through an increase in iron-carrying proteins in the blood, known as iron transferring. Nevertheless, poor absorption as well as inadequate diets are the key reasons for deficiency.

As is the case with calcium and zinc, iron absorption can be quite a problem. Your body absorbs only a mere average 8–10 per cent of all the iron you consume. Vegetable sources are particularly poorly absorbed, and you stand a much better chance with beef and liver, where up to 30 per cent absorption occurs. Thus, getting adequate supplies of iron is especially a problem for vegetarians. However, there are ways to increase iron absorption in the intestines and enhance the maintenance of proper levels.

Absorption always improves when there is a need for the mineral, such as during pregnancy, breastfeeding or after blood loss. The presence of hydrochloric acid in the stomach, as well as ascorbic acid (vitamin C) in the small intestine, changes ferric iron to the more conveniently absorbable ferrous iron. Since citrus juices and various fruits and vegetables naturally contain good doses of vitamin C, they can assist in the body's iron absorption. Beef and liver comprise easily absorbed iron, while these foods also provide amino acids and stimulate production of hydrochloric acid in the stomach. Iron absorption can be further aided by cooking with iron utensils and by ensuring that there are adequate amounts of copper, cobalt and manganese in the diet.

On the other hand, low amounts of stomach acid or the use of antacids will drastically reduce iron absorption. Phosphates found in meats and, especially, in soft drinks tend to create insoluble iron salts that cannot be absorbed. The same is true for spinach and other vegetables containing oxalic acid and whole grains containing phytic acid. There is a suspicion, but not a definite determination, that soy protein may also contribute to problems of iron absorption. But without question, the caffeine and tannic acid in coffee and tea reduce iron absorption, as do very high concentrations of calcium, which compete with iron. To complicate matters further, iron absorption becomes more difficult as we age.

Unused iron is eliminated by the body through the faeces. But the body retains iron quite well, with the exception of blood loss in women. The average individual tends to lose 1 mg daily.

So, how can you tell if you are getting enough iron? Well, for starters, your circulation will be quite good. You will have rosy cheeks, pink earlobes, a pink tongue and adequate stamina. A pale tongue generally means anaemia, which should persuade you to try a more iron-rich diet. As with other minerals, iron-poor soil is an all-too-common occurrence, and can result in produce that does not contain as much iron as it should. If cattle graze on iron-poor feed, they, too, will not produce high-iron beef. But real problems arise during the milling of grains; in wheat and oats this can cause a 75 per cent reduction of iron. 'Enriched' breads and cereals contain the practically non-absorbable ferric variety of iron. The best possible way to obtain the most iron is through a varied, wholesome diet that consists of unrefined foods as close to their natural state as possible, and includes beef, liver and other organ meats, whole grains, green vegetables, pulses, nuts and seeds, and brewer's yeast.

Iron surely does provide us with the look of health. Rosy cheeks, warm hands and feet and an energized feeling can belong to all of us. If you are feeling weak and tired and lack stamina, the first safe bet may be to improve your iron level. By the time anaemia sets in, you will have become immensely deficient. But in addition to anaemia, a lack of iron can impair respiratory activity, and coronary artery ailments and vascular insufficiency can be seriously worsened. However, it is important to note that an excess of iron can actually contribute to hardening of the arteries and heart disease. As mentioned earlier, a delicate balance remains the key to optimal health.

Energy and iron seem to go hand-in-hand. The mineral is often referred to as an endurance booster. Iron-poor blood is often the cause of chronic fatigue and sluggish performance. Since iron resides in red blood cells and transports oxygen to working muscles, the lower your level of iron, the less oxygen your muscles receive. Thus, your muscles become less efficient, produce more lactic acid and fatigue more quickly.[16]

Perhaps it appears that you have an adequate supply of iron and you still feel as if you're not performing at peak level. In other words, if you're not anaemic, can your iron level still be low? The answer is: yes. By increasing your diet to include more iron-rich food or by taking supplements, you can improve your performance.

Researchers compared the improvement in fitness of two groups of women who had sufficient iron levels. The study was carried out during a seven-week training programme and came up with some encouraging results. One group was given iron supplements during training, while the other group took placebos (dummy pills). When the study was concluded, both groups had improved their fitness levels, but greater gains were made during the last two weeks of the programme by the women who had supplemented their diets with iron. Further, unlike the control group, these women possessed healthier blood levels of various iron indicators.[17]

Better performance results from a higher-iron intake because iron is a necessary component of haemoglobin, myoglobin and several enzymes and is critical for oxygen utilization in exercising muscles. Iron deficiency or depletion may lead to poor physical performance, but it can also critically affect the iron stores in already iron-depleted adult women, who exercise according to Dr Charlotte Pratt at Virginia State University.[18] In a recent study of adult women, she says, it was demonstrated that the level of ferritin in blood plasma, a measure of iron stores, decreased between the 6th and 13th weeks in women engaged in fitness-type exercises, suggesting that reduced iron stores may result from moderate exercise. The US Department of Agriculture has concluded that women who have below-normal blood stores of iron may start feeling cold before they experience tiredness, the usual side-effect of iron deficiency anaemia.

MANGANESE: FREE-FLOATING FAT

The body contains a total of about 15–20 mg of the trace element manganese, of which nearly half is found in the bones and the rest in the liver, pancreas, pituitary gland, adrenal glands and kidneys – the active metabolic organs. It plays a role in the activation of numerous enzymes and the synthesis of cholesterol, L-dopamine, muco-poly saccharides, and sex hormones. In tests on male laboratory animals, low-manganese levels caused a lack of interest in sex and, eventually, sterility; most improved, however, with a supplementation of this mineral. Manganese is also necessary for blood clotting, the formation of bone and the development of connective tissues. It is important in insulin action and in the metabolism of proteins, carbohydrates and nucleic acids. Manganese makes possible the proper use of blood fats, a function which prevents heart and artery ailments; it helps to metabolize these so that they can be employed to make cells walls and protective nerve sheaths. When you are deficient in this trace element, fats float throughout the circulatory system, collecting in increasingly larger particles which then adhere to the linings of arteries.

Manganese is found in plant tissues, but especially in nuts, seeds and whole grains, as well as dark leafy green vegetables. It is quite difficult to absorb, however, and a deficiency can occur, generally as a result of eating too many processed foods and/or excess calcium and phosphorus, and from iron deficiency.

Manganese deficiency is usually a serious business. Nervous instability, convulsions of pregnancy, bone disorders, sterility, diabetes, rheumatoid arthritis and even cancer are among the possible destructive outcomes of a low-manganese diet. Although manganese is one of the least toxic elements, the key operating term remains 'balance'. An overconsumption can drastically reduce your appetite as well as cause psychiatric disorders and neurological symptoms and slow down your thinking, among other problems.

A study conducted at the State University of New Jersey concluded that manganese-deficient laboratory animals, when compared to controls, had less insulin receptor affinity. The researchers suggested that a deficiency of manganese affects glucose metabolism by inhibiting the number of glucose carriers that are available for transport or perhaps by altering the affinity of the carrier for glucose in fat tissue.[19]

Thus, a manganese deficiency can cause diabetes. Repeatedly, studies have shown that diabetics of all ages had low levels of the mineral, and control groups with no history of blood sugar problems have consistently been shown to have manganese levels that are twice as high. When diabetics are given manganese over a period of time, their condition improves.

Manganese used as a therapeutic nutrient has been known to be successful in treating fatigue and poor memory (by protecting brain tissue and helping oxygenation), as well as nervousness, irritability and dizziness. Although it is not known why, manganese can help reduce some of the symptoms of Parkinson's disease such as muscle rigidity and twitching. Researchers have also discovered that tardive dyskinesia, a disorder characterized by the uncontrollable twitching of the lips, tongue and/or jaw, is often corrected by additional manganese and B-complex vitamins, especially nicotinic acid and choline.

Some epilepsy sufferers have also gained relief from this mineral. Common symptoms such as muscle convulsions and mental lapses are now being linked to improper manganese blood levels. Animal experiments have suggested that low-manganese levels in the blood may be a key factor in this frequently violent disorder. When manganese is taken in combination with B vitamins, it has been able to alleviate fatigue and weakness by enhancing nerve impulses.

Researchers have also noted a direct correlation between manganese and most tumours and cancer cells. The trace element helps prevent cancer by synthesizing RNA. When manganese deficiencies occur, cells are improperly made and some of these may become destructive cancer cells. In the future, this mineral may play an important role in preventing cancer cell production as well as the spread of the disease.

Manganese, as a part of the super-oxide dismutase enzyme system, protects against the cell damage and ageing caused by free radicals. It works with a wide variety of nutrients to keep us in optimal health. For example, vitamin C could not do nearly as much as it does without the assistance of manganese. This crucial nutrient further protects us from ammonia that develops in our cells during the production of energy and heat when protein is broken down. Ammonia is so powerful an agent that a thousandth of a milligram in a quart of blood can kill you.

ZINC: HEALING TIMES

Zinc is a component of numerous enzymes involved with digestion and metabolism. It is vital in the synthesis of nucleic acid and in the development of the reproductive system. It can work properly only with the right balance of other minerals and vitamins, and these other nutrients cannot do their jobs without the aid of zinc. Food processing and poor soil quality due to agricultural techniques have made zinc very difficult to obtain from food. Processing eliminates much of the zinc as well as manganese, chromium, molybdenum and the B vitamins. Cooking methods can further reduce the availability of this important nutrient.

Absorption becomes a problem when phytic acid and excessive calcium and phosphorus are present in your diet. High levels of copper, excessive fibre, inadequate vitamin D in the body and the ingesting of coffee and canned foods also reduce zinc absorption. But zinc is required for more than 100 enzymes and is believed to be a part of more body functions than any other mineral. Besides the immune system, it is essential for proper growth and development, the maintenance of body tissues, sexual function and detoxification of chemicals and metabolic irritants. It is further required for the synthesis of DNA. Healing after burns, cuts and surgery is speeded up with the aid of zinc, as is the resolution of skin disorders and male prostate problems.

Yet the body contains only about 2.0–2.5 g of this water-soluble mineral. It is found in the retinas of the eyes, the heart, spleen, lungs, brain, adrenal glands and skin, with some minor deposits in organ tissues, hair, teeth and nails. In men, it is most concentrated in the prostate gland and in semen: impotence can often be traced to low levels of zinc. It is easily and rapidly eliminated by the body via the gastrointestinal tract, in the faeces. It is also eliminated through urine and perspiration, and such stresses on the body as burns, surgery and weight loss can lead to an increased need. Hair analysis provides a quite accurate reading of zinc levels, as does red blood cell measurement.

The best way to obtain zinc from your diet is through animal foods. Like iron, the zinc in these is bound with proteins and so is absorbed far better. But when it's bound with the phytic and oxalic acids in, respectively, vegetables and grains, it's much more difficult for the body to absorb. The greatest amount of zinc is found in oysters, but these are certain to contain a relatively large amount of copper and, unfortunately, far too many of the poisonous metals and chemicals that today pollute our oceans. Other good (and, it is hoped, pollution-free) free sources include fish, poultry, pecans, brazil nuts, pumpkin seeds, mustard, chilli powder, black pepper and cocoa.

Most recently, zinc has been found to be greatly beneficial to women who suffer from PMS (pre-menstrual syndrome). Those awful debilitating symptoms such as crying spells, irritability, cravings for sweets, depression, breast tenderness, fatigue, mood swings, head and muscle aches can all be attributed to PMS. But now it is known that teenage girls who are zinc-deficient often have delayed menstruation and suffer from menstrual problems as they get older. In addition, researchers at the Baylor College of Medicine in Houston have concluded that zinc deficiency may be related to this monthly dilemma. They claim that, since small amounts of zinc regulate the secretion of female sex hormones, including progesterone, a lack of the nutrient may exacerbate problems associated with PMS.[20]

Progesterone is secreted by one of the ovaries following the release of an egg which occurs roughly two weeks before menstruation begins. The Baylor researchers took regular blood samples of women with and without PMS, and discovered that those who suffered from PMS had much lower zinc levels in their blood. They concluded that this might have led to a decrease in progesterone and certain natural opiates, or endorphins, produced by neurons in the brain.

At the University of Kentucky at Lexington and at the University of Alabama Medical Center, medical experts have found an even more amazing use for zinc. They are using this nutrient to promote recovery from serious head injury.[21] Over a period of three years, 60 head-injury patients were supplied with either the normal amount of zinc found in intravenous formulas and hospital foods or, through supplementation, some five times that quantity. A standard test known as the Glasgow Coma Scale, used by neurosurgeons to assess mental function following head injury, showed that a month after their accidents, the zinc-supplemented patients were performing exceptionally better and recovered much faster. These brand new findings give researchers reason to believe that zinc will deliver promising results in several areas of impaired cognition and neurotransmission.

Recently, a role for zinc has been found in the treatment of AIDS.[22] A depressed immune system is frequently caused by zinc deficiency. A weakened immune system clearly leaves a person susceptible to a variety of life-threatening illnesses, AIDS among them. At the New Jersey Medical School, researchers found that, of the 26 AIDS and AIDS-related complex (ARC) patients they studied, 30 per cent were zinc deficient. In fact, it has been well documented that those with AIDS and LAS (lymphadenopathy syndrome, a pre-AIDS condition) have considerably reduced serum zinc levels. Children with AIDS have been found to show all the signs and symptoms of zinc deficiency.

When children are generally low in zinc, they have poor appetites and abnormally slow development. Learning disabilities and short attention spans are also common. Eventually, acne, hair loss and delayed sexual development occurs. With these symptoms come constant fatigue and, in some severe cases, dwarfism and a complete lack of sexual function.

A progressive zinc deficiency, which becomes increasingly more common as we get older, is believed to be a serious factor in the gradual breakdown of the ageing immune system. Researchers have documented that zinc supplementation can increase the number of circulating T-lymphocytes, white blood cells that fight infection and improve antibody response.

The New York Academy of Sciences reports studies in which patients with different inherited malfunctions, as well as haemophiliacs who were at risk of developing AIDS, all had a serious problem with zinc. The deficiency is believed to be the result of either poor absorption or an excessive excretion of the mineral.

It is important that you always have a good supply of zinc in your system and never do without it. According to recent US Department of Agriculture surveys, the average intake of zinc by American women between the ages of 19 and 50 was less than 75 per cent of the government's recommended daily allowance of 15 mg – which is notoriously famous for being too low in the first place. Men, however, consumed about 95 per cent of the requirement. In the UK, the reference nutrient intake (RNI) for zinc for women of the same age group is even lower than the US RDA: just under 4 mg/day. Men are supposed to need just over 5 mg.

COPPER: A BIT NEUROTIC?

Copper is found in all tissues of the body. It interacts with iron and zinc and is a part of numerous enzyme systems. It's also essential for the production of haemoglobin, the oxygen-carrying molecule. The full amount of copper in the body totals about 75–100 mg, but despite this relatively small quantity, it is responsible for performing many necessary functions. It is an important part of the cytochrome system for cell respiration, an energy-releasing process. Further, it assists vitamin C in oxidation and works with this vitamin to create collagen, particularly in the bone and connective tissues. Too much copper can create too much collagen and result in stiff and less flexible tissues.

Copper deficiency is frequently associated with, among other ailments, hardening of the arteries, cirrhosis of the liver, infectious hepatitis, dermatosis, a slowing down of growth, and osteoporosis. But too much copper in the body can have equally detrimental effects, such as aplastic anaemia, nephritis, schizophrenia, eczema, rheumatoid arthritis, toxaemia of pregnancy and sickle cell anaemia. Unlike zinc, overconsumption of copper, as well as deficiency, is of general concern.

Many mental problems arise as a result of high-copper/low-zinc levels. Depression, hyperactivity, some symptoms of PMS, schizophrenia, learning disability and senility have been linked to this. Some people with high copper levels have also experienced anxiety attacks, joint and muscle pains, mental fatigue, manic depression, insomnia, autism, high blood pressure, stuttering or postpartum psychosis. Some medical researchers insist that copper/zinc levels be checked for all those with the above-mentioned complaints, and they encourage alcohol and cancer sufferers to have the same investigations. Nevertheless, the World Health Organization continues to claim that copper is nontoxic.

Women who take birth control pills suffer ill effects. Many attribute this to increases in oestrogen hormone levels, which can increase serum copper levels to more than twice the normal amount. At the same time, the red blood cell count, where copper is crucial, tends to be decreased. The same chain of events can take place during pregnancy, which may explain a variety of psychological and other symptoms that women experience while pregnant or on the pill.

Mild symptoms of copper toxicity may cause your doctor to diagnose you as a bit neurotic or a hypochondriac. After all, how many of us don't occasionally feel fatigued, irritable, nervous or depressed? However, self-treatment is not difficult. An overdose of copper can generally be treated with supplements of zinc and manganese. They compete with copper for absorption and assist in copper elimination through the bile and urine.

CHROMIUM:
THE CHALLENGE OF ADEQUATE LEVELS

Scientists did not actually isolate chromium in the body until 1959, although it has been established as a mineral since 1797. This essential trace element is found in many parts of the body, including the skin, fat, brain, muscles, spleen, kidneys and testes. It also received widespread attention recently as it is considered an essential part of glucose tolerance. Chromium assists in the regulation of carbohydrate metabolism by enhancing the action of insulin to control the utilization of glucose in your body. An outrageously small amount of chromium is required to do this vital job. Our blood contains some 20 parts per *billion* of this trace element – far less than one microgram (one-millionth of a gram). Any excess is quite easily cleared by the kidneys.

People living in the United States have much lower levels of chromium than residents of other nations. They also have high rates of atherosclerosis and diabetes, and some scientists think that there is a link between these two facts. Asians, for instance, have the least artery disease, and their chromium levels are five times higher than American ones. The people of Africa have levels that are double those in the US, and they also have a much lower incidence of diabetes. The higher levels of chromium result from the consumption of far less refined foods than that consumed in the US, and foods that have been grown on soil that has not been depleted of its minerals.

It is believed that adult-onset diabetes is a direct result of chromium deficiency since the amount of the trace element generally decreases in our bodies as we get older. The past several decades have seen a seven-fold increase in this disease in the US and similar increases in other industrialized countries. Again, manufactured foods and poor soil quality can be blamed. Natural sugarcane is a rich source of chromium, for example, but by the time it reaches our tables as refined sugar, 93 per cent of this vital mineral has been processed out. When whole grains become white flour, 40 per cent of their chromium disappears. To make matters worse, white flour, sugar and fats actually deplete your body of the chromium already stored. Thus a poor diet and ageing can, together, cause serious chromium deficiency. Hence, when we become chromium deficient, blood sugar metabolism becomes a problem that may lead to another leading cause of death – diabetes mellitus. This is all quite extraordinary when you consider how absolutely simple it is to diagnose and treat chromium deficiency.

In addition to regulating blood sugar, chromium is quite capable of reducing blood cholesterol levels, even providing the benefit of slightly increasing HDL (high-density lipoprotein), the 'good' cholesterol. Re-searchers have been able to bring down levels of LDL (low-density lipoprotein) cholesterol – the 'bad' sort – by nearly 15 per cent by supplementing people's diets with inorganic chromium daily. This cer-tainly reduces a person's chances of getting heart disease.

It is rare, indeed, that anyone suffers from too much chromium. With low absorption and high excretion, getting adequate chromium into the body can be quite a challenge.

Athletes and those who work out regularly are another special risk group. Exercise results in an accelerated excretion of chromium, zinc and copper.[23] Those who exercise quite intensely experience repeated losses of these minerals. When high losses occur at the same time as low dietary consumption, the body suffers.

It is estimated that between 25 and 50 per cent of Americans have levels of chromium that are far too low. The same is true of other nations that have diets consisting mainly of processed foods. Most of us receive about 90 mcg (micrograms) of this nutrient daily, but only a mere 2 per cent of it (i.e. 1.8 mcg) is absorbed. The blood requires about 2 mcg to maintain healthy tissues. In other words, our diet should supply us with a minimum of 100 mcg of chromium each day.

Scientists have been able to duplicate biological and pathological changes – e.g. adult-onset diabetes, clogged arteries, fatigue and anxiety – under experimental conditions simply by introducing a chromium-deficient diet. 'When you consider that atherosclerosis can be induced experimentally by creating a chromium deficiency, it is only logical to conclude that a definite relationship exists between chromium deficiency and atherosclerosis,' says one leading authority.[24]

SELENIUM: HEAVY METAL FIGHTER

Hypertension, or sustained high blood pressure, is yet another condition that leads to heart failure or stroke. A number of preventive and curative nutritional measures have so far been substantiated in the fight against this condition. But there is another, albeit little known, nutrient that scientists have discovered can control hypertension as well.

Researchers at the Cleveland Clinic have reported that Americans living in an area where the soil has a low concentration of the trace element selenium run a three times greater risk of death from hypertension-induced strokes, aneurysms and heart attacks than people living in areas with high soil concentrations.[25] In one angina study, for example, researchers documented reduced symptoms in almost all of the patients who took daily doses of 1 mg of selenium and 200 IU of vitamin E.

Selenium's precise action in controlling blood pressure is not yet known, but studies on lab animals have produced the same results as the Cleveland survey. Researchers at the Community Cardiovascular Council in Savannah, Georgia may have provided another clue. When 10,000 high school students were tested in this low-selenium region, far too many of them were found to have abnormally high blood pressure for their age. In addition to low levels of selenium, the students had very high levels of the toxic heavy metal cadmium (*see later in this chapter*). Since cadmium has been proved to increase blood pressure when it builds up in the kidneys and liver, the researchers concluded that selenium prevents cadmium-caused hypertension, since selenium fights cadmium for the body's cell binding sites.[26]

Selenium offers many other health benefits. Besides controlling blood pressure, scientists have found it to be an important factor in cancer prevention and vital to the restoration of the immune system. Additionally, it assists in the elimination of environmental toxins from the body.

Scientists at Cornell University discovered that people with low blood selenium levels had four times the rate of skin cancer than those with high levels of the mineral. Others have concluded that selenium supplementation guards against breast cancer, especially when vitamin E is included. But selenium plays so many other roles. It helps the body resist infection from the yeast *Candida albicans*, guards against tissue damage from oxidation and contributes to male potency and fertility.[27]

How does selenium work? It is a component of the enzyme glutathione peroxidase (GP), a crucial factor in antioxidant function, which explains its role in preventing such modern diseases as cancer and cardiovascular conditions. GP is also an asset in red blood cell metabolism, and it prevents chromosome damage in tissue cultures.

Selenium appears to be especially effective in this respect when it is combined with vitamin E. Along with some other nutrients, these two are powerful weapons against ageing and what are today considered age-related diseases. This is directly attributable to the nutrient's antioxidant properties since tissue oxidation by free radicals is a contributing factor in degenerative diseases.

Soil with a poor content of selenium has also been directly linked with increased rates of cancer. Regions that have high concentrations of selenium in soil report extremely low rates of cancer, especially of the breast, colon and lung.

Considering the extraordinary function of selenium, it is astonishing to find that the body contains less than 1 mg of it. It's found in the liver, kidneys and pancreas and, in men, in the testes and seminal vesicles. Men require more selenium since it is involved in sperm production and movement. Fortunately, the body finds it far easier to obtain selenium than most of the minerals we already mentioned: this trace element has an absorption rate of about 60 per cent.

Selenium may best be obtained by eating brewer's yeast and wheat germ. Liver, lamb, fish and butter are also good sources. Additionally, whole grains, brown rice, nuts, vegetables and shellfish are quite rich in this mineral. Nutritionists believe that safe dosages for selenium supplementation should be 50 to 200 mcg. In the UK, the RNI stands at about 30 micrograms.

Overall, selenium can help prevent disease by increasing our resistance levels. Numerous exciting possibilities for selenium's use may come to light once more studies get under way. Today, it is known that it (along with other minerals) is effective in treating many inflammatory conditions, and it is showing great promise in alleviating problems associated with arthritis and certain autoimmune dysfunctions.

BORON: ON THE THRESHOLD

Another mineral on the threshold of great potential is the barely known boron, still technically classified as a 'possible essential trace element'. The bulk of it is found in the parathyroid glands, while it is believed to assist in the maintenance of calcium, thus further warding off osteoporosis. As a result, boron is also possibly linked to magnesium and phosphorus balance. If research continues in the direction it is already headed, boron may be found to be vital in the prevention of hypertension, atherosclerosis and arthritis. But considerably more evidence is required for validation.

Most of us are acquainted with the traditional use of boric acid for the skin and eyes in the form of an astringent and antiseptic. But its total physiological effect is yet to be understood.

Recently, however, researchers have discovered that boron deficiency causes changes in brain-wave patterns. This clearly shows a decline in alertness, according to experts at the US Department of Agriculture's Human Nutrition Research Center. Apparently, when you reduce dietary boron, you also get a drop in alpha-wave activity and an increase in the theta-wave activity on electro-encephalograms (EECs). That is the same kind of change you see when people become drowsy and less alert.

The subjects in this study ate meals containing no fruit or fruit juices and very few vegetables, so that they received approximately 0.25 mg of boron each day. Half of the group received an additional 3 mg supplement. Researchers noted that fast food, even if accompanied by vegetable toppings, is extremely boron deficient.

Other studies have further substantiated boron's effects on motor function. When boron-deficient individuals' reaction times were tested, they performed quite poorly. It appears that, during such a deficient state, activity is more coherent among some brain regions than in others. This can affect you in different ways, depending on what you are doing at the times you are particularly deficient. In other words, if you're taking a leisurely stroll, boron deficiency really won't affect you, but if you're driving a car, typing or monitoring a computer, that's quite another story.

Today, in the light of boron's low toxicity and our possible deficiency, estimates of adequate levels range between 3 and 5 mg. It has been suggested that a healthy diet of wholesome foods would provide about 3 mg of boron daily. But an excess of this nutrient, primarily through the use of boric acid, can cause nausea and vomiting, as well as anaemia, hair loss, skin disorders, seizures and nervous reactions. However, this is only likely if boric acid is actually ingested or you develop a high sensitivity to it.

The best sources of boron are foods grown in boron-rich soils, which includes most basic wholesome foods. Apples, pears and grapes are excellent choices, as are leafy green vegetables, pulses and nuts. Refined foods, again, will cause a serious boron deficiency just as they will with other nutrients.

ALUMINIUM: FROM POTS TO DEODORANTS

We have been looking at the minerals that our bodies require for optimal health, but there are also minerals we ingest that can have devastating consequences. Aluminium is one of these. Aluminium cooking utensils have been linked with the development of Alzheimer's disease, and British researchers have suggested that aluminium-rich drinking water may be a leading factor in its onset. Today, about 0.75 million people in

Britain suffer from some form of irreversible dementia, and of these, 60–70 per cent have Alzheimer's disease. Researchers have discovered extremely high levels of aluminium – 10 to 50 times normal are not uncommon – in the brains and nerve tissues of Alzheimer victims.

It may also be that aluminium reduces vitamin levels or that it binds DNA. In addition, it has been blamed for the weakening of the tissues of the gastrointestinal tract. Further, when antacids are taken, the aluminium contained in them has been known to bind pepsin and weaken protein digestion. Its astringent qualities can also dry tissues and mucous linings, as well as promote constipation. Additionally, the persistent use of deodorants (most of which list aluminium as the No. 1 ingredient) can actually clog underarm lymphatics and lead to breast problems such as cystic disease.

Aluminium is not easy to avoid, however, since it is the third most common element on Earth. The majority of us ingest 1–10 milligrams daily from food sources such as fruits and vegetables grown in aluminium-tainted soil. In the past, food additives were also a leading source, frequently used for the preservation of fruits and pickles and as an anti-caking agent. However, the EC now restricts the use of aluminium and its compounds to the external coating of confectionery and a few liqueurs. Still, it is quite easy to consume some 100 mg of aluminium daily, which is primarily stored in the brain, lungs, kidneys, liver and thyroid without us ever being aware of the problem.

You may be surprised to learn that the most abundant concentrations of this dangerous mineral are found in buffered aspirin and antacids containing aluminium hydroxide, as well as in cosmetics. Aluminium from these sources alone can add a staggering 500 to 5000 mg to your body each day. This fact makes the controversy over aluminium cookware laughable when you consider that it contributes a mere 0.7 mg of aluminium to your system.

The best way to determine toxic states of aluminium is a combination of hair, blood and urine analysis. Because most of us are often in contact with aluminium, we are all susceptible to its ill effects. Signs of aluminium poisoning include constipation, colicky pain, loss of appetite, nausea, gastrointestinal problems (including a reduction in the absorption of selenium and phosphorus from the gut), skin disorders and low levels of energy. As aluminium builds within your body, additional ailments may occur, such as muscle twitching, numbness, paralysis and fatty degeneration of the kidneys and liver. Aluminium toxicity can cause the loss of bone matrix and may result in osteomalacia, a softening of the bone. Many of the 20,000 residents of Camelford in Cornwall experienced at least some of these symptoms in 1988, when 20 tons of aluminium sulphate was accidentally dumped into their mains water supply.

Of course, becoming aware of how frequently aluminium enters your body is the first line of defence. Once a build-up does take place, there are effective ways of eliminating it. Oral chelating agents such as tetracycline are useful, as is calcium disodium edetate (EDTA) which clears out excess aluminium. Additionally, an iron chelation, known as deferoxamine, helps the body rid itself of the mineral. In one study with Alzheimer's patients, about 40 per cent experienced a significant improvement after deferoxamine therapy.

LEAD: HARM IN A COFFEE MUG

While aluminium consumption is of grave concern, lead's poisonous contributions can be lethal. Lead can cause serious harm to just about every organ in your body: the heart, liver and kidneys and the immune, reproductive, gastrointestinal and nervous systems. Each year, about a quarter of a million American children acquire lead poisoning, often through ingesting flakes of lead-based paints. Especially alarming is the quantity of lead found in reconstituted baby formula, which is accentuated when water from lead pipes is added to it. Simple exposure to lead can result in a lower IQ, low concentration levels, stunted growth and quite impaired learning and thinking abilities. With each study, researchers have found that levels of lead that used to be considered safe are way off the mark.

Like aluminium, lead finds its way innocently into our bodies. Tap water, decorated glassware, lead crystal, ceramic ware (including coffee mugs), foil wrappings and some food cans are all common sources. Although government guidelines exist for lead safety in the products we buy, manufacturers don't necessarily follow them. In the United States, the Environmental Defense Fund, in cooperation with the California attorney general, has taken legal action against ten ceramics manufacturers that distribute in that country, including such well-known names as Wedgwood, Lenox and Pfalzgraff.[28]

Lead is created so deep in the Earth that it has only surfaced in the past 4000 years as a by-product of silver smelting. Scientists believe it may have led to the downfall of the Roman Empire! The Romans decided lead was the perfect mineral for water pipes and drinking vessels. This practice may very well have resulted in decreased mental function and birthrate and an increase in deaths. But we didn't learn from the Romans' experience, and in the modern era, lead soon found its way into paint, petrol, insecticides, tin cans and other products. The higher-octane additive in petrol has been the most consistent and devastating source of environmental pollution ever known.

As the world's greatest lead contributor, the United States has passed some legislation to help curb its overabundance, but the problem is still widespread. Many older homes have lead paint on their walls, and while unleaded petrol is now increasingly common in America, the harmful effects of carbon monoxide and hydrocarbons continue to poison the environment and, eventually, us. Lead cannot be got rid of easily; when it gets into the soil, it does not degrade. Scientists who have examined centuries-old skeletal remains have concluded that, today, we have some 600 to 1000 times greater levels of lead in our bodies than our prehistoric ancestors did. The US uses about 1.3 tons of lead a year in petrol, paint, pottery, batteries and pigments, among other products. Some 400,000 to 600,000 tons is released into the atmosphere and, thus, into our food and our tissues.

Lead poisoning has, like aluminium contamination, also been successfully reduced with EDTA therapy, and other, more controversial therapies exist. However, the safest way to reduce high levels of lead in your body is through a high-calcium diet. Some physicians accomplish this through injections of calcium chloride in combination with vitamin D. Vitamin C and the amino acids cysteine and methionine also assist in the detoxification of lead and other poisons. Foods that contain these amino acids – for example, beans and eggs – are excellent sources for lead elimination.

These measures are important to take since this heavy metal is the most common toxic mineral and the No. 1 contaminant of the environment and the body. It rates third in toxicity, right behind cadmium and mercury. Nevertheless, high levels of lead can be fatal.

CADMIUM: OVERLOAD AND TOXICITY

There is widespread environmental poisoning with cadmium, too. Like lead, it is a mineral found deep within the Earth, but it became a significant part of our air, water and food when it was brought to the surface during the mining of zinc.

Cadmium can be a cause of high blood pressure that may lead to heart disease. In animal studies, high levels of cadmium produced an increase in the size of the heart, high blood pressure, atherosclerosis and poor kidney function. It tends to be stored in the kidneys and may cause serious tissue damage there, as well as calcium kidney stones. This mineral has a close relationship with zinc; thus, cadmium's toxicity is more powerful if you are zinc deficient, and it can be kept under greater control if you are adequately supplied with zinc.

Your immune system can also suffer as a result of cadmium overload. Bacteria and viruses can easily grow in a high-cadmium system. Lung and prostate cancer may result as well. Most recently, cadmium toxicity has been associated with prostate enlargement. An excess of cadmium also causes bone and joint aches and pains. It can actually weaken bones, resulting in easy fractures and breaks, or deformities of the spine. Very often, high levels of cadmium in the body are fatal.

With increasing daily exposure to cadmium, many experts claim that this is already resulting in an increased incidence of emphysema and anaemia. But much more research is required to substantiate its complete ill health.

At present, the best way to ward off cadmium contamination is by avoiding processed foods, cigarette smoke, shellfish, coffee, tea and salt water. Coal burning also lends a good deal of cadmium to the environment. Additionally, you should eat foods high in zinc such as whole grains, pulses and nuts.

In grain, cadmium latches on to the core of the kernel; zinc, on the other hand, is in the germ and bran. So when grains are processed, the zinc is eliminated and cadmium preserved. As a result, refined flour, rice and sugar are relatively high in the toxic mineral and low in the essential one.

The average smoker inhales about 20 mcg of cadmium daily, nearly half of it going into his or her lungs and the greater portion into the atmosphere which poisons second-hand smoke breathers. The body eliminates some of the cadmium, but some of it is stored in the tissues every single day.

But even if you are careful about your diet and environment, cadmium can find its way into you via your water pipes – the mineral is frequently used to guard metals from corrosion. In areas of 'soft' water, which is a corrosive, cadmium and other minerals are released when the pipe metals deteriorate. 'Hard' water, which contains calcium and magnesium salts, coats metal pipes and guards against the leaching of additional, possibly toxic minerals.

Soil becomes cadmium-rich due to water and sewage contamination, air pollution and high-phosphate fertilizers. As a result of all this cadmium, damage to the body tissues by free radicals is greatly increased.

MERCURY

Mercury is also highly poisonous. As with lead and cadmium, modern humans contain far higher levels of this toxic mineral than their ancestors did. It has been around for some 2000 years, and is still being used as a medicine! Dental fillings are also still frequently laden with this dangerous element, as are some cosmetics and some of our food, since fungicides and pesticides containing it are commonly used in agriculture. Industrial waste contaminated with mercury has poisoned our water, fish and plants.

We can ingest mercury from air, food and water. When mercury fumes are inhaled, they pass through the lungs and find their way into the blood. The kidneys store about half the body's mercury, while the blood, bones, liver, spleen, brain and fat tissue hold the rest. Central nervous symptoms often result since mercury attacks the brain and nerve tissues. It is also believed to interfere with the proper functioning of selenium. A major fear is that this toxic mineral is an immunosuppressant.

Acute symptoms of mercury poisoning include fever, chills, coughing and chest pain. Lower exposures generally cause fatigue, headaches, insomnia, poor coordination, anxiety, emotional distress and lack of sex drive. These ailments may be followed by nervous symptoms such as dizziness, tremors and depression. As poisoning continues, numbness and tingling of the hands, feet or lips, followed by greater weakness and loss of memory as well as hearing and speech problems and, in some cases, even paralysis and psychosis may occur. Some experts have linked mercury toxicity with multiple sclerosis. In extreme cases, brain damage and birth defects have been reported. Although the extreme symptoms are rare, unfortunately the subtle and nervous system problems that result from low but constant exposure to mercury are far more common than we would care to admit.

As stated at the beginning of this chapter, some 60 minerals have been found in the human body. The aim here has been to offer a glimpse of their importance and to give you reason to investigate further as your particular needs require. In the years to come, nutritional medicine will rely far more on minerals than it has to date, and they may even be valued more highly than vitamins. Since our bodies do not manufacture minerals and they are more difficult to obtain from foods due to low levels of absorption, deficiencies are far more common than we may realize.

CHAPTER SEVEN

NEW AGE
STRESS

'**C**an you read my mind?' was the cheeky question posed to a holistic healer by a nuclear physicist who had travelled from Chicago to Phoenix in search of any solution for his chronic pain.

'Why on earth would I want to wander in that mess of confusion?' was her reply.

Constant backaches, headaches and joint pains had led David to the United States' leading medical experts in search of the cause of his pain. But, after four years of extensive investigation, all tests had shown absolutely no abnormalities and David was sent to orthodox physiotherapists for exercise, ultrasound and water therapy. This had mild benefits for David, but most of his aches and pains persisted. He then flew to New York and saw one of the world's leading orthopaedic surgeons, who mercilessly scrutinized his medical records from the beginning and thoroughly examined David himself.

The long-awaited diagnosis finally came, but it was just about the last thing David wanted to hear. The good doctor had come to the conclusion that David's physical pains were self-inflicted by mental chaos and emotional anguish. His 'triple-A personality', as the doctor called it, had put David into overdrive, and his body could no longer function with the constant 'flight or fight' demands that David slavishly placed on it.

David went ballistic! He told the doctor that he did not pay him exorbitant fees only to be patronized, belittled and humoured, nor did he intend for his case to amuse the surgeon. He stormed out of the office. His anger, resentment and disappointment grew as he began to calculate all the time, effort and money that had gone into his four-year quest for pain relief. As David tensed up even more, his pain intensified. He swallowed a maximum dose of painkillers and muscle relaxants and tried to get some sleep on the plane home, but as he put it, 'I couldn't shut down the activity between the ears.'

Weeks passed. David simmered down a bit and began to think about what the surgeon had said. He even began to discuss the issue with close friends – a first for David, since he usually felt that revealing emotions was a waste of time *and* a source of entertainment for those who had the luxury of engaging in 'pity parties'. A strange thing happened when David repeated bits of the doctor's analysis. One by one, his friends each said more or less the same thing: 'Oh, I could have told you that!' 'You've been burning both ends of the candle ever since I've known you.' One even said, 'You're brilliant at your career, but at times I think you must be mad to drive yourself as hard as you do.'

David was floored, but still he tried to rationalize his situation. All his actions and efforts were legitimate, he told himself, required, necessary, crucial! 'Few bricks short of a load,' replied a colleague.

Over the next months, David tried to assess this new-found awareness. He began closely to monitor the events in his life and the occurrence of his pain. Sure enough, a correlation existed. He located an osteopath who recommended mind control techniques. David had once considered such methods – creative visualization, meditation, biofeedback, hypnosis and other therapeutic relaxation techniques – to be somewhat akin to voodoo. This time, however, he gave himself permission to try one or two. He would engage in some mind control activities but wouldn't really expect any results. A bad start, but better than none at all.

This led to David's encounter with the healer in Phoenix. He was appalled by her response. He was equally amazed that she didn't appear to be sufficiently impressed with who he was. 'My mind is filled with complicated matters,' he said, 'which, to the lay person, may appear to be confusion.'

'Right,' she said, ignoring his pompous explanation.

And so David's exploration of the mind/body connection began, a connection that many experts have already established and whose value they are substantiating with each passing day. Many aware individuals are already making use of this vital information, while countless others, like David, are either unaware of it or have consigned it to the realms of science fiction.

Today, however, even the strictest of orthodox practitioners accept that the mind has the power to heal. Disease is a total body response. Approaches such as visualization, biofeedback and meditation, among others, allow stress to be eliminated from the body before it can accumulate and cause physical disorders. The ability to bring about self-healing, increased energy and a state of peace is all within our grasp, just waiting to be utilized.

Dr Gerald Epstein of the Mount Sinai Medical Center in New York City is a believer. He has come to the conclusion that we can literally 'wish' our emotional and physical problems away. He talks about a 'waking dream therapy' in which 'you can learn to use images [visual and intellectual portrayals of your emotions] to change old emotional experiences and create new ones.' Dr Epstein believes that, 'instead of simply reacting or adjusting to past experiences, you build fresh ones by changing stagnant beliefs. There's no such thing as a physical illness that doesn't affect the mind, or an emotional problem that doesn't get translated into body language or pain.'[1]

CREATIVE VISUALIZATION

Visualization, in particular, is currently a widely used discipline, especially among athletes and people suffering a multitude of medical conditions. As you begin to rid yourself of limits to what you think is possible, a whole new world begins to open up. In creative visualization, you simply relax deeply and picture the state you wish to be in, leaving all other thoughts behind.

The success that élite athletes have had with visualization encouraged a team of researchers at the University of Louisiana in New Orleans to see if it could actually be used to increase strength. They concluded that such a mental workout boosts and strengthens a physical one, and recommended that mental practice be included in physical rehabilitation programmes such as those after surgery or prolonged immobilization, to speed up recovery.[2]

Athletes have known about and successfully practised creative visualization for years. When you think of an Olympic training session, a picture of an athlete sitting or lying down quietly does not usually pop into the mind. Yet those at the top of their respective fields realize that mental training is a crucial part of physical conditions. American gold medallist Dick Fosbury describes the effect it had on his performance as a high jumper some 20 years ago:

I BEGAN TO DEVELOP MY STYLE DURING HIGH SCHOOL COMPETITION, WHEN MY BODY SEEMED TO REACT TO THE CHALLENGE OF THE BAR. I BECAME CHARGED BY THE DESIRE AND WILL TO ACHIEVE SUCCESS. THEN I DEVELOPED A TOUGH PROCESS IN ORDER TO REPEAT A SUCCESSFUL JUMP. I WOULD PSYCHE MYSELF UP, CREATE A PICTURE, FEEL A SUCCESSFUL JUMP – THE PERFECT JUMP – AND DEVELOP A POSITIVE ATTITUDE TO MAKE THE JUMP. MY SUCCESS CAME FROM THE VISUALIZATION AND IMAGING PROCESS.[3]

Visualization, or imaging, can greatly enhance whatever you wish to achieve. Getting started appears to be the most difficult part for most people, although actually practising visualization is ridiculously simple. The first thing you need to do is to make yourself comfortable and concentrate on your breathing. Feel every sensation as you inhale and exhale in a rhythmic fashion. Create a steady rhythm as you breathe. Next, it is vital to clear your mind. This may appear challenging at first, but ridding yourself entirely of all thoughts will become much easier as you progress.

Now, what is it you wish to achieve? Say, you have to give a speech. Plot out a detailed, specific and realistic mental script depicting yourself actually giving it. Imagine walking up to the podium looking confident, assured, cheerful, enthusiastic, well groomed, well dressed, your speech well prepared and rehearsed, the audience waiting to greet you. Anticipate a bit of the nervous energy that you'll experience as you begin to address your audience and see yourself gaining control as well as their confidence. Now hear and see yourself speaking intelligently and authoritatively, yet in an entertaining way. See your audience's enthusiastic reactions and feel their welcome. Now think about coming to a successful conclusion. Relish your relief and satisfaction. When you actually do give the speech, you will recall these images and good feelings, and this will guide you past any tough moments while you maintain grace under pressure.

In the above exercise, you got yourself started. Now you can begin to master your emotions. Always begin in a comfortable physical state, with rhythmic breathing and an emptied mind. Now examine everything about the place where you will give the speech. Imagine yourself exploring the room foot by foot. Back row, front row, aisles, exits, noting the location of the podium, loudspeakers, water glass and so on, and being aware of the lighting, temperature and all the rest. Give yourself permission to feel nervous tension, anxiety, stage fright and all the emotions that go into a performance. If you wish, even allow yourself to feel the desire to cancel the whole darn thing and move on to something else.

Now go over the entire scenario once again and give the speech, but rewrite the script. Relish the parts of the experience that you enjoy, such as the lines you know will generate great interest or a roaring laugh from the crowd. Savour the knowledge that certain important members of the audience will find you intelligent, well informed and devastatingly attractive. Imagine your adrenaline rising and your body becoming weightless as you deliver this splendid speech. See your confidence and authoritativeness fill the room.

Be certain that every imaging procedure you perform is satisfactory to you. You really can't fake emotions or lie to your body. But dealing with your emotions beforehand can help you work through difficult areas. You can experience a genuine sense of selfmastery that will prove invaluable in all your endeavours.

After you practise these three exercises, you may move along even further. At this point, you want to find your optimal level of alertness for a super performance. About half an hour before your speech, find a quiet place and regulate your breathing while you clear your mind. Now think about your feet. Are your shoes creating any tension in them? If so, see yourself blowing the tension out of your feet as you exhale. As you take a deep breath, feel revitalizing energy occupying your inner space. Repeat exhaling tension and inhaling energy step by step throughout your entire body until all nervousness, anxiety and tension has been replaced by vitality, strength and energy.

THE POWER OF THE RIGHT BRAIN   The success of creative visualization can be attributed to the mind's unique ability to think in two distinct ways. Half of the brain's process is logical, which allows us to compute mathematics and master language; this takes place in the left hemisphere. (Computers perform similar logical functions, but do so at speeds beyond our capacity.) Our right brain, however, performs holistically – that is, all information is examined at one time as a whole. This type of awareness controls our visual, emotional and intuitive thinking. In many ways, the holistic-functioning right hemisphere is superior to the sequential mode of the left brain. No computer exists today that can 'think' or function like the right brain. In fact, neural network research is *the* field of computer design right now.

Undoubtedly, the power of the right brain holds great promise for those who know how to utilize it. Experts say there are three basic methods for obtaining right brain superiority: Think visually, draw pictures and sleep on it.[4] If this sounds a bit unrealistic or simplistic, it's because you are thinking with the left brain now.

Creative visualization and positive imagery permit the right brain to go to work for you. For example, when you drive a car, sew a garment or fix a bike, the right brain is performing. When driving, you don't calculate distances with mathematical formulae; instead the right brain usually analyses the road ahead and automatically tells you which way to go. Regardless of the task before you, visualization will allow for a better outcome.

Your right brain can provide you with creative solutions if you allow it to do so. First of all, think deeply about your problem. For best results, gather all the information required and consider it consciously. If no solution presents itself and you are at your wits' end, then simply let it go. Forget about the problem and let your right brain take over. If you wish to resolve the problem badly enough, the right brain will provide a solution. In due time, you may get a flash of insight when you least expect it.

Regardless of what you may be doing or thinking at the time, the right brain will forward its information to the left brain and your solution will be at hand.

DRAWING AND DREAMING   One method for sharpening right-brain function is to draw pictures, which greatly enhances your brain's visual capacity. The saying that a picture is worth a thousand words reflects right-brain powers. For instance, when you wish to remember someone's name or would like easily to recall information you are hearing or reading, it is important to make a visual association, to draw pictures of it in your mind. This can also work in a literal sense – create actual drawings, diagrams, flow charts, maps, stick figures, whatever the situation calls for at the moment. Virtually any visual representation of specific information will increase your powers of recall and further assist you in understanding it.

Additionally, creative thinking can result through right-brain awareness. Drawing pictures works here as well. The right brain and creative thinking go hand in hand, but since our communication abilities occupy the left brain the right brain is at a loss for words when trying to communicate its thoughts. Imagine having such a treasure house full of solutions and innovative ideas which cannot be unlocked in the traditional way – i.e. verbally – but is there, just waiting for you. You can deal with this dilemma quite easily. Simply communicate with your right brain visually. 'Idea sketching' has been employed by creative individuals throughout time. Sketch freely any ideas as they pop into your mind. Putting your ideas on paper allows you to contemplate and modify their meaning.

That master of the right brain, Leonardo da Vinci, communicated virtually through sketching alone. In notebooks comprising thousands of pages, he explored anatomy and created numerous mechanical devices by engaging in detailed sketching and further refining of his ideas. By transferring the pictures from his mind to paper, Da Vinci employed the powers of his right brain which allowed him to recognize patterns and gave him the ability to associate and assemble in a creative manner what must initially have appeared to be unrelated items.

As Aristotle so accurately stated: 'The soul . . . never thinks without a picture.' Imagery is really the basis of our thought processes. Much evidence exists to support the claim that we thought in images long before we developed language. Even today, as we enter this world as newborns, before we learn to speak, we primarily experience the world visually. Soon enough we learn language to describe what we see, think and feel, and many of us even lose the natural instinct to see, think, and feel on a sensory level. It has been claimed that the genius of Shakespeare resides, in large part, in his massive vocabulary which he constantly utilized to evoke sights, sounds, textures, smells and tastes that wake within us that which we once possessed and now have lost.

Yet another means of strengthening right-brain performance is, quite literally, to sleep on it. Indeed, the unconscious state is a time when the right brain can perform quite well. Sometimes ideas pop into your head out of nowhere, and you may even receive a solution to your problem through a dream.

Some of us rely more on the 'sleeping solution' than others. We are in very good company. Einstein dreamed of his theory of relativity, Niels Bohr dreamed of the model of the atom and Friedrich Kekulé von Stradonitz saw the chemical structure of the benzene ring while asleep.

This is not to imply that you should not fully utilize the logical powers of your left brain. But when it fails to produce results effectively and rapidly enough, switch gears and eventually master the use of both brains simultaneously.

MEDITATION

The power of the mind to control and heal is multifaceted. Along with creative visualization, millions of people have found life-enhancing qualities as a result of meditation. Simply put, meditation is a state of restful alertness and heightened awareness. If you ask a hundred people to explain what meditation does for them, you will most likely get a hundred different answers. Meditation is a most personal and subjective experience that takes place solely in your mind. It is unique to you. When you sit down to meditate, you can, with practice, actually close out the entire world and live only in 'the moment'. Imagine not being distressed over the past or anxious about the future, to have your mind and all of your emotions bathed in stillness, in absolute peace! You come to a state of simply 'being'. There is something incredibly rewarding to the mind, body and spirit when you are able to reach this state of complete restfulness, and advocates swear that it can help lead you to a more productive life.

For thousands of years in the East, meditation has been a powerful tool for personal growth, but in a mere two decades, it has become a daily way of life for millions of Westerners, too. It is recommended and practised by medical doctors to combat stress and aid in the prevention and healing of a multitude of stress-related illnesses, from heart problems to cancer, ringing in the ears, chronic back pain and AIDS.

Recently, the University of Miami Medical School revealed an extraordinary finding, claiming that aerobics and relaxation techniques such as meditation may equal the benefits of the drug AZT (zidovudine) used to treat HIV infection and AIDS. These two therapies alone seemed actually to increase T-cell counts for people with HIV infections.[5] Researchers reported that HIV-positive men who practised relaxation techniques or aerobic exercise had higher blood levels of CD4 cells and remained healthier longer. The increases in helper cells were about the same as if the patients had taken AZT. In addition, Michael Antoni, the psychologist who directed the study, said that it was evident that the more the subjects practised a relaxation exercise over the first five weeks of the study, the less depressed and anxious they were and the higher their helper cell counts. Thus, although relaxation and exercise do not cure this tough disease, they can certainly help to improve the quality and duration of life.

Much discussion and exploration in the medical community has centred on the concept that all diseases are somehow linked to a weakened immune system. Hence, anything that you can do to enhance the strength of the immune system is of benefit for people with HIV as well as those with other health concerns.

Other recent reports point out the contribution that meditation can made to the alleviation of back pain. Dr Jon Kabat-Zinn, founder and director of the Stress Reduction and Relaxation Center at the University of Massachusetts Medical Center in Worcester, says that sufferers of chronic back pain can learn to control their pain through deep breathing and meditation techniques derived from Eastern philosophies.[6] This has also been the finding of pain clinics in the UK. At one, the Centre of Pain Relief at the Walton Hospital in Liverpool, hundreds of those suffering from chronic back pain, as well as other types, are taught meditation, creative visualization and self-hypnosis to help them manage their pain.

It's no longer hearsay that psychological factors and mental states have a profound effect on pain and recovery. There is now clear evidence that fear, worry, depression and tiredness increase pain, while joy, calmness, confidence and goodwill have the opposite effect. Therefore, whatever the source of pain or discomfort, the ability to control it would be a powerful quality to possess. One study showed that 72 per cent of meditating patients experienced at least a 33 per cent reduction in pain, while 61 per cent showed at least a 50 per cent reduction.[7]

Meditation can also have benefits in disease of the circulatory system, particularly high blood pressure. According to a number of well-designed studies, regular meditation can reduce blood pressure significantly in many people with hypertension,[8] and can have other effects as well. This research was carried out by the cardiologist Dr Herbert Benson of the Harvard Medical School, who is also the director of the hypertension and behavioural medicine departments of the Beth Israel Hospital in Boston, Massachusetts. Dr Benson has been investigating the effects of meditation on blood pressure for many years; as long ago as 1980 he publicized his findings in the popular book, *The Relaxation Response*.

Since the severe heart muscle pain of angina occurs when there is not enough oxygen to meet the heart's requirement, Dr Benson decided to find out if meditation reduces the rate of the heart and, thus, its oxygen requirements. He found that as a result of meditation, the oxygen consumption decreases by 10 to 20 per cent, becoming effective within the first three minutes of meditation. This is exactly what happens when angina sufferers take the drug Inderal (propranolol), but minus the harmful side-effects, which can include tiredness on exercise, intestinal upsets, dry eyes and skin rashes. Dr Benson discovered that meditation brings a far deeper state of relaxation than does sleep, which decreases oxygen consumption by only a mere 8 per cent and then only after some five hours.

Dr Benson's studies further showed that meditation can help control arrhythmias (irregular heartbeats). One type of these – ventricular fibrillation – can lead to sudden death, when the heart quivers instead of beating and cannot pump blood adequately. Hence, by reducing the occurrence of abnormal heartbeats, you may be literally saving your life.

At the Brigham and Women's Hospital in Boston and the Harvard School of Public Health, meditation is taught to numerous patients with arrhythmias as a complementary therapy to their medication. The results show that 30 per cent of the participants actually decrease the frequency of irregular heartbeats – at times, dramatically. Two of three patients with ventricular tachycardia (an acutely accelerated heartbeat) established a normal heart rhythm within three minutes of meditation.[9]

FROM THE OLD TESTAMENT TO MODERN-DAY CHICAGO

Meditation techniques are not reserved only for practitioners of Eastern religions. The oldest form of meditation in Christianity involved taking a word or phrase from prayer and carrying that word or phrase with you, letting it repeat itself in your mind and on your lips until it lived in your heart. Jewish tradition also incorporates meditation. In the ancient mystical branch of Judaism known as cabbala, there is a ritual involving meditation on the four Hebrew letters that make up the name of God; through this, one was to attain a union with the divine.

Indeed, in the Scriptures, there are numerous references to meditation. In the book of Joshua it says, 'This book of the law shall not depart out of thy mouth, but thou shalt meditate therein day and night . . .' (Joshua 1:8). Psalms 46:10 literally exhorts: 'Be still, and know that I am God.' Later, the psalmist writes: 'My mouth shall speak of wisdom; and the meditation of my heart shall be of understanding' (Psalms 49:3).

Recently, a group of parents in Chicago were in an uproar when they found out that their children were being taught meditation in school. They said they had their own Christian prayers and did not want their offspring to receive this ungodly teaching. But, clearly, God's word endorses the idea of meditation.

Jesus was certainly known to withdraw from the public on occasion, to reach God through prayer and meditation. Whether it is referred to as meditation or contemplative prayer, Christians throughout the ages have engaged in it. St John and St Paul both experienced the heights of Christ-consciousness; St Paul wrote: 'I live; yet not I, but Christ liveth in me' (Galatians 2:20). Towards the end of the 4th century AD, St Augustine, in his *Confessions*, examined the meditative procedures that stirred his spiritual being. Other great thinkers resorted to the practice. Dante and Meister Eckhardt, writers and scholars of the 13th and 14th centuries, combined biblical insight and meditation with great intellectual ability. In the 16th century, the Spanish saint Teresa of Avila was intensely engaged in direct communication with God through meditation. Her friend St John of the Cross produced a wealth of works on Christian meditation.

By now, you may be thinking that meditation is the monopoly of Catholic saints. Not so. Martin Luther and John Wesley were both great practitioners of meditation, with the aim of gaining greater awareness of the presence of God. The Protestant Jacob Bolheme wrote extensively about meditation, and George Fox, the founder of the Society of Friends, taught followers to listen to the 'still small voice' from within. Peter Poiret and the English mystical poet William Blake further explored and wrote about the powers of meditation.

This may lead some to think that meditation is an intellectual activity. Quite the contrary. It is an increase in the quality and depth of our complete awareness. Others may consider meditation to be a form of escapism. This is false. Meditation is a tuning in, not a tuning out. Many of those who have experienced a high state of awareness with meditation have unquestionably lived lives of greatest service to humanity.

LIVING IN THE MOMENT   Today, there appears to be plenty of things to become stressed about and a greater need than ever to have some sense of order in our lives. You can't pick up a newspaper or turn on the television without being reminded that all is not well with the world. But the worst source of stress is not actually the result of the atrocities and difficulties we see and hear about. The worse source of stress is in our own minds. All our talk about world peace is quite insignificant if we do not have peace in our own lives.

With so many stimuli fighting for our attention from external sources as well as from within, it becomes quite difficult to concentrate on any one thing for any length of time. Our thoughts seem to leap from one subject to the next, and we appear to have no control over them. You know the scenario: 'Is this really what I should be doing with my time now? . . . I know the report is due on Friday, but I just can't work on it now even though I know I should. . . . If I don't make an appointment to have the cat fixed, that damn neighbour's cat will have her pregnant again. . . . I really have to keep that lunch appointment with Elizabeth, although that report is due on Friday!'

We all have thoughts about things we can do nothing about. We all have thoughts about what we should be doing right now. We all have thoughts about the future – usually worries about things that never actually see the light of day. We dwell disproportionately on these sorts of things and rarely have a sense that all is well with the world. The end-result: stress, confusion, loss of control, illness.

But try to remember a time when you were totally absorbed in the moment. This is very easy for children to do. It comes naturally to them. But somehow we lose this ability when we become adults. Imagine that you took a walk on a brisk winter day, and the beauty of a dark grey barren tree against a powder-blue sky caught your attention. You gazed at it for several moments and felt yourself sigh, the tranquillity of the sight entering you for a moment. It was a relaxing experience, wasn't it? By the time you walked back home, a sense of peace and even happiness possibly came over you. What you experienced was a breath of fresh mental air. For those few moments, your mind was free. You were not contemplating any important decisions. You were not sitting in judgement over anyone. You weren't concerned about the job, the mortgage, the kids. Imagine having this sort of experience for 20 minutes, half an hour or a full hour, once or twice a day. The end-result – true relaxation – can work wonders in your life.

Thus, 'living in the moment' becomes the key to success. But how do we achieve such a state of mind? First, you need to learn how to quiet yourself down. You need to bring about a state of deep physical relaxation, coupled with a highly alert mental state. As a result, you will experience a lowered metabolism rate, a slower heartbeat, decreased respiration, reduced levels of lactate (a waste product) in your blood, and changes in brainwave patterns. This state of relaxation is very different from calm sleep, sitting in a quiet corner, or even hypnosis. One might assume that the mind would go 'wobbly' under these circumstances, but quite the opposite is true. Imagine habitual freedom from anxiety, restlessness, tension and depression. That is the result of regular meditation.

Although physical changes are an obvious outcome of meditation, among the other subjective sensations that eventually occur after you've been meditating for a while is an overall feeling of well-being, a sense of lightness, ease and tranquillity. Your senses seem to have awakened, colours appear brighter, food tastes better, your movements are more graceful and you possess greater energy.

A clear association has been made between our state of mind and our health. Hence, if physical illness can be caused by tension, emotional turmoil, deep-rooted resentments, fears, guilt and anxiety, then learning to control them can certainly bring you closer to a state of well-being.

You can break the worry-tension-illness cycle by combining physical exercise with regular meditation. We tense up far more than we realize. Just about any thoughts or actions produce some level of anxiety. But when you consciously relax muscular tension, you are less likely to continue holding on to negativity and stress. This is especially true when you find yourself in an irritating situation. What happens when you get angry? Well, you generally clench your jaw and tense up your neck and shoulder muscles, your stomach may begin to churn, you breathe faster, press your lips together, squint your eyes and clench your fists! Now it would be quite difficult to react this way if you were relaxed, wouldn't it?

In others words, you have a choice. You can allow turmoil to rule your life, or you can control the turmoil. You really have to make a conscious decision to find a better way of handling your stress or it will win by default. But it's not enough simply to tell yourself how you would react; you must condition and prepare yourself for it as do athletes for their sports or students for their exams. Once or twice a day, you must simply eliminate stress through meditation and regain control over your mind and body.

Some may have difficulty believing in a practice, the benefits of which they cannot actually see at first. After all, an athlete's conditioning has quite visible results. But think of energy for a moment. There is not one centimetre of the universe that is not occupied by it, but there are very few signs of it. For instance, our eyes have the ability to see less than one-millionth of all the radiation around us, but we accept the fact that the invisible energy is really there. Some scientists even accept the hypothesis that, during meditation, a life-force is released that is more significant than nuclear energy.

After a time, those who meditate regularly are delighted to discover that they have a choice in how they will act and react in all situations. You are not a speck of matter destined to be tossed about aimlessly by external forces. You are a vehicle in control of those forces, and you can use them to gain greater strength.

It can be said that the stress of living today claims more lives than the plague did in the 14th century. Lifestyles had to be altered to deal with the plague, and now we must resort to measures for dealing with stress.

FOCUSING AND REFOCUSING   Perhaps the best way to begin a meditation session is first to do a few warm-up and deep breathing exercises. When you sit down to meditate – on the floor or in a chair, or even lying down, whatever is most comfortable for you – you'll feel more relaxed if you have done some gentle stretching and isometric exercises. A walk or warm bath or gentle massage beforehand can also get you into the right physical state. Deep breathing requires you to fill your lungs completely, with as much air as possible. As you inhale, slowly mentally count down from eight. Then hold the air for another eight counts, and then exhale for eight seconds more. You may repeat this half a dozen times.

By now you should feel sufficiently warmed up and relaxed to begin meditating. It's important to note that there are a wide variety of meditation types, but for purposes of introduction, we shall cover only the basics here.

Initially, you should choose a simple word or phrase – perhaps one from your faith, or you could follow Dr Benson's advice and simply say 'One'. Whatever you choose, repeat it silently to yourself, in sync with your steady rhythmic breathing. At first, random thoughts will surely cross your mind, but you should focus and refocus on the work or phrase you are saying. Soon, you will genuinely enjoy this brief state of calm and restfulness. You can begin this simple meditation practice with ten-minute sessions about two or three times a day.

This simple daily event will give you a sense of tranquillity, not just while meditating but throughout the day. The continual daily practice will help you to learn how better to maintain your equilibrium most of the time.

Another way of meditating is to calm yourself, do the relaxation and deep breathing exercises, then sit down straight and still in a quiet place, closing your eyes and try to think about absolutely nothing except for one object for focusing. (e.g. a rose petal – not the smell, touch, size, colour, etc., just the image of the petal). You carry on focusing on this for as long as you feel comfortable – from five minutes at first to even hours as you become more advanced. Usually, 20 minutes twice a day is quite sufficient. But the more time you can remain focused while in a meditative state, the greater the rewards. Advanced meditators can actually become so absorbed in the present moment that they lose all track of time.

You may think at first that this is too much of a luxury of time, considering your hectic schedule. But that's precisely why you need to take the time to recharge yourself and resharpen your senses. It will give you more mileage for your energy. Think of all the minutes in your day that are actually wasted, through waiting, anxiety, indecision, coffee or cigarette breaks, unnecessary phone calls, or simply through sloppy use of time. Somewhere in your day there are definitely 20 minutes you can use to serve yourself. After all, when the rewards from doing so include increased efficiency and a reduced sleep requirement, you will more than compensate for the time you have allocated to meditation.

Don't forget that the experience of meditation is quite different for everyone. It is crucial to approach the practice with an open mind and allow it to unfold in its own way without direct effort or guidance from your conscious mind. Don't set yourself up with preconceived ideas about what you should or wish to experience. The meditation will guide you; you should not guide it. It's enough to know that simply learning to clear your mind of all thoughts and focusing on one word or on one object will provide you with enormous relaxation and will thus result in great benefits.

It's also important to note that meditation is an ongoing changing experience, and the adventure may be quite different from day to day. Sometimes you will feel sheer joy and happiness, that all's well with your world. At other times, it will be difficult to clear your head of all the distracting thoughts that are fighting eagerly for your attention. Attempt to rid yourself of all the emotions provoked within you simply by imagining that each intruding thought dissolves as it crops up. If you don't acknowledge and engage in communication with the interrupting thoughts, you can easily and slowly return to your meditative state.

If you are just beginning to meditate, make a firm decision not to be judgemental or hard on yourself if it doesn't go as smoothly as you expected. You may want to try out different types of meditation and find the one that suits you best. There are no definite rules and you are not in competition with yourself or others. Meditation is simply your own private, quiet domain that provides you with a release from the hectic experiences of your day. It's your recharging system. Your reward.

Visualization and meditation are thus excellent contributors to our emotional, psychological and physical well-being. After all, when you control your mind, you have the ability to achieve great things. When your mind controls you, you are a slave to your ego and your emotions. By learning to visualize and meditate, your mind learns how to quiet down and, as a result, elevates your consciousness.

BIOFEEDBACK

In modern times, our attention spans have suffered a severe reduction. This makes the practice of mind control techniques quite unappealing to many people at first. Most of us have the desire to improve, to gain control of our lives, but we are short on perseverance. However, when you experience that extraordinary feeling of great peace and calm, there will be little that can hold you back. For centuries, Eastern mystics have claimed that this should be our natural state of being. Imagine feeling and functioning in this state of peace and tranquillity at all times!

Today, physicians are beginning to prescribe some control techniques to go along with orthodox care and, in some cases, when orthodox treatment has failed altogether. This is especially the case with biofeedback. Biofeedback training involves the use of electronic devices to tell people how their bodies are functioning and teaches them how, by trial and error, they can influence organs or systems that are generally not under conscious control, such as blood pressure and brain wave activity. At times, this technique is used to regain control of what has been lost as a result of injury or illness. Biofeedback may be used clinically to treat many conditions, such as hypertension, insomnia, migraine, incontinence, chronic pain, stress, tinnitus, anxiety disorders and Raynaud's syndrome.

How biofeedback actually works has been much debated, but surprisingly this hasn't prevented its broad use by many mainstream physicians. The esteemed Mayo Clinic, Cleveland Clinic and the House Ear Institute in the United States all rely on biofeedback. More recently, researchers have begun to use this technique to help people with diabetes learn how to control their blood sugar levels.

They first attach sensors to areas of the diabetic's body where muscle tension is greatest when the person is under stress. This generally means the forehead, jaw, neck and shoulders. The sensors signal the amount of muscle tension to the machine, which records the degree of tension on a meter, expressing this either as numbers or by producing a varying sound. High numbers and low sounds equal very tense muscles.

Stress is an important factor in diabetes. When you are particularly stressed, your body produces hormones that can raise the amount of glucose (a simple form of sugar) in the blood. This is precisely what diabetics try to avoid. But a balance has to be achieved. There are also times when hormones will decrease the amount of sugar in the blood, resulting in, an unwanted and potentially dangerous low blood sugar, or 'hypo' attack.

Biofeedback and relaxation techniques have also been used at the Medical College of Ohio. They are currently experiencing success with helping insulin-dependent diabetics deal with stress, and they suggest that the same approach could be used by people with non-insulin-dependent (or mature onset) diabetes.[10] It is important to note that biofeedback and relaxation training do not eliminate stress. Instead, these techniques allow you to cope better under stressful circumstances and let you manage stress more effectively.

HEADACHES AND BIOFEEDBACK About three quarters of the people who take up biofeedback training do so to learn deep relaxation skills. Of course, such relaxation can be learned without electronic monitoring, but oddly enough, migraine sufferers fare much better with biofeedback than with any other type of relaxation training. Blood pressure, on the other hand, can be just as easily controlled with most relaxation therapies, including biofeedback.

Anyone who has ever experienced migraines can attest to their severity. Unlike other headaches, they are usually accompanied by nausea, perhaps vomiting, and an aversion to bright light (photophobia). At times a migraine attack may further result in visual disturbances and sensory malfunctions such as arm numbness as well as speech difficulties, movement restriction, drastic mood swing, appetite suppression, constipation and/or water retention.

It appears that attacks are the result of changes in the blood vessels of the head. It is thought that there is such a constriction of the vessels that brain flood blow becomes grossly insufficient for normal neurological functioning. Stress and diet have been labelled as contributing factors to the development of migraine attacks.

To treat migraine, a small electronic probe is placed on the forehead (in children) or at the nape of the neck (in adults), which measures the tension of the underlying muscles. A tiny cuff covering a finger records the pulse rate, and another finger is an electronic thermometer. While you sit back, you monitor your body's inner workings on a television screen and try to bring your muscles to the deepest relaxation state possible. As your pulse slows and skin warms up, this is reflected on the screen. Experts claim that skills are learned that help people reduce the activity of skeletal muscles that, when tense, contribute to the headaches, and reduce the activity of the sympathetic nervous system (the nerves associated with adrenaline and its physiological effects). The ability to warm the skin of the hands at will depends on learning how to achieve a kind of relaxation that diminishes the output of the sympathetic nerves throughout the body. This has been proved to be a highly effective way to abort migraine headaches.

Skin temperature biofeedback has been used quite successfully. Researchers discovered that once their patients learned temperature control, the severity of their headaches was severely reduced, and with more practice, they could actually prevent migraines from coming on in the first place. In one study, 47 per cent of the participants derived substantial clinical benefit as a result of temperature biofeedback.

Tension headaches are not quite as disabling as migraines, but can still be extremely painful and debilitating. The pain is described as a tight band around the head or a weight pressing down on the top; occasionally the back of the head and the neck muscles are equally painful. A good amount of evidence blames tension headaches on psychological stress; victims of this seem to suffer from these sorts of headaches frequently.

Tension in skeletal muscles can be very easily assessed by measuring the electrical activity in them using an electromyograph (EMG). The readings from this device can then be used for purposes of feedback. The very first study of biofeedback involved five patients with severe and persistent tension headaches. Within two months, all of them reported relief. After a three-month follow-up, the benefits they had derived were still with them; three had rid themselves of headaches completely, while the other two continued to get them but with a far lesser degree of pain.

TASTING BRAIN WAVES   Biofeedback is experiencing acclaim in other areas. Individuals with peptic ulcers, abnormal heart rhythms, epilepsy, Tourette's syndrome and Parkinson's disease have had success with more specialized and sophisticated applications of the technique. Typically, biofeedback works because it helps us to learn how to control muscle tension, skin temperature and rate of perspiration, which in turn allows us to manage many stress-related ills.

But, at the end of the day, biofeedback really helps people achieve one thing: relaxation. Training can take from as long as a few weekly sessions to more than 20. Thereafter, the majority of participants can relax on their own without the use of the machines. However, before anyone considers using biofeedback, physical problems must definitely be ruled out first.

You really do need to learn coping strategies to minimize stress in your life in the first place, but if everything else fails, biofeedback is an excellent mind-over-body therapy.

Our bodies usually give us very little indication of what is happening inside them. We may be aware of pulse, temperature and perspiration. We may notice muscle function and heart action by intensively focusing our attention on them. But overall, we know next to nothing about our inner functioning. Have you ever heard, tasted, smelled or felt your brain waves, blood pressure, muscle cells? Each one of these, however, can be detected and displayed on a monitor which will allow you to experience them, learn about them and, eventually, control them.

In reality, biofeedback uses quite simple devices to read minor physiological activity. After all, we have used thermometers to measure our temperatures, we are familiar with the gadget our doctors use for reading blood pressure, and some of us will have had our hearts monitored by an electrocardiograph (ECG). And, of course, there are numerous other instruments that can record deeply hidden or elusive body activities that are virtually impossible for us to experience ourselves. Today, the technology exists that makes the monitoring of nearly every obscure internal activity entirely possible and is, in fact, regularly used for medical and research purposes.

Biofeedback empowers you to read and interpret certain inner functions and gives you the control to correct them. Your fate is thus literally in your hands and not in those of physicians. They may teach you and guide you, but they cannot 'fix' you. That is your responsibility.

An estimated 70 per cent of our medical problems are actually induced or worsened by psychological factors such as fear, anxiety and depression. Mind control can make a great impact on these, and will certainly help lead one back to a state of well-being. Biofeedback in particular has applications that are important to a great many medical, psychosomatic, psychological and behavioural problems.

Biofeedback is an odd combination of stark simplicity and obvious complexity. It appears deceptively simple: just locate certain functions inside the body and find a way to display them externally; then manipulate the findings by directing the power of the mind at the body and thus causing change. But biofeedback is uncomplicated in concept only. How can we even begin to consider what is involved in using a device that literally shows us how the mind can control its own and the body's state of well-being? The complexities of the mind/body machine are manifold. Biofeedback involves countless interactions with surface and deep-rooted emotions, the higher mental functions of understanding and the dynamics of very complicated physical processes. Simple? And amazingly enough, most people can learn this aspect of mind control after just a few sessions, although some may need a couple of dozen. Many of the ill-informed still believe that biofeedback must be carried out life-long if it is to work. This is not the case. Study after study has proved that, once the biofeedback technique has been learned, it has very long-lasting effects.

Most scientists, like the rest of us, are ignorant about the phenomenon of internal self-control. Just knowing how to make something work and knowing how to create desired outcomes does not explain exactly *how* it all took place. But, despite this, biofeedback's effectiveness in an increasing number of human health conditions continues to be discovered. It has literally made the mind and the body one and the same.

BIOFEEDBACK AND BLOOD PRESSURE   Biofeedback's first triumph was in the control of blood pressure. Hypertension affects millions of people throughout the world, mostly in Western societies, and can lead to stroke and heart attack. In many cases, there are no detectable causes, so researchers finally came to the belief that mental stress is the chief cause of high blood pressure. Drug therapies for hypertension are less than satisfactory, with unpleasant and sometimes serious side-effects. Besides, no drug can actually 'cure' hypertension; it can only 'manage' it for as long as you take the drugs. With biofeedback training, however, you can learn to raise or lower your blood pressure at will. Hypertensive individuals who have carried out this training have consistently achieved clinically significant changes.

Besides hypertension, biofeedback scores successfully in another area of cardiovascular pathology – namely, arrhythmias. There are two heart function irregularities in particular where it has been especially effective: premature ventricular contractions (PVCs) and tachycardia. With PVC, the ventricles contract irregularly and ineffectively, which can bring about a heart attack. The very rapid heartbeat of tachycardia may be due to a number of abnormalities. The heart can actually beat so fast that it can result in a heart attack or sudden death. Electrocardiology makes heart rate easy to monitor, and biofeedback can be used to control the beat-to-beat variations in the rate. Studies have consistently shown that patients with these conditions and using biofeedback all developed a fair degree of heart rate control, while the reduction in PVCs can be quite dramatic in an average of four out of five patients. Follow-up evaluations with the PVC sufferers up to 21 months later showed that the benefits continued for those who had achieved success with biofeedback.

Researchers have also reported terrific results with tachycardia patients after only as few as four biofeedback sessions. One patient was able to reduce his regular heart rate by 17 points after some two months of training and was found to have maintained that count when he was examined 18 months later. As a result he managed to carry on a normal life-style and greatly reduce his use of tranquillizers.

Electromyographic (EMG) biofeedback is also being used to help people with neuromuscular dysfunction – e. g. paralysed muscles or those with damaged function due to hemiplegia (one-sided paralysis), peripheral nerve damage, spasmodic torticollis ('wry neck') and cerebral palsy. For instance, biofeedback produced good results in hemiplegics twice as successfully as traditional physiotherapy, but the best results occurred when biofeedback was followed by physiotherapy.

Cerebral palsy, in which a variable number of sensory and motor malfunctions are the result of non-progressive brain damage, is another condition that has shown improvement with biofeedback. In one study, a group of 18 affected school children received biofeedback training a few times a week for between 2 and 12 months. Those who used a head device learned to control their head stability; the ones who used an arm-position monitor gained a great deal of arm mobility. There wasn't a single child who did not make serious improvements in muscular performance.

When biofeedback was first introduced in the 1960s, it held great promise for great problems. But today, it has been re-evaluated and refined, and better controlled studies are beginning to find even more beneficial uses for this mind-to-body linking system.

HYPNOSIS

While biofeedback is very much a modern phenomenon, the same is certainly not the case of an age-old method of mind control that is currently receiving widespread medical application. Hypnosis has found broad-based acceptance among orthodox physicians – it was even given a seal of approval by the American and British medical associations more than three decades ago.

This should not be surprising. After all, studies show that nearly 95 per cent of receptive people who undergo hypnosis receive some benefit as a result. In both the United States and Britain, physicians are currently combining hypnotherapy with orthodox treatments to help patients with migraines, arthritis and burns. Mainstream medical journals frequently report ways in which hypnotherapy helps people to use their bodies' own powers to heal. Sick children have been able to control their immune systems, and adults with ulcers have learned how to control the secretion of stomach acid. Researchers have also found that hypnosis can reduce inflammation and can also help patients to widen their own blood vessels (to reduce high blood pressure) and airways (to reduce the effects of asthma).

However, experts are at a loss to explain exactly how this works. A few have suggested that hypnosis allows direct access to the limbic system, the brain centre associated with emotion and involuntary activities such as digestion and hormone regulation.

Cancer patients who have undergone chemotherapy have been able to avoid the expected nausea after being hypnotized. Burns victims who have been hypnotized right after the incident that caused their injuries recover much faster and with less medication than those who are not hypnotized. Surgeons report that post-operative healing takes place much more quickly when their patients are hypnotized beforehand. This is not to say that there aren't still many disbelievers in the medical community, but even if you take the most pessimistic view and believe that hypnosis produces a strictly placebo effect, you can't argue with the successful outcome of relieving pain and fear.

Recently, the Stanford Hypnotic Susceptibility Scale was administered to a group of female university students who were diagnosed as bulimic. Oddly enough, researchers discovered that bulimics make highly susceptible hypnosis subjects. They also, in general, respond quite well to hypnotic suggestions that allow them regain control over their eating habits.

Hypnosis can be used regularly to help people break bad habits, conquer fear and deal with pain. The hypnotic state isn't a zombie-like trance that allows you to move into a unexplored part of your mind, says Dr David Spiegel, professor of psychiatry and behavioural sciences at

Stanford University and a leading researcher on hypnosis and its effect on personal health.[11]

IT'S MORE LIKE BEING SO CAUGHT UP IN A GOOD MOVIE THAT YOU FORGET IT'S A MOVIE – YOU DON'T JUDGE IT, YOU GO WITH THE EXPERIENCE. YOU'RE NARROWING YOUR FOCUS OF ATTENTION AND PUTTING OUTSIDE, OR DIS-ASSOCIATING, YOUR AWARENESS OF YOUR BODY, THAT YOU'RE IN A THEATER, THAT YOU'RE GOING TO HAVE TO DRIVE HOME AFTER IT'S OVER. YOU ENTER THE IMAGINED WORLD.

FROM MESMERISM TO LEGITIMACY   Hypnosis has had a cyclical history of acceptance and rejection. Descriptions of how to bring about what is now known as a hypnotic trance appear in Egyptian writings of more than 3000 years ago. The Druids, Incas and many other peoples used trances to do battle against illness. In the late 18th century hypnosis found its way into Western society when it was administered as a medical therapy by the German physician, Franz Mesmer.

While Mesmer received both applause and ridicule for the technique that was first dubbed 'mesmerism' and only much later called 'hypnosis', the lack of scientific evidence at the time did not prevent others from putting it to use. In the United States, Phineas Parkhurst Quimby (1802–66) employed it to cure an invalid who later achieved great fame as Mary Baker Eddy, the founder of Christian Science. Those who resorted to hypnotism at that time were amazed at the success they had with relieving pain during surgery. In 1834 the English surgeon John Elliotson (1791–1868) described many surgical procedures that were performed painlessly when using hypnosis as anaesthesia. Twelve years later Dr James Esdaile of Scotland reported on 345 major surgeries conducted in India with hypnosis as the sole anaesthetic. In the same year, 1846, ether became available and, a year later, chloroform. With the introduction of these chemical anaesthetics, strong opposition to hypnosis literally killed its use.

But it was another English physician, Dr James Braid, who rid hypnotism of the dubious connotations of 'mesmerism' and introduced the 'hypnotherapy' that we know today. He used it in a variety of cases, especially in the treatment of pain; he even treated himself, through self-hypnosis. Finally, after World War II, psychiatrists and dentists decided that there was some merit in hypnosis. The British Medical Association and the American Medical Association both passed resolutions that allowed hypnosis training in medical schools. Government agencies and private foundations funded research laboratories at prestigious univer-sities. Hypnosis was at last on the road to legitimacy and acceptance.

COUNTERING PAIN   Today, hypnosis is still widely used to control pain. For people who can be easily hypnotized, many studies have concluded that hypnosis can be as powerful a painkiller as morphine. Those who are less susceptible still manage to gain benefits as part of a comprehensive pain control programme to help them learn how to relax and counter anxiety.

With chronic pain and stress so common today, it is no wonder that Dr Henry Clarke of the Oregon Health Sciences University has long used hypnosis to relax anxious patients. About 5 per cent of people grind their teeth at night and may develop serious pain and complications as a result. Stress is believed to be the most common inducer of such subconscious activity. By employing hypnosis, along with other treatment where necessary, such as the wearing of jaw splints, Dr Clarke has been able to bring about a decrease in teeth grinding in about 40 per cent of his patients. This has also greatly reduced the patient's jaw, facial, neck and shoulder pain, which is associated with teeth grinding. [12]

Smokers and dieters can also achieve success with hypnosis since it has been found useful in behavioural change programmes. It's not an instant magic solution, but rather an aid in the building up of will power that can help you stop smoking or eat less.

What exactly happens to you when you are hypnotized? Hypnotherapists can direct you into a hypnotic state by one of several methods. The idea is for you to become as relaxed as possible and for your attention to become focused. The narrowing of attention causes you to ignore your surroundings and any distractions and to pay direct attention to the issue of concern. Therapists usually speak in a monotonous and rhythmic voice, asking you to think about your heavy eyelids and very relaxed muscles. Or they may paint a tranquil picture for you, like floating on a cloud or lying on a beautiful deserted beach. By now, you should have forgotten where you are. At this point, therapists can make suggestions to help you deal with your problem. If you are, say, a night-time tooth grinder, they may say 'Lips together, teeth apart,' as well as additional statements that will bring you to a normal behaviour pattern. They may further encourage you by saying, 'You may want to grind your teeth to deal with stress, but you won't'. They will end your state of hypnosis simply by telling you to open your eyes. You remain aware of everything that has transpired and there are no mysteries.

Hypnosis has been described as a kind of sleep, but it's not. You are always aware of what is being said to you; it can be thought of as a state of receptive, responsive, attentive concentration. Some considered it a transference of power involving submissive, instinctual behaviour, but you do not have to be submissive – you can be as alert as you choose to be. The Russian physiologist Ivan Pavlov (of 'Pavlov's dogs' fame) wrote that the hypnotic state is a neurological change caused by psychological suggestions, but there is not a shred of evidence for this. Dr David Spiegel, quoted earlier, says that hypnosis may actually heighten your ability to control what is going on in your body – hence its success.

In the hands of trained professionals, hypnosis is harmless, useful and very relaxing, but it is not altogether without risks. There is a possibility that improper hypnotic suggestions could make the condition being treated worse instead of better. Because of this, you need to be as cautious when searching for a hypnotherapist as you would be when looking for any other medical specialist. In Britain and the US, anyone can call themselves a hypnotherapist; there are no laws requiring formal training or certification. Your best bet is to request a referral from your family doctor, and then make certain that the hypnotherapist is a licensed physician, psychiatrist or dentist or, if a psychologist or other type of counsellor, that he or she belongs to a recognized professional association. In Britain, these are: the Association of Hypnotherapy Organizations (contactable via the British Complementary Medicine Association), the British Society of Medical and Dental Hypnosis and the British Society of Experimental and Clinical Hypnosis. All these will also provide you with the names of hypnotherapists in your area.

The techniques discussed in this chapter bring us closer to understanding the meaning of the phrase 'the patient as a whole'. The foremost healthcare specialists of today accept this concept as the guiding principle of treatment. The physical, mental, emotional and spiritual aspects of each individual are intertwined and cannot be viewed separately when you consider the well-being and optimal health of that individual. The physical body only represents the visible part of our being. It is the outer result of a chain of unseen events that take place within the spirit and the mind. Thus, when you think about a person as a 'whole', you should mean the mind, the spirit and the body collectively, not separately.

Modern medicine has accumulated an enormous amount of evidence regarding the physical body. But the true value of the inner person, the consciousness that utilizes the body, has failed to receive its due.

Physicians who view their patients as 'whole' individuals tend to concentrate on the fundamental causes of their illnesses while assisting them back to good health, unlike others who concentrate on superficial manifestations of disease and look for ways to 'cure' them. Modern medicine can and does suppress most symptoms of illness to an extraordinary degree, but this doesn't mean that you have been cured. Aspirin may rid your head of a headache, but the origin of the pain has not been located and dealt with. Eventually aspirin may become ineffective and you will require stronger medication, which could lead to other complications. You may soon find yourself in a cycle of ill health that can be quite vicious.

The current emphasis on preventive medicine is admirable as far as it goes. It's just that when you consider the cold, hard realities of medical, environmental, dietary and lifestyle conditions, this form of prevention isn't worth much. Our current system of healthcare is hell-bent on seeking quick and easy solutions to diseases instead of recognizing the fundamental destructive forces that have caused them, and utilizing rational thinking and common sense to deal with such problems.

However, modern medicine could be on the threshold of a new era, when it will achieve its true purpose: to treat patients as unique individuals and not just as bodies and minds that are somehow independent of the expression of their spirit. This should lead us to a new definition and understanding of health and healing that incorporates the vital need of humanity to be at peace with itself and in harmony with its environment.

Many great healers of this world say that the life force is always within us. Like many concepts foreign to our conditioned way of thinking, a precise, scientific definition of this 'life force' eludes us, but you might think of it as an active energy that is present at all levels of our existence. It can be moved, derailed or blocked within us, usually without our conscious awareness. It is unseen and usually unrecognized. And, most often it is the circumstances within the individual that disturbs it and violates its essential purpose.

CHAPTER EIGHT

REVITALISING YOUR BODY

he quest for optimal health involves not only what you put into your body but what you do to it. As a result, the 1990s are seeing a shift in the purpose of exercise. Our aim is not simply to be thin, muscle-bound Fonda-types, but to ward off chronic illness and to obtain maximum energy for optimal health.

The actor Arnold Schwarzenegger and his colleagues on the US President's Council on Physical Fitness and Sports came up with a plan to mail blank exercise prescription pads for doctors to fill in and pass along to their patients. The back of each sheet would say:

EXERCISE IS EFFECTIVE FOR THE PREVENTION AND TREATMENT OF A WIDE VARIETY OF MEDICAL CONDITIONS. AMONG THESE ARE: HYPERTENSION, VASCULAR DISEASE, HIGH CHOLESTEROL, OSTEOPOROSIS, HEART DISEASE, PULMONARY DISEASE, DEPRESSION, STROKE, OBESITY, BACK PAIN AND DIABETES.[1]

According to the most recent evidence, bowel cancer should be added to that list.

No longer just a general preventive measure, exercise today is being prescribed by type, intensity and duration. And with good reason. We have strayed far from our biological blueprint and are now paying the price with needless mental and physical suffering. Nowhere is this more apparent than in the United States. The modern American way of life has resulted in brain chemistry changes in the majority of sedentary people, leading to extraordinary rates of various levels of depression. Scientists have determined that the rate of depression in the US has increased nearly 20-fold in the last 100 years, and especially since 1950. In addition, American children under the age of 12 weight 50 per cent more today than those of a mere 30 years ago, and the Centers for Disease Control report that only some 8 per cent of the US population exercises adequately enough to maintain minimal cardiovascular fitness.

The British cannot afford to mock their American cousins. The Royal College of Physicians, in a report entitled *The Medical Aspects of Exercise*, stated that the levels of habitual physical activity in the general British population are so low that merely walking for a short time at a normal pace may be more than many people can comfortably tolerate. By the age of 40, half of all British men and three quarters of all women spend the vast majority of their waking lives in chairs. The British Heart Foundation, in a report headed *Exercise and the Heart*, said that less than one in five British people take enough exercise to benefit their hearts. In sedentary people, muscles actually start wasting away from the mid-20s, after which about half a pound of muscle is traded every year for half a pound of fat. The undesirable changes in blood fat chemistry that eventually result in heart disease can even be found in the arteries of inactive primary school children.

The US Centers for Disease Control report that inadequate exercise has about the same effect on the body as smoking a pack of cigarettes each day. They further claim that inactivity is the single most dangerous risk factor in heart disease – greater than high blood pressure, cholesterol or smoking.

Even though exercise and the heart have been closely correlated for quite some time, evidence clearly shows that people are far more disciplined about taking medication over the long term than they are about exercising. Research at the University of California has revealed that exercise is just as effective as drugs in lowering moderately elevated blood pressure[2] – and with a great many other benefits and none of the side-effects. More than 60 million Americans have high blood pressure that can be largely managed without the use of drugs. In Britain, where most of the population is chronically inactive, 65 per cent of all women over the age of 50 have above normal blood pressure. A mind-boggling 90 per cent have elevated cholesterol levels, which too can lead to heart disease. It has been concluded that regular dynamic exercise of moderate intensity can reduce the incidence of coronary events (e. g. heart attacks) and deaths from heart disease by up to 50 per cent. The *British Medical Journal* has said that the impressive contribution of exercise as secondary prevention should not be underestimated. But even if heart disease occurs as a result of such poor lifestyle choices, you're still not at an end – that is, if you survive.

In the past two decades, numerous studies have concluded that exercising after a heart attack, open heart surgery or even a heart transplant greatly improves rehabilitation and decreases the chances of significant disease progression. The best results came from patients who continued regular exercise workouts with strength and flexibility exercises.

'A WONDER DRUG'

Depression, like heart conditions, occurs in modern men and women with staggering frequency, and it, too, is often brought on by physical inactivity. Lifestyle, of all possible factors, is the leading concern for epidemiologists, the scientists who study how we live and die – and lifestyle is directly related to mental health. Researchers decided to take a close look at a group of people who live their lives very differently from most of us: the Amish people of Pennsylvania who follow a strict 19th-century lifestyle devoid of electricity, cars and most modern tools and appliances. The researchers found that the Amish suffer a rate of depression that is one fifth to one tenth that of American urbanites. In fact, the majority of non-industrialized societies lack the modern afflictions that plague us, and some cultures have no comprehension of depression and suicide.

Research has shown that depression is directly associated with recreational drug use and television-watching time. Those who regularly participate in sports, however, rarely have episodes of depression. Therefore, depression and a lack of physical activity appear extremely well linked. Recently, it has been documented that depression is the single most definitive personality factor that distinguishes physically active from sedentary middle-aged American men. On the other hand, it has been consistently found that healthy, inactive adults show significant decreases in depression after they begin to exercise.[3]

Even if one must rely on psychotherapy to resolve emotional problems, exercise has been proved a valuable adjunct. It is a much preferred substitute for antidepressants, tranquillizers, sleeping pills and other drugs. After all, exercise and antidepressant drugs produce similar effects on the brain neuro-transmitter systems, which regulate mood, and both usually reduce symptoms. However, biochemical treatments don't always work – not to mention the side-effects, which can include (depending on the drug), drowsiness, agitation, loss of sexual function, skin rashes and constipation.[4] Exercise, on the other hand, not only lifts most depressions, or better yet, prevents them from coming on in the first place, but *its* side-effects include weight loss, alertness, sounder sleep, stronger bones, lower blood pressure, normal fat and carbohydrate metabolism, a reduced risk of heart disease and a longer happier life, to name just a few.

Dr William Morgan, a former president of the American Psychological Association's division of exercise and sport psychology, has said that 'Running should be viewed as a wonder drug, analogous to penicillin, morphine and the tricyclics.'

Exercise is most effective in the reduction of stress and depression when it involves prolonged, rhythmic exertion and controlled breathing. Long-distance runners refer to the exercise-induced psychological changes the experience as the 'runner's high'. This is the result of their bodies producing endorphins, natural opiates. Endorphins have been proved to block pain and to create a feeling of well-being. Those who exercise regularly show a measurable, reproducible increase in their blood levels of endorphins. Exercise may also favourably alter brain levels of various neuro-transmitters such as norepinephrine, serotonin and dopamine.

Scientists have discovered that physically active people improve their brain function and the nervous systems as much as their circulatory systems. An extraordinary medical review that scrutinized more than 80 studies concluded that 70 per cent of them revealed the important gains to be made in mental health when a person becomes physically fit. Many experts today theorize that the brain may be similar to muscles, in that it, too, could lose its capabilities when not used.

BACKS, BONES AND BLOOD VESSELS

As you have already read, backache affects 80 per cent of us. Musculoskeletal disorders, particularly low back pain and arthritis, benefit from exercise enormously. Again, you can prevent yourself from ever getting to this point of pain by taking regular exercise.

Oddly enough, exercise is possibly the most over-publicized yet under-utilized treatment for the far-too-common problems of backache. Many doctors simply offer lip service regarding the great value of physical activity, and their patients aren't actually encouraged to exercise regularly. Most experts feel that, no matter how severe the pain, there is always some type of exercise that can be done, even if it's only gentle stretching or brief daily walks. It's quite typical for backache sufferers to be sent for lengthy physiotherapy sessions where they receive electrical therapy, hot packs, ice, massage – but absolutely no exercise.

Between 70 and 90 per cent of all back pain is directly due to muscle or ligament disorders, generally associated with lower back weakness. In most cases, back pain can be got rid of in a few weeks with or without medical intervention, but it is more likely to return if the underlying weakness has not been corrected. As soon as you return to your normal way of living, the pain comes back. Once you have been injured, your back is four times more likely to be hurt again. The secret is not to lie back and take it easy, but to diligently stretch and strengthen your back muscles.

We should approach back pain in much the same way that we handled heart problems in the 1970s, when doctors warned patients against physical activity. Today, we know such advice was and is nonsense – and even detrimental to heart patients. And as it was for them, physical activity has been shown to be far more beneficial to back pain sufferers than drugs and rest.

The majority of back pain results from muscles going into spasm; the slipped disc so many people refer to occurs in less than 5 per cent of cases. The *New England Journal of Medicine* recommends that no more than two days of bedrest should be allowed; any more than that would further weaken the muscles. When you consider how many millions of people suffer from back pain and that less than 1 per cent of them require surgery, it says a lot about how much you should share in the control, elimination and prevention of your own back pain.

Perhaps no one understands this better than the employees who have injured their backs while at work. In both the US and the UK, work-related back injuries are the No. 1 occupational health hazard. Some half a million members of the American work force injure their backs every year.[5] The National Safety Council in the US reports that the cost of every single back injury runs to about $18,000 (£12,000), and together they total between $30 and $60 billion (£20–40 billion) a year.

Thus it comes as no surprise that American companies have decided to do something about this. At several of its plants, Coca-Cola began injury-prevention and rehabilitation programmes, which focused on screening for back problems and helping identified employees to strengthen them. This resulted in a 32 per cent decrease in back injuries and a 78 per cent gain in worker days, which would normally have been lost to recuperation. On the other hand, the back injury rate at the Coca-Cola plants that did not have such programmes in place increased by the same percentage as the decrease elsewhere, while days lost on the job skyrocketed by more than 300 per cent.[6]

When DuPont realized that their employees' back problems were costing the company $40 million (£26.7 million) a year, they too jumped on the bandwagon and took control. Within a year, they had saved $10 million (£6.7 million) and today they are able to pocket $50 million a year (£33.3 million) extra from their worldwide operations.

The back is an extraordinary piece of architecture, but our way of life is simply far too destructive. Physical inactivity, excessive stress and bad footwear all contribute to the problem. The result is weak muscles that go into spasm, leading to a chain of events that can leave you in a disastrous state. The entire muscular system can be harmed as a result of a single muscle injury, and the pain spreads. But if you strengthen your back muscles, your body's balance can be restored and pain alleviated.

While back pain is an equal-opportunity condition, this is not the case with the bone-loss disease osteoporosis. While a small percentage of men get it, a massive 45 per cent of women over 50 suffer significant bone loss and almost 40 per cent will fracture their hips, spines or forearms as a result.[7] The disorder can, in large part, be prevented. For instance, weight-bearing exercise often slows down the loss of bone minerals, and even women over the age of 70 can build up bone mineral with low-level weight training. Hence, by walking and taking part in some weight training, women can decrease their loss of bone minerals while increasing their strength and endurance. At the same time, they will also improve their stamina, balance and coordination, which should help prevent the falls that can lead to broken bones. Even the least amount of exercise can help prevent osteoporosis. Research suggests that three 20- to 60-minute sessions a week are capable of arresting bone loss and even promoting bone building in older women.

Equally important is the association between exercise and diabetes. Both insulin-dependent and non-insulin dependent (mature-onset) diabetics can benefit enormously from regular exercise. Mature-onset diabetes can actually be controlled with exercise. Research has shown that almost 85 per cent these types of diabetics and many of their family members are obese. A good workout programme actually has an insulin-like effect on the body and also has a positive effect on blood lipids. Although insulin-dependent diabetics will continue to need injections of the hormone in most cases, there is the possibility that the amount can be reduced when exercise becomes a routine part of the person's lifestyle.

Regular exercise can also reduce your chance of developing diabetes. The *Lancet* reported a study of 122,000 American nurses, who were divided into two groups: one took weekly exercise (brisk walking, jogging, cycling and so on), with the other group did none at all. Twice as many of those in the second group developed diabetes as those in the exercising group.[8]

Another condition that can benefit from exercise is peripheral vascular disease, when the arteries and veins, particularly in the legs and feet, become diseased. Until recently, drugs were the only treatment, but now slow-paced walking and water exercises (hydrotherapy) are often recommended instead to improve blood flow.

OBESITY, CANCER AND AIDS

One condition that is not usually referred to as a disease, but is considered as such by many experts, is obesity – definitely a lifestyle factor and a very dangerous one at that. Dieting has become a multi-billion dollar business, with diet foods and drinks alone costing $23 billion (£15.3

billion) a year in the US – not to mention the money expended on commercial diet plans, clinics, health spas and all the other things that comprise the weight-loss industry. Today there are more than *30,000* different diets[9], all claiming to be the sure-fire way to lose weight and keep it off. Although a huge number of people – a quarter of the American population, for instance – are dieting at any given time, very few of them actually lose poundage, and if they do, even fewer manage to keep it off for long.

A sedentary lifestyle is believed to be one of the key reasons for such an epidemic of obesity. The combination of sedentary work, television watching and the consumption of high-calorie junk food is lethal. The average American eats about 44 tonnes (40 tons) of food in a lifetime, including 57 kg (125 lb) of sugar a year. A person may actually be eating fewer calories yet be far more overweight than someone else. Studies show that, in such cases, physical activity is the determining factor.

The problem with obesity is that it often leads to many other potential health problems, such as high levels of cholesterol in the blood (hypercholesterolaemia). Scientists have proved that exercise lowers LDL cholesterol (the bad kind) and increases the HDL cholesterol (the good kind), particularly in combination with weight loss.

Recently, researchers from around the world have been examining the association between exercise and various types of cancer. Bowel cancer – the second most common cancer in the UK (after lung cancer in men and breast cancer in women), which in England and Wales affects one in every 100,000 people between the ages of 40 and 45 and one in every 250 between 80 and 85 – is the first for which scientists have been able to determine a serious link. A study from Harvard University scrutinized the cancer history of 17,000 men for up to 23 years and discovered that those who were moderately to highly physically active had a 50 per cent lower risk of bowel cancer than those who participated in minimal amounts of physical activity. 'Moderately active' is defined as the burning of more than 1000 calories per week in recreational activity. This can translate into jogging or playing tennis two hours a week or simply walking ten miles a week.[10]

In addition, a 21-year study of 8000 Japanese men in Hawaii showed that the ones who were physically active at home or at work were up to 70 per cent less likely to develop bowel cancer than the sedentary men. Similarly, studies of Swedish men and women have shown that being sedentary may triple the risk of this type of cancer.[11]

With so much attention being focused on the immune system today, we are learning that exercise also has a positive effect on those with HIV and AIDS. The University of Miami found that it improved immune

functioning in men following a positive diagnosis for HIV. At the end of a
four-year study, the control group showed a decline in natural killer cells
and a steep rise in psychological distress. In contrast, the men in the
aerobic exercise group showed only a slight drop in natural killer cells.[12]

THE DANGERS OF DOING NOTHING

According to the *British Medical Journal*, exercise is emerging as a key
element in most national health promotion recommendations and strategies. This is because, says the journal, exercise can provide a feeling of
well-being not only in those who are well, but in those with illnesses that
restrict their performance.

However, population studies show that very few of us get anywhere
near adequate exercise. Even if we participate in it enthusiastically for a
while, drop-out rates are enormously high. For instance, less than 12 per
cent of British women maintain a fitness routine for more than a year. Yet,
when it comes to the human body, the worst thing you can do to it is to do
nothing at all. Unlike most machines, the body actually falls apart from
lack of use, not overuse.

The 'disease syndrome' is a new term coined by health practitioners. It describes succinctly how our sophisticated physical system
falls prey to various unnatural conditions because of a sedentary lifestyle.
Most of the illnesses we associate with the ageing process are brought on
by our lack of respect for our bodies. Most cases of heart disease,
arthritis, mental disorders and so on are not a result of misfortune but of
poor management.

Fortunately, such a sad state of affairs can not only be arrested, but
reversed. The body responds appreciatively to use and it won't be long
before it lets you know just how grateful it really is. In a matter of weeks,
your heart rate when at rest will become lower, your fat will begin turning
into muscle, your bones will become stronger and you will sleep better,
among numerous other benefits. A Royal College of Physicians report
claims that, following a mere eight weeks of regular exercise, sufficient
and demonstrable biochemical adaptations take place. Some experts
even say that you will become cleverer!

But do these advantages impress the sedentary majority? It can be
safely stated that, if people were given the choice between a supplement,
a drug or exercise in order to extend their lives, maintain their bodies,
keep their good looks and chase away the blues, most would choose a
supplement or a drug.

WALKING BACK TO HAPPINESS . . .

One simple, yet highly effective, way of getting enough exercise is
planned daily walking. It is hard to believe that such a simple, common

action can produce some extraordinary results for our physical and mental well-being. However, the ordinary act of normal walking has been proved to give most of the benefits that runners achieve but without the knee, hamstring and back problems.

This most natural of human physical activities achieves marvellous benefits. It rids the body of extra weight, decreases blood pressure, helps maintain normal cholesterol levels, regulates blood sugar, prevents osteoporosis, keeps back pain at bay, helps strengthen the immune system and boosts emotional well-being.

More good news is that you don't have to alter your life drastically and exercise yourself into a frenzy to improve your heart. Making a routine of walking will do. In a large study of more than 12,000 men, researchers at the University of Minnesota School of Public Health discovered that, among the least active men, death from heart failure was 30 per cent greater than in those who were moderately active. As little as a 30-minute brisk walk every day could improve or even save millions of lives.

Walking and other aerobic activities have also been shown to help our hearts deal with psychological stress. If you're under mental stress and you're not as physically fit as you should be, your heart will overreact to 'fight or flight' biochemicals such as adrenaline.

Indeed, walking can be a powerful antidote to depression. It has been known for ages that the mind affects the body, but we are just on the verge of understanding how much the body affects the mind. A brisk 20-minute or longer walk every day can greatly improve emotional stability, according to researchers at Indiana University at Bloomington. They concluded that the psychological benefits of exercise are comparable to gains from standard types of psychotherapy. When depressed individuals were assigned to do exercise, relaxation therapy or psychotherapy, researchers found that, after 12 weeks, all three activities reduced depression, but nearly a year later, the depression of those who had chosen exercise and relaxation techniques showed the greatest improvement, while the psychotherapy groups did not fare as well.[13] Some experts say that regular exercise provides us with a sense of control over our bodies, allowing us to feel better about ourselves overall.

Brown University reports of yet additional benefits that exercise has on the brain. Patients with Alzheimer's disease, who walked 30 minutes three times a week for ten weeks, showed dramatic improvements in their ability to communicate. They were able to express themselves far better than a group that had been assigned to engage in conversation at the same time as the others were out walking.[14]

A BOOST TO THE SYSTEM

Doctors at the Loma Linda University School of Public Health in California say that the quickest way to boost the immune system is to take a good walk. When a group of sedentary women walked 45 minutes a day, five days a week for 15 weeks, their immune systems underwent changes similar to those that take place at the onset of an infection, as the body prepares to fight against invaders. Their levels of antibodies – which help combat infection – increased by 20 per cent, and when they came down with colds and the flu, their ailments lasted less than half as long as those of a sedentary control group.[15]

Physically active women are also far better at managing the symptoms of premenstrual syndrome (PMS). Scientists at the Human Performance Laboratory at Ball State University in Muncie, Indiana, studied two groups of PMS sufferers: one group walked or jogged regularly, and the women in the other group were largely sedentary. Within only four months, the exercising group reported a significant reduction in PMS symptoms, mainly the absence of great mood swings, increased appetite and crying spells, but also a reduction in anxiety, breast tenderness, cravings for sweets and fluid retention. The researchers concluded that the anti-PMS effect of regular exercise is possibly due to an increase in the levels of endorphins, the chemical messengers in the brain that produce a feeling of well-being.[16]

But all ills aside, what society appears to be obsessed about today is weight loss. It is unfortunate that the older we get, the less physically active most of us become and the heavier we get. Obesity is an epidemic with no end in sight, but as we have seen, dieting is not the answer. But there are ways of losing weight without dieting. The *Journal of the American Dietetic Association* reports that a ten-week walking programme can reduce body fat without any special diet.[17] Other researchers have discovered that, by simply walking a few hours a week, you can trim inches from your measurements without necessarily losing any weight. At Baylor University in Waco, Texas, scientists studied a group of dieters and a group of walkers. When investigated a couple of years later, it was found that the dieters had initially lost weight quickly, but had gained most of it back. The walkers, on the other hand, had taken a longer time to lose weight, but their loss had been steady and permanent.

It appears that walkers use up fat for energy. When you walk, your body increases the concentration in the cells of specific enzymes required for fat metabolism. Hence, walking and other forms of exercise improves the body's ability to use body fat for fuel. Furthermore, walkers utilize what are known as 'slow-twitch' (as opposed to 'fast-twitch') muscles. Birds have slow-twitch muscles in their wings; so do our legs. This is the best fat-burning type of muscle, and so walking is ideal for weight loss.

THE ART OF WALKING

Many of us view walking as merely a means of moving from one place to another, just a part of daily functioning, so it can be difficult to accept that it confers any special benefits. It may be even harder to see it as an art, but that is just how walking was viewed by the American philosophers Henry David Thoreau and Ralph Waldo Emerson, the German poet Goethe and the British novelist Charles Dickens. They were in good company. Plato and Aristotle both claimed that walking purified the spirit, cleared the mind and improved thought and creativity, and poets, philosophers and novelists through the ages regularly engaged in the 'art of walking'. Thoreau possibly had the best view of walking: he disregarded all the physical benefits and simply did it because it 'is itself the enterprise and adventure of the day'.

The American physician-writer Oliver Wendell Holmes says, in *The Autocrat of the Breakfast Table* (1857–58), that in all forms of exercise there are three powers simultaneously in action: the will, the muscles and the intellect. Each of these predominates in different kinds of exercise. In walking, he wrote, the will and the muscles are so accustomed to working together and perform their task with so little expenditure of force, that the intellect is left comparatively free. The mental pleasure in walking is the sense of power over all our moving machinery.

Holmes and the other literary walkers lived at a time when the convenience of modern transport did not exist. Therefore their enthusiasm for and pleasure in walking far exceeded ours since they already walked so extensively in their normal, everyday lives.

Walking can be considered your ultimate fitness routine from almost the beginning to the very end of your life. Initially, it builds up your body strength. Then it maintains a certain level of physical and mental fitness, and towards the end of your life, it slows down the ageing process so your later years can be much more enjoyable. Far too much of what has been attributed to ageing may, in reality, be a result of the progressive inactivity that frequently goes along with it. Therefore, if you prevent inactivity, you will also prevent the numerous physical and mental problems associated with the passing of years.

Since your entire body atrophies if your walking muscles atrophy, it is simple enough to assume that walking aerobically (i.e. with the maximum oxygen intake) is one of the greatest forms of exercise. After all, more muscles are used while walking than during just about any other type of activity. You simultaneously improve your leg and thigh muscles, abdominals and buttocks. Walking works the shoulders, triceps and forearms. Even your skin improves, making it stronger, thicker and more elastic. Walking can be a life-long basic conditioning programme regardless of the level of intensity. In addition, most sports and other physical activities tend to develop only certain groups of muscles, thus leaving you physically unbalanced. Walking develops all muscles equally.

We may think that professional athletes are in great shape, but we would be wrong. The truth is that many ordinary, regular exercisers – electricians, accountants, secretaries, teachers, lawyers – are actually in better overall shape than some top athletes. Many world-class weight lifters, for example, have devastatingly poor cardiovascular systems.

To begin a sport such as running or tennis, one has to be already at a certain level of fitness in order to benefit and stick with it. You literally have to walk before you can run. With regular walking, you can prepare your muscles, lungs and circulatory system for the more challenging aspects of greater physical activities. You will also develop better breath control, body coordination and endurance. The greater body awareness you develop from walking will, in itself, give you the needed confidence to build on and expand your exercise programme.

While most sports are seasonal and many exercise programmes extend over a fixed period of time, walking has no such limitations. The benefits don't come and go; they are delivered with each passing day as you continue to walk. Because sports and others forms of exercise tend to leave so many gaps in our physical conditioning, walking really must be a part of any workout, or the sole exercise choice if time, effort and ability are limited.

With the right attitude, regular walking can be not only excellent for our optimal health but also a pleasurable part of life. Perhaps Plato expressed it best when he wrote that walking is so relaxing 'it could almost relieve a guilty conscience.'

Since many of us walk every day, we may be confused about how much extra walking is required to benefit our health. Take Thoreau: he walked 250,000 miles during his lifetime – that's almost four hours a day. Johann Gottfried Senne walked from Germany to Italy and back; then he walked to Russia, Finland and Sweden. Edward Payson Weston, at the age of 70, walked from New York to San Francisco (2930 miles) in just over three months; then he trudged from New York to Minneapolis (1217 miles) in a month. More recently, David Kunte walked around the world in four years, and a decade ago, an Englishman, George Meegan, walked nonstop for some seven years. In 1984, my friend's grandmother began walking and today we have no idea where she is!

But don't get nervous. This much walking is far more than is required for good health. Initially, your goal should be to increase your mileage gradually each day and to walk aerobically for a set time and set distance. In addition to set walking times, you can increase the amount of walking you do each day by walking to and from work as much as possible (or, if you take the bus, get off one or two stops before your destination), take the stairs as opposed to the lift, walk to do your errands and incorporate lunchtime walks and evening strolls into your routine. A friend who is an agent in the entertainment industry makes a point of slowly walking across his office while on the phone for hours on end. He brought a telephone headphone set and rarely sits down while conducting his daily business. It is a creative solution to a lower back and shoulder problem he developed after two years in the business with a telephone jammed between jaw and shoulder.

Your aerobic walk should consist of 20–30 minutes at 4–5 miles per hour at least two or three times a week. This can be very easily achieved on a treadmill if you're in the city, but many people prefer doing it in the fresh outdoor air. If certain days present obstacles to your walking routine, you can certainly make up for the shortfall later on or over the weekend. If you incorporate a long weekend walk or a hike, you're well on your way to better health. The key is to be consciously aware of how sedentary you've become so that you can do something about it before problems result.

WEIGHTLESS EXERCISE

Besides walking, the next ideal exercise is swimming. Like walking, this is virtually a risk-free physical activity. If you don't like sweating, straining, pounding and jarring, swimming provides you with a nonsuffering way to become fit. After all, if physical exercise is not enjoyable, you simply won't stick with it.

Working out in water provides extraordinary benefits under marvellous conditions. Too much stress and too little exercise usually results in weight gain, high levels of anxiety and a weaker mind and body. Swimming causes your heart and lungs to pump oxygen to all the major groups in your body. Thus, its aerobic benefits equal those of running, cycling or skiing. It is a wonderful exercise for maintaining flexibility, since you use long stretching movements. Further, the fine toning and strengthening of muscles results from the natural resistance of water.

Water naturally supports and relaxes muscles and joints. Working out in water has a way of making you feel instantly relaxed and comfortable. It calms the mind as it strengthens your body. When it comes to joints, muscles and bones, swimming is possibly the best all-inclusive exercise, with very low injury rates.

Your body weighs only one tenth as much in water as it does on land. In other words, if you weight 95 kg (15 stone) on land, you will weigh 9.5 kg (1½ stone) in the pool! It's the best way to defy gravity short of going into outer space.

Two thirds of our bodies consist of water. The Romans wisely utilized the healing powers of water, as the Japanese do now. Hydrotherapy – water used medicinally to treat injury and illness – is a beneficial way to treat ailments, and today physiotherapists have their patients exercise in water to strengthen and relax muscles as well as improve their function.

Water's support and buoyancy allows you to exercise at maximum level without the physical stress that occurs when you exercise on land. Just a mere decade ago, doctors warned the ill and the injured to stay put and rely on bedrest, but this, we now know, is possibly the worst advice an injured person can be given. The muscles waste away while the loss of physical conditioning actually contributes to anxiety and depression. Water exercise thus becomes the ideal vehicle for rehabilitation or maintenance of muscles and bones, when land activity is difficult or too painful to perform. Water naturally cushions the body.

Experts find swimming particularly suitable for the elderly to prevent the loss of bone mineral and to help replace it. Those with arthritis especially know how difficult exercising can be, but swimming is an excellent choice for them particularly when the knees are afflicted. Your whole body needs to be functioning optimally for good health, so, regardless of your ailment, you need as much exercise as the next person. An arthritic condition that leads to a lack of exercise can be detrimental to your cardiovascular system, for example. While engaging in any exercise may add more pain to your already well-established aches, the weight-lessness you feel in water means that no additional stress is placed on your joints, and you will experience the least amount of pain while you are getting your whole body into shape. Water exercise has emerged as the physical activity that benefits virtually everyone, lending itself to weight loss, cardiovascular fitness, muscle tone, and general conditioning.

Swimming alone exercises the entire body, maintains the heart rate at a high level, lowers blood pressure, exhilarates and refreshes, and rehabilitates weakened or injured muscles. Rhythmic exercise in water increases blood flow, especially in your limbs, while swimming at 60 to 80 per cent of maximum capacity fulfils the criteria for cardiovascular fitness. Exercising in water is drastically different from exercising on land, since in the pool you work against a universal resistance that can't be matched by an activity on land. In other words, you cannot overextend your back, knees or ankles.

Although water exercise can do great things to maintain healthy individuals, it also provides a new freedom for amputees and those with scoliosis (spinal curvature), muscular dystrophy, multiple sclerosis and paralysis, among other conditions. It's also one of the few workout programmes that can be done safely during pregnancy.

The benefits of water exercise are quite extraordinary. Water pressure, buoyancy and resistance all work simultaneously for a total body-and-mind effect. Water pressure does great things to help stimulate your body's circulation and bring your respiratory system into better condition. You feel water pressure the moment you step into the pool and automatically your breathing rate increases. Hence, even a minor water workout soon has positive effects. Buoyancy, on the other hand, supports the body in water, making movement very simple indeed. This is especially of benefit to those with special medical restrictions or those who are quite overweight. A law of physics known as Archimedes' Principle makes this possible. It states that a body immersed in a fluid is buoyed up by a force equal to the weight of the fluid displaced by the body. This explains why we float in water.

The improvement in your muscles that occurs during water exercise is primarily due to water resistance. Simply by walking slowly in water, you experience resistance that works toward conditioning your body. Obviously, the harder you work and the more movements you incorporate in your water workout, the greater the overall benefits.

An exercise programme that includes a gentle massage will probably tempt even the more virulent of exercise haters. When water resistance and pressure affect your body as it moves through water, it provides a soothing effect while enhancing surface circulation. This is what makes you feel calm and alert at the same time. When you take all these things into consideration, you should see that water exercise gives total body fitness minus the sore and stiff muscles, questionable results, perspiration and just plain hard work.

Many water enthusiasts say that working out in water gives them a mystical sense of freedom. They perform in a state of altered sensory perception. The pure enjoyment of being in water that most people experience eases their minds, eliminates stress and allows their minds and bodies to become harmoniously united.

TAKING TO THE WATER

So where would you begin? First of all, it's important to note that swimming is only one of many water exercise options. Swimming exercises about 90 per cent of your upper body muscles. Running is just the opposite: it works out the lower body. But you can run in water – albeit not as fast, but the benefit will be greater. Water aerobics classes have become quite popular in the United States, with nearly every health club and fitness facility offering them, and they are becoming increasingly common in the United Kingdom.

Swimmers must first focus on skill rather than on endurance. They should also alternate the swimming strokes they do – side stroke, backstroke, free-style and breaststroke – to balance and workout different muscle groups. When swimmers have learned how to perform these strokes properly and confidently, distance and endurance can be expanded.

But if you are just beginning water exercise, walking in water does wonders for building up endurance. Walk as many widths of the pool as you can for half an hour each day. You should walk as briskly as you can in waist or chest high water. Physiotherapists highly recommend this activity for those who suffer from heart problems or have difficulty with blood circulation in the legs.

The next step might be tethered swimming. Many rehabilitation centres use this form of water workout for those who could benefit from hydrotherapy but cannot swim. Ballet-type bars are used for holding on while kicking the feet. This can be done in just about any position. You get a fantastic workout without having to worry about going under.

A major reason why so many of the people who are most in need of exercise stay out of health clubs and fitness centres is that they feel they have to look good and already be quite physically fit before they can join. Many aerobics classes are simply too demanding for your average sedentary type, and most of the participants appear to have god-like bodies – so the heavy, the elderly and the not-so-fit stay away. But once health clubs begin adding water aerobics to their roster of activities, this trend begins to reverse itself. I was amazed to see what a group of 80-year-olds can do in water and how much more pleasurable it made their lives on land.

Water aerobics can range from play time and calisthenics in chest- or waist-high water to using equipment that increases the resistance of arms and legs to water. A good workout lasts between 45 minutes and an hour. But you don't have to be a part of a class. You can engage in water aerobics on your own by doing the motions that feel best suited for you.

There are some basic rules to remember if you opt for exercise in water. First, don't get into the pool right after eating; wait at least two hours after a large meal. Make sure the pool is kept clean and is properly (but not overly) chlorinated; bacteria and other pathogens can thrive in water. Also, if you're feeling particularly insecure, ensure that the pool has a lifeguard on duty while you're working out. Initially, you should exercise in the shallow end anyway and have a flotation device handy at all times until you become very confident with your new exercise programme. Last but not least, note the pool's temperature. Most pools are heated between 26 and 29°C (78–84°F). The harder you exercise, the cooler you'll want the water, but anything lower than about 26°C, like a lake or mountain stream, will feel bracing but will be too cold to engage in prolonged exercise comfortably. If the pool gets above 32°C (90°F), the heat may be too much for you.

From most of those who don't exercise regularly, one can almost hear the cry, 'I don't have time for all of this.' But where exactly does all the time go? Have you ever watched something on television that you could have done without? How many telephone conversations have you had that could have been cut short or eliminated altogether? Have you gone out to buy the groceries and spent an extra hour simply window shopping? There are countless ways in which we all waste time, yet all that is required for exercise is an hour, three times a week.

If the time issue can be resolved, the next hurdle that must be overcome is the thought of sore muscles and potential injuries or just the idea that exercise is hard work. With water exercise, we have eliminated these concerns. Then some may feel beyond the age of exercise or may be concerned about medical conditions that might prevent it. However, the fact is, the more exercise you get, the younger you feel. But you don't have access to a pool, you say? Well, you actually have many options if you stop and think about them. Most councils run at least one indoor pool and there are health clubs with pools and YMCAs and YWCAs; perhaps a local college or university will allow you access. If your aim is to get into a pool, you'll find a way.

THE LIGHTNESS OF BEING

I'm reminded of my friend Liza, who is both quite heavy and has some troubling medical problems as well. She weighs 102 kg (16 stone) and suffers from lower back pain, irritable bowel syndrome and constant allergies; at times, she also tends to get quite depressed. Her collection of Park Avenue doctors kept her heavily medicated but her troubles showed no desire to depart. After years of no results, Liza, with the help of trusted friends, finally began to look to herself for solutions to the conditions that had virtually paralysed her normal way of life. Although she was not prepared to part with traditional Western medicine, she was willing to look at her diet and begin an exercise programme. Unfortunately, her new diet involved only an elimination of fat and salt, but it was a beginning. To find an exercise programme, however, was much more challenging since Liza's ability to move her muscles and joints was limited. 'I can't do anything on land' was her standard reply. Then she found a fitness centre in her Manhattan neighbourhood that offered water exercises. Never one to turn down an opportunity to go shopping, she promptly bought an extensive 'water wardrobe' and went to the workouts three times a week.

Initially, all her friends were a bit concerned because the exercising, she said, increased her appetite! But a change soon took place. Liza began to really look forward to water aerobics because she could do what everyone else did in the pool – this certainly was not the case in the gym. Moreover, she began to experience a newfound 'lightness' afterwards, and also what she referred to as a 'manic state'. After only six weeks, water exercise had had an effect on her body and mind.

With dieting still a dilemma, Liza noticed that she had lost several inches off her waist, thighs and arms even though she had actually lost no weight. But this was encouraging enough to cause her to join Weight Watchers. Progress was slow but she stuck with it, and after two months, she had lost 5 kg (11 lb). Since this was the most she had lost in years, Liza was elated.

'Julie,' she said over the phone one day, 'I'm ready to try something on land.' I suggested walking to her appointments each day instead of taking the usual taxi. She did, and she increased her water workouts to an hour and a half, four times a week. This was a year ago. Today, Liza weights 73 kg (11 1/2 stone) and has reduced her medication by more than a half. She still eats an abundance of artificial diet foods, the 'non-foods' we talked about earlier, but she is slowly on her way to better health.

Tiffany had a problem quite the opposite of Liza's. She is tall, anorexically thin, works at a demanding job while attending college full time. She refuses, as she puts it, to poison her body with medications, although she is understandably exhausted all the time and feels constantly sleepy. Although she is fairly good about her diet, she thought that exercise in addition to her frantic daily schedule just might do her in. She had an epitaph for anyone who suggested a regular exercise programme for her: 'Here lies Tiffany. She had no cellulite.'

But exercise for Tiffany was not about weight loss or cellulite, it was about energy. Jogging or a step aerobic class certainly might have added to her level of physical stress, considering her lifestyle. But swimming or water aerobics, her friends told her, would have a most soothing and calming effect on her, which is what she needed most. Convinced this was going to kill her, Tiffany gave in, got up at 5.30 every Monday, Wednesday and Friday morning and did a water aerobics class at her university. Then a strange thing happened. On Tuesday and Thursday mornings, she went to the pool just to swim. Something crazier was to follow. Tiffany finally graduated from college, got a less-demanding job with a local law firm and yet she still continued to sign up for the early morning water aerobics class. And last month, she got her boyfriend and her mother involved in them, too. She never got around to actually admitting to her friends that the workouts helped her, but these days, she's more rested, complains far less of aches and pains, her skin has cleared up and she is a lot more pleasant to be with.

OXYGEN AND EXERCISE

It may surprise you that both walking and swimming are considered good types of aerobic exercise, since these days, when we talk about aerobics,

LIFE FORCE

an entirely different sort of exercise comes to mind. Mostly we think of aerobic dancing, which was pioneered in the early 1980s and popularized in various forms by Jane Fonda. But the term 'aerobic' simply means 'with oxygen', and 'aerobic exercise' is any form of physical exercise that requires additional effort by the heart and lungs to meet the increased demand for oxygen from the skeletal muscles. The exercise generally requires heavier breathing than passive muscular activity and results in increased heart and lung efficiency with a minimum of wasted energy. As well as walking and swimming examples of aerobic exercise include running, jogging, vigorous dancing and cycling.

To be fit is to have a strong, lean body, muscular endurance, a healthy heart and lungs and, above all, lots of energy. Aerobic exercise works the whole body, hence it benefits the whole body. After a good workout, you feel as if you have more energy since exercising aerobically makes you use more energy. Consequently, you may feel less tired throughout the day and may even have energy left over for other activities without feeling exhausted by day's end.

When you are both sedentary and under mental stress, adrenaline builds up in your heart and brain. As a result, when you become exhausted, your entire system is loaded with adrenaline. The best way to counteract such an effect is with aerobic exercise, which will revive and revitalize you all over again. When your body is given the opportunity to process and deliver oxygen rapidly and efficiently, you will naturally have more potent vitality and energy. With a great aerobics dancing class, you will also have fun and enjoy yourself in the process.

Yet most of us don't exercise at all. The US President's Council on Physical Fitness says that 95 per cent of Americans are out of shape. Today, an average 20-year-old man has the body capacity of a 40-year-old: he cannot climb a flight of stairs or run a city block without exhaustion. Thus it is quite true when they say that man does not die, he kills himself. But conditioning the cardiovascular and pulmonary system – the heart, blood vessels and lungs – can change all that. Aerobic exercise can do this through endurance activities of greater intensity and duration than you are already used to.

Regular aerobic exercise does more for the heart than any other activity. It strengthens the heart muscle, decreases blood pressure, reduces heart rate, lowers blood cholesterol and triglycerides, reduces the likelihood of developing arrythmia and improves collateral circulation (when new blood vessels form to take over the circulation of blocked vessels).

Recently, aerobic exercise has been found to be an effective way of managing diabetes. In Britain, about a quarter of those who have had diabetes for 30 years develop kidney disease, 7 per cent go blind and quite a few have heart attacks, strokes and gangrene from narrowed arteries. Regular aerobic exercise, as we have seen, can improve the heart and the circulatory system, which can reduce these risks of diabetes. The famed Mayo Clinic in Rochester, Minnesota reports that, of the 10 million Americans with maturity-onset diabetes, more then 80 per cent are overweight. But simply managing one's diet to control this disease is not enough. Exercise, it is now believed, directly affects your body's need for insulin.

Insulin's key function is to control glucose (blood sugar) by making possible the transfer of glucose from the bloodstream to the cells of the brain and muscles, where it is utilized for energy. But when people become diabetic, their pancreases produce an inadequate supply of the insulin or their body's tissues are unresponsive to the insulin. When either of these occur, the glucose level in the blood rises while the cells starve. Aerobic exercise, however, can come to the rescue. It causes your body to utilize insulin more efficiently so you don't require as much of the hormone to transport glucose from the bloodstream into the cells.

BURNING CALORIES

Generally, it takes about one-and-a-half months of an hour of aerobic exercises three to four times a week before a firmer body and fewer inches are noticeable. Weight loss will occur if you combine calorie reduction with aerobics. This may be naturally facilitated since regular exercise usually regulates hunger. A good aerobic hour can burn around 600 calories and is equivalent to a seven-mile jog. A marvellous bonus is that you continue to burn calories at twice your normal rate *after* you stop exercising. Up to six hours later, while you are watching TV, eating or sleeping, you are still burning excess calories at a greatly increased rate.

The great benefit of an aerobic class is that you work at your own fitness level but continually challenge yourself to improve. Soon, as you become more fit, your body will demand a greater volume of oxygen over a longer time. You will be able to work harder and longer without shortness of breath and a loss of energy. Additionally, as your body becomes far more efficient and finely tuned, you will recover in no time at all after a vigorous session and will have greater stamina throughout the day. Furthermore, you will benefit from improved circulation which will not only contribute to healthier organs but a better complexion. Finally, you will improve your flexibility, balance, coordination and body control in general, which will be evident in your everyday life.

One of the main reasons why people stick with aerobics more than with any other form of exercise is that it can be highly expressive and personally gratifying. 'Aerobic addicts' become hooked on the energy gained and pleasure sustained by a regular workout.

A well-rounded aerobic programme is not solely a matter of aerobic dance sessions at a health club or leisure centre a few times a week. As well as those, it should be accompanied by perhaps an early morning jog a few times a week, cycling over the weekend, a brisk walk some evenings and some regular swimming a day or two a week. Of course, you should ease gradually into increased activity. A neighbour of mine, Sherry, began her aerobic workouts with a brisk hour-long walk at 6.00 a.m., before work, three times a week. When this was no longer challenging enough, she increased the walks to five and soon six days a week. Later, she opted for climbing seven flights of stairs to her office instead of taking the lift, and then, when she went out, she began to park her car as far away as convenient, in order to increase her walking distance. Eventually, she incorporated a Sunday afternoon mountain climb, which she rode to and from on her bike. Come next month, she has promised to start an aerobic dance class to further fine-tune her respiratory system.

A proper aerobic workout needs to last a consistent 12 to 20 minutes or longer, preceded by a 15-minute warm-up and followed by a 15-minute cool-down. You will know that your right level of exercising has been reached when you begin sweating. Sweating is a normal and needed function that allows your body to cool down when it needs to.

Now you can work hard and produce a good sweat playing tennis, basketball, even golf. But these are not aerobic activities. In fact, they are anaerobic – 'without oxygen'. Anaerobic exercises are stop-and-start activities. They are excellent sources of exercise all right, but the oxygen factor is not there. Like a great meal, massage, date or holiday, it just doesn't last long enough. Aerobic exercise simply forces your body to take up a great deal of oxygen. The entire purpose of sustained aerobic activity is to increase the maximum quantity of oxygen that your body can utilize within a given period of time. In other words, your body is brought to the point where it can quickly take in a great deal of oxygen and vigorously circulate a lot of blood, resulting in an effective delivery of oxygen, via the bloodstream, to all the cells of the body.

No weakling can perform such a task. Powerful lungs, a strong heart and a healthy vascular system are required. Your aerobic capacity is possibly the best indicator of your overall well-being. You cannot have optimal health if you are not physically fit.

To improve your aerobic fitness, you need to work at it. But by doings things you like, doing them with people you like and liking the results, the work will seem more like play. Therefore, you will stick with it.

One of the key factors that will help you stay with an aerobic programme is learning how to minimize post-exercise aches and pains. If you have been quite sedentary, some discomfort will certainly be an initial byproduct of aerobics if you do too much too soon. The idea is not to feel stiff and exhausted the following day but gradually to increase your energy as a result of aerobic exercise.

First of all, be absolutely certain that you have the proper sport shoes. Aerobic shoes with sufficient arch support and heel cushioning must be worn to protect feet and joints. This may seem obvious, but it isn't to everyone, no matter how grand. An aerobic instructor told me how recently the Duchess of Kent and her entourage visited a Florida spa, and most of the ladies turned up for an aerobics session dressed in shirts with sarongs and were either barefooted or wore thongs. Imagine doing the treadmill in thongs! But that's exactly what some of them did. Aerobic shoes are designed for forward and lateral movement to allow you a wide range of activity.

You may be causing yourself unnecessary harm if your body is not properly aligned during the workout. Good posture is absolutely essential. If you 'think tall', you will eliminate much muscle strain and fatigue while gaining maximum respiratory benefits. It is also important to do aerobics flat footed with your knees slightly bent, not leaning forward on the balls of your feet. Of course, without warming up and cooling down properly, you are asking for serious trouble. Muscles must be adequately stretched and deep breathing begun before you can enter an aerobic state safely.

A good aerobics instructor will guide you through the entire process, but there are several things that it is up to you to remember. Do not eat a large meal or drink anything alcoholic for at least one hour before your workout. It's equally important not to overload with food right after exercising. I've seen many women eat excessively or indulge in normally forbidden foods simply because they have worked off some calories and feel free to reward themselves. This can be quite counter productive, needless to say. The only thing you should be filling your stomach with before, during and after exercise is water, and lots and lots of it.

HIGH IMPACT, LOW IMPACT, NON-IMPACT

Far too many people used to feel that they needed to be already fit and with a body beautiful before embarking on aerobic workouts that (so it seemed) were dominated by young attractive women and men. But this is clearly not the case today. In the 'old days', all aerobics classes were high impact – quite fast and furious. But when the staggeringly high rates of injury caused by this were revealed – a nearly 80 per cent injury rate among instructors and 45 per cent among participants – things began to change. Soon, well-cushioned aerobics shoes, resilient flooring and certified instructors became the order of the day. But what truly liberated aerobics was its reinvention into low-impact and non-impact.

With high-impact aerobics, beginners trying to keep up with the pace suffered impact-related injuries to the back, hips, knees, legs and ankles. However, you'd be hard pressed to find a high-impact class at any health club today, for aerobic exercise has become much safer and user friendly. The bump and grind has for most part been taken out of aerobics, and the feet are generally kept on the ground. Aerobics today involve not jumping around furiously but working with gravity. You move fluidly, rhythmically and at your own speed, for which your body will be grateful.

In addition to low-impact and non-impact aerobics, there is a new phenomenon in aerobic exercise. Step-training (also called bench or step aerobics) involves stepping on and off a bench that can be elevated to your own level of fitness, while you make a wide range of arm movements in time to popular music. Step-training exercises both upper and lower body muscles at the same time, and if carried out correctly, it places no more stress on legs, ankles and knees than walking.[18] The phrase 'carried out correctly' is very important, however. In 1993, British osteopaths reported a flood of people injured by step-training. It seems that they had all been using home equipment, had not been warming up with stretching exercises, and were 'stepping' too often, too high and/or too fast. The consumer magazine *Which? Way to Health* recommends seeking your doctor's advice before taking up step-training, and ensuring that, before beginning, you are reasonably fit. Once you begin, use good equipment, follow instructions carefully and don't do too much too quickly.[19]

Step-training is a high-intensity, low-impact power workout minus the stress on the joints. It burns fat and calories and conditions the heart and lungs while also toning up legs, hips, buttocks and thighs. Like regular aerobics, step-training must be done in sessions of 10 to 20 minutes, with a gradual warm-up first and a gradual cool-down afterwards. You should not step-train more than three or four times a week; instead, try other aerobic activities such as walking, swimming or cycling on alternate days.

Many people in their middle years feel they are too old to take part in such aerobic workouts. But this really makes no sense at all. In reality, the older you are, the more you need to exercise aerobically. You reach your physiological middle age in your mid-20s at the latest, not the appointed age of 40, and after the age of 25, your body begins to decline, primarily because of lack of use. Those who don't exercise regularly simply lose the optimal use of their bodies and age more rapidly.

A woman reaches her physical maturity by the age of 18 or 19. If she is sedentary, that's when ageing begins to creep on her. The heart loses its ability to pump blood at a rate of 1 per cent every single year past physical maturity. Additionally, the chest wall stiffens and the body is less able to take in oxygen. Muscles become weaker, the metabolism slows down, bones lose calcium and nerve impulses travel more slowly.

If you are sedentary, your blood vessels will be constricted by some 30 per cent, which will naturally affect your heart. By the age of 30, you will lose nearly 5 per cent of your muscle fibres. By the age of 60, up to 30 per cent of your muscles will be replaced by fat. Worse yet, the blood flow from arms to legs can slow down by up to 60 per cent. Eventually, your body's flexibility and bone mass deteriorate. All this doesn't occur instantly, but by the time you are 40, all will be evident. Before you realize it, life as you once knew it is over.

Aerobics will not solve all of the problems. Many other factors must be taken into consideration. But aerobic exercise is one of the best ways known for slowing down the ageing process.

THE OLDEST EXERCISE

While aerobics is the newest trend to better health, yoga is the oldest, and it has made a remarkable re-entry into modern society as the ideal workout for millions. In the 1990s life has become more hectic than ever, so it seems only natural that such a gentle yet all-inclusive form of exercise would reach popularity now. Stress, tension and anxiety have led us to physical and mental burnout, so people have sought an exercise programme that incorporates relaxation and soothes both the body and mind. To eliminate muscle tension, develop physical strength and vitality, rejuvenate mental abilities and balance emotions, many have turned to the ancient exercise of hatha yoga.

This, the simplest form in a system of physical, mental and spiritual development, is only the beginning of yoga. Originally, yoga was an art and science developed for the realization of full human potential, including extensive practice of mental training and a basis that reflects the world's oldest and most sublime philosophy. Hence, for individuals whose aim is to be the complete masters of their own bodies and minds, hatha yoga – the yoga of the body – is merely a path leading towards the yoga of the mind.

Those who loathe the very thought of exercise may feel quite differently when introduced to yoga. In a short time, without the need for special equipment, clothes, shoes or locations, practising a few yoga postures can rid the body of tension, bring about greater flexibility and ease a weary mind. And if you bore easily, there are 84,000 posture variations to keep you going. I know of no other form of physical exercise where you can choose to do so little and gain so much. The benefits of yoga are so comprehensive that you cannot easily recognize all the progress you will make. It's like looking at an iceberg – what's visible is only a tiny portion of the whole thing.

The amount of stress that is inflicted upon us, and which we inflict on ourselves, is epidemic today. Alcoholism and drug addiction have become primary health problems, and many of us haven't got a clue about what it means to relax. We should remember Newton's third law of motion: for every force, there is an equal and opposite force, or reaction. Because we live in an era of high stress that leads to physical and mental distress, we must learn techniques to combat the effects of stress.

Hatha yoga provides us with a natural and effective way of doing just that. It chiefly consists of exercises known as 'postures', but also includes controlled breathing, diet and relaxation. The purpose of the postures is to limber up every muscle in your body. If you think that other forms of exercise can do this, such as calisthenics, you would be partially correct. But that is like having the best and most finely tuned car in the world and then putting a drunk driver in it. Yoga's postures not only tune up your muscles but have an effect on all of your body functions, such as circulation, digestion, elimination and the nervous system. Over the centuries, a rare few yogis of India have been able to control all bodily functions at will.

Yoga, in its most primary form, is the disciplining of the intellect, the mind, the emotions and the will. One of the major works on yoga, the *Kathopanishad*, says:

WHEN THE SENSES ARE STILLED, WHEN THE MIND IS AT REST, WHEN THE INTELLECT WAVERS NOT – THEN, SAY THE WISE, IS REACHED THE HIGHEST STAGE. THIS STEADY CONTROL OF THE SENSES AND MIND HAS BEEN DEFINED AS YOGA. HE WHO ATTAINS IT IS FREE FROM DELUSION.

There are at least ten different kinds of yoga. Hatha yoga, the popular physical variety, which is the most commonly practised type in Europe and America today, helps to free the body from physical tensions which are reflections of tensions in the mind. It teaches you how to utilize the body and mind to gain relaxation and physical fitness. With regular practice, yoga results in strength, stamina and flexibility.

Today, yoga is taught at gyms, health clubs, YMCAs and YWCAs, and council-run leisure centres, and there is a wide range of books and videos on the market as well. One does not get easily discouraged by yoga because it can be quite simple, even though, of course, as with many disciplines, levels of difficulty can be very high for the most advanced practitioners. Although you can learn from books many of the basic postures yourself, it is best to receive instruction from an accredited instructor. Even children can benefit from certain forms of yoga. The exercise revives rather than tires the body. You virtually stimulate the glands, nerves and muscles without causing any fatigue.

For those of us who engage in tennis, jogging or aerobics, it may appear quite odd that such a drastically different exercise can have such far-reaching benefits. Let's face it, most exercise today is frantic, furious, demanding and quite violent to our muscles. With yoga, however, the exercise is slow, fluid and gradual, while you focus on relaxation and proper breathing rather than on point scoring and mile- and clock-watching. This makes it such an ideal exercise for people of all ages and all levels of physical fitness.

We exercise to increase our circulation and take up more oxygen. We already discussed just how, in aerobic exercise, you need to raise your heart rate to achieve this goal. But with hatha yoga, this can be accomplished with the easy movements of the spine and various joints of the body, through deep rhythmic breathing and systematic stretching, tensing and relaxing of the body's muscles. When you perform yoga postures with deep rhythmic breathing, you draw blood to the spine, which tones up the nerves emanating from the spine. Certain postures deliver blood to the brain and stimulate other organs of the body. For example, sufferers of arthritis of the spine can alleviate pain enormously by doing rhythmic bends and twists which result in greater mobility. Additionally, nerve pressure caused by subtle misalignment and vertebral maladjustments can be relieved by yoga postures.

GORILLAS VERSUS SWANS

An increasing number of professional athletes, fitness enthusiasts and physiotherapists are turning to yoga to complement their regular routines and standard forms of treatment. The sweaty, hard and painful approach to exercise of the 1980s is quickly giving way to the relaxed and tranquil methods of the 1990s.

'There is no way I could have played as long as I did without yoga,' Kareem Abdul-Jabbar told *Men's Health* magazine.[20] After 20 years in professional basketball in the US, Abdul-Jabbar said that it was yoga that made his training complete. He took up yoga at the age of 14 to gain suppleness, concentration and more effective breathing. 'As a preventive medicine, it's unequalled,' he explained. 'Once I started practising it, I had no muscle injuries during my career.'

Men's Health also reports an interesting phenomenon. According to the magazine, many athletes regularly go through yoga postures while training but refer to them as 'stretches' and not as yoga. It's part ignorance, part embarrassment on the part of the athlete. Remember when it was revealed how many football and rugby players practised ballet in secret? It improved their flexibility, and the results were evident on the playing field, but how unmasculine! I suppose it's more acceptable among that set to move like a gorilla than like a swan.

These athletes would feel quite differently if they knew the impressive history of this ancient ritual. In earlier times, the teaching of yoga was reserved for the élite, and to keep the common people away from this cherished art, it was surrounded by mystery and cloaked in obscure formulae. Today, however, science has unravelled most of the mysteries and 'common' people are learning to accept yoga's benefits.

No one can reach optimal health if their heart, lungs, brain, liver, kidneys, eyes and hearing are not in perfect order. Although many forms of exercise will bring about strong muscles, this in itself does not produce a healthy person. It is healthy organs *and* healthy muscles that make for a healthy individual. Yoga postures always aim at producing internal effects – they influence the condition of the organs and secretory glands.

The yoga postures are intimately connected with a prescribed method of breathing. Hatha yoga incorporates a number of respiratory techniques and each posture must be considered with a specific breathing exercise if the desired effect on nervous balance is to be achieved. If we learn how to breathe correctly, it can greatly affect our stress levels. Nerve centres of the brain can be influenced with proper breathing, which induces relaxation by having a sedative effect.

Our living habits have caused an impairment of our breathing. Naturally, we all breathe because we couldn't live without air. The way we breathe keeps us alive but not thriving. It is extremely shallow. It comes from the upper chest, bringing in a very small quantity of oxygen, certainly not enough for our lungs to function at full capacity or enough to fuel our body's cells properly. The greater part of our lungs lie dormant. If breath is the energy of life, the living force, then we don't have much of it. We derive more energy from oxygen than from anything else.

Yoga breathing is slow, deep and rhythmical. It exerts a gentle pressure on the liver, stomach and digestive tract, which in turn stimulates other organs. It strengthens the diaphragm, reduces the flood of 'fight or flight' symptoms, drops blood pressure, brings down the pulse rate and calms tense muscles. When you are under stress, you tend to gulp short and fast breaths and 'over-breathe'. This creates extra anxiety, and doesn't allow enough oxygen to get to the brain, which results in dizziness, light-headedness and confusion. Your vision can even become blurry. This lack of oxygen forces the heart to beat faster and pump more blood as perspiration breaks out. At the same time, the constriction of blood vessels makes your hands feel as if they are frozen. Pain control clinics and psychiatrists are teaching breath control techniques to help their patients. Yoga practitioners have done this for thousands of years.

Constant practice is the secret of yoga's success. As oil seeds must be pressed to yield oil, and wood must be heated to ignite it and bring out the hidden fire within, you too need to practise the proper forms of exercise to bring about optimal health. The practical approach of yoga is aimed at enriching the health and consciousness of people going about the complicated, stress-beset activity of modern living. A few years ago, it was necessary to 'sell' yoga to the West, but this is no longer true. People got the message that 'yoga works' and the number of converts is growing daily. It is rewarding at any level, even for the average middle-aged person who has got out of touch with his or her muscles and joints, which have stiffened up and lost tone and elasticity. It is possible to take up yoga at any age, even if your ankles, knees, hips, wrists, elbows and shoulders are stiff, your spine is inflexible, your hamstrings have shortened and your coordination, balance and muscle tone are poor.

You can practise yoga for life, unlike certain physical activities and competitive sports that become too difficult or boring once your strength, energy and drive-to-succeed diminish with age. The biggest problem people have with yoga is getting started, but unlike other types of exercise programmes, yoga has a very low drop-out rate – a testament to its efficacy and value. After all, who wouldn't want to stay with a formula that enriches both the body and the mind? The postures allow us to attain a steadiness of both body and mind, a feeling of lightness, suppleness, psycho-physical poise and overall optimal health. The benefits to the nerves, glands and vital organs, as well as to the muscular-skeletal system, are enormous. If further incentive is needed, consider this: yoga can rejuvenate flagging sexual performance. It's truly one of the best anti-ageing formulas known to humanity. By eliminating tension, reducing weight, resculpting your body, reducing facial wrinkles and improving memory by increasing circulation to the brain, yoga can lead you toward peace of mind as well as a healthy body. You are never too old, tired, tense, anxious, overweight and out of condition to be helped.

Yoga provides us with the techniques and thus the opportunity for knowing our minds and bodies. In the process, we increase our will power and mental strength. We learn to concentrate better and gain greater confidence. In the final analysis, we establish mastery over our thoughts and, thus, our bodies.

THE TREE, THE FROG AND THE COWFACE

If you were to give yoga a try, what may you actually expect? Initially, you will probably learn the four basic postures: the Adept Seat, the Lotus Seat, the Powerful Seat and the (unfortunately named) Swastika Seat.[21] You begin by doing the following:
1 Body straight, sitting crosslegged with one heel at the anus, the other at the front, chin on breast.
2 Legs folded with feet, soles upward, on opposite thighs; arms crossed,

hands on thighs (or arms may be crossed behind, hands holding big toes); tongue pressed against teeth; chin on breast or held up; gaze on tip of nose.

3 Legs stretched out, apart; waist bent; head held in hands and placed on knees.

4 Sit crosslegged with feet between calves and thighs, body straight.

Some yoga postures have unusual names, such as lotus, tree, frog, cowface, Egyptian or modified fish. The stretches should never be painful, for you only go as far as it feels comfortable; the minute you feel pain, ease up. All the techniques of yoga aim to bring about tranquillity.

Although the previous instructions describe a common starting posture, there is another extremely simple one you can try, a resting pose. Lie flat on your back, legs stretched out with heels apart and feet falling limply outward. Place your arms alongside your body, allowing them to rest on the floor. Turn up the palms of your hands, keeping the fingers limp and slightly curled. You may place thin cushions under your neck and knees. Now, breathe only through your nose and do not control your pattern of breathing. Simply be aware of your breath. Then, take two deep abdominal breaths, exhaling completely. As you inhale, let your abdomen rise as high as it can possibly go, then, as you exhale, feel it sink all the way to the spine. Release your abdominal muscles, and once again, simply be aware of your normal breathing. You will soon notice that your breathing is now quiet and smooth and has an even rhythm. At times, you may feel the urge to inhale deeply or even yawn, causing you to sigh upon releasing the breath. Somewhere in your muscles, tension is melting away.

Now that your breathing is under a well-established pattern, begin to pay special attention to the rest of your body. From feet to scalp, examine it for signs of tension. As you run across areas that seem 'rigid', consciously let them go. You can literally command a tense part of your body to relax by saying 'Let go' while firmly focusing on the problem site. With each release, your will feel the muscles become heavier as they rest with their full weight and go limp like a sleeping cat. I am always amazed how, after my cats, Bob and Marceau, make a lethal bee-line for an unsuspecting baby lizard and deliver it to me, they go as limp as water balloons. I can virtually mould Marceau like a ball of putty without him tightening a single muscle. It is this level of relaxation that you should be aiming for.

With so much to gain with so little effort, one can't help but wonder why it has taken so long for us to catch on to yoga. In many respects, it's largely due to ignorance. There are people who still believe that yoga is a religion, that they'll have to stand on their heads, walk on coals or lie on a bed of nails; that they'll have to become a vegetarians; that yoga consists of sitting in an odd position and thinking; or, simply, that yoga takes far too long to achieve any results.

If you want to call positive thinking and meditation a religion, fine. But most people would agree that these are part of the basis of all religions. As far as standing on your head is concerned, certainly you might eventually do that – it is the most advanced position in hatha yoga. If you did it at the start, it would be like picking up a basketball for the very first time going up against Kareem Abdul-Jabbar! Now what are your chances of success if you did that? As for thinking that yoga takes far too long, it's like saying that you'll never take up swimming because you can't compete at Olympic level.

As far as being a vegetarian is concerned, yoga does encourage a healthy way of living which includes healthy food. But have you ever exercised your body and then believed that you could simply – to use a less-than-scientific term – 'pig out'? Common sense tells you that you should not engage in practices that cancel out your good efforts.

Further, yoga is about 'concentration' which is worlds away from 'thinking'. Whoever said, 'Sometimes I sits and thinks and sometimes I just sits,' never practised yoga. It can be quite difficult for most people to shut out the frantic activity between their ears and concentrate inwardly. To develop a calm, controlled and disciplined state of mind is a learned behaviour.

Finally, a word to those who desire a quick-fix from their workouts. A quick-fix has never fixed anything. Lots of frequent quick-fixes generally lead to a major problem down the road. It's like shabbily patching an unstable roof: one day the rain will come and the roof will collapse. Sporadic, high-energy exercise will not do for you what steady yoga practice can achieve. Those who perform yoga postures regularly are actually quite surprised at how quickly they do see results. As they gain strength, stamina and flexibility, it not only improves their lives overall, but allows them to enjoy and excel more at forms of exercise and sports than they had previously thought possible.

MEDITATION IN MOTION

Another ancient activity has also made a comeback and is about to become an important and widely practised form of exercise. It is called t'ai chi chuan and it is here to stay. Regular practitioners of t'ai chi say it rejuvenates them, motivates them to stay with the exercise programme and brings them closer to optimal health.

T'ai chi is actually an ancient martial art, and before the 19th century it was a guarded secret among select Chinese families. It consists of a formal series of slow, graceful, continuous movements that are performed in a supple and relaxed manner. The philosophy behind t'ai chi is that you can reach a point where the mind and body are in sync, working mutually to achieve total well-being. 'Intelligence over force' is t'ai chi's hallmark. The carefully executed moves are performed with a straight and upright posture that encourages the flow of energy, and the relaxed state of the body allows the shifting of its weight to the legs. Achieving relaxation and a perfectly straight posture simultaneously sounds a lot easier than it is in reality. The legs can become so heavy as to cause pain, which in turn causes a tightening of the muscles. Hence, most of us are quite unaware of how difficult it is to obtain true relaxation.

When t'ai chi is performed correctly, its benefits include improved blood circulation, the loosening and limbering up of joints, and mental relaxation. It can be distinguished from most other forms of exercise primarily by its ability to promote deep mental relaxation. In this respect it's like yoga, and, indeed both yoga and t'ai chi have been referred to as 'meditation in motion'. Softness, pliability and complete relaxation are the goal of both disciplines. In essence, the aim of both yoga and t'ai chi is to unite the body and mind harmoniously.

To achieve through t'ai chi the same results of serenity that can be gained from yoga, you practise slow, orchestrated movements that are integrated and continuous throughout the entire exercise session. You never stop one posture and then do another. The whole process is smooth, slow and on-going. Some explain it by saying the movements are like pulling and releasing a rubber band at different levels of intensity – never snapping, never going wobbly. Like yoga, this too brings about flexibility and relaxation.

Where the two differ, however, is that yoga utilizes proper breathing methods to gain good biorhythms, while t'ai chi zeros in on flowing movements to produce the good biorhythms, which results in proper breathing. Therefore, mastering proper biorhythms by engaging in continuous motion and by not holding a static posture is the key difference between t'ai chi and yoga. Yoga is an internal exercise which results in external relaxation; t'ai chi is an external exercise that brings about internal harmony.

T'ai chi can take as little as ten minutes to perform, but a half-hour t'ai chi session gives you the same exercise benefits as a three-hour game of golf. T'ai chi enthusiasts say they always feel good, relaxed, refreshed and exhilarated after a workout. In addition, they claim to inherit a few of the values the Chinese prize highly – patience, perseverance, tolerance, discipline and confidence.

Chi is energy. Energy is power. While you practise t'ai chi, you are relaxed, but at the same time, you are fully aware of your energy flow. You must pay constant attention to what your body is doing. Usually when we exercise, it's common to let the mind wander because it takes you away from the pain that brings us gain. But with t'ai chi, you cannot perform the movements properly or achieve the health benefits if you don't concentrate intensely. In this case: no brain, no gain.

Properly executed, t'ai chi movements feel good to the body and bring about grace and control, while many people even speak of the sense of empowerment that it gives them. But what t'ai chi practitioners primarily gain is cardiovascular fitness, strength, endurance, flexibility and self-confidence.

Prevention magazine even reports that this 2500-year-old workout can boost the immune system. They say that t'ai chi may actually increase the amount of T-lymphocytes in your body. These 'T-cells' are the samurai of the immune system, white blood cells that destroy bacteria and possibly even tumour cells.

In a study reported in *Prevention*, 30 healthy volunteers who practised t'ai chi had their T-cell counts compared to those of 30 who didn't. During a resting state, the T-cell count of the t'ai chi group were higher than those of the control group, and after a 20-minute session of t'ai chi, the t'ai chi group's T-cell counts went up by an additional 13 per cent.

A session of these 'slow-motion calisthenics', as some have called t'ai chi, can consist of as few as 20 graceful, fluid movements, but the martial art's full range comprises 108 movements. It is divided into several levels of training. Initially, the moves are gentle, slow and soft, but gradually, the workouts become more intense and vigorous. T'ai chi is considered an ideal form of exercise for the out-of-shape, the elderly and those recovering from illness. Athletes have learned that it enhances their ability to focus and that they have an improved sense of balance and speedier recovery between workouts. Others have resorted to t'ai chi to work through ME (myalgic encephalomyelitis), also known as chronic fatigue syndrome.[22]

Scientists are today proving what the Chinese have known for ages. A group of Australian researchers have concluded that those who practise t'ai chi regularly can effectively reduce blood levels of stress hormones after experiencing stressful situations.[23]

Sophia Delza, who, in 1940, became the first American to teach it in the US, said that t'ai chi

NOURISHES MUSCLES, FACILITATES JOINT ACTION AND STIMULATES THE NERVOUS SYSTEM, ALL WITHOUT INCREASING THE ACTIVITY OF THE HEART OR BREATHING RHYTHM . . . NO MUSCLE JOINT, LIMB, NO PART OF THE BODY IS EVER OVERTAXED OR UNDERACTIVATED.[24]

And according to Ying Lehua, a renowned teacher of t'ai chi:

PRACTISING T'AI CHI CAN RAISE THE DEGREE OF INTENSITY OF THE CENTRAL
NERVOUS SYSTEM, ACTIVATE OTHER SYSTEMS AND ORGANS AND IMPROVE
THE COORDINATING FUNCTION OF THE CEREBRUM, CREATING CONDITIONS
FOR PREVENTING ARTERIOSCLEROSIS AND OTHER HEART DISEASES.[25]

As new and foreign as this form of exercise may seem to us, t'ai chi is
actually the most widely used physical training system in the world. In
China alone, more than 200 million people do t'ai chi regularly.

With t'ai chi, there is no limit to what you can accomplish. Since force
is never exerted, your body never has to do more than it is capable of.
Therefore, you do not waste strength and energy but rather increase your
endurance. The pinnacle of success with t'ai chi is obtained when images
are used to deal with immobile body areas. As we saw in the previous
chapter, your mind affects your body; physical responses can be activated
by your thoughts, feelings or visualization. It has become evident that all
bodily systems are intertwined in one brain-regulated network. Stress
and poor thought patterns can bring about illness, but the opposite also
holds true. Effective thinking, breathing and body maintenance can
maintain or restore your health. After all, an inflexible body is rigid, and an
inflexible mind is grim. Rigidity and grimness eventually destroy good
health and shorten your life. T'ai chi as a total system improves your
health by allowing you to perform movements that emphasize the
strengthening and conditioning of both the body and the mind.

CHAPTER NINE

KNOWING YOUR MIND

In times of great change, rapid expansion, constant readjustment and general transition, as we are experiencing today, enormous stresses almost force us to re-evaluate our modes of thinking. In modern medicine, this has resulted in altered interpretations of the nature of health and illness and of human beings themselves. Such a transition does not happen overnight, however. Yet although the added weight and variety of stresses that we endure as part of a complex society take time to manifest themselves in illness and new types of diseases, the changes in our attitude towards medicine must be accelerated if we are to catch up with the new ideas regarding human nature. We need a greater understanding and acceptance of psychological conflict, in which our physical body plays a secondary role.

This was the all-too-real situation in which a middle-aged woman I met during an overseas flight found herself. Frances, serene, attractive, sat comfortably sipping a cup of tea while becoming mesmerized by the quiet antics of a little boy across the aisle. She chuckled softly and began to talk to me about the simpler joys of life. Our conversation had a most tranquillizing effect on me. I couldn't help but ask, 'Have you always had such a sunny disposition?"

'Heavens, no!' she replied. 'I had to learn how to live all over again about ten years ago. My views on life had to change drastically.'

Well, this statement certainly wasn't going to be left unquestioned. Frances began to tell me about her past life in Philadelphia. Then, she was a single mother and a critical-care nurse with more stress in her life than she cared to recall. She never felt really well and had simply learned to live with her constant tiredness, fatigue, mild depression, anxiety and uncertainty about the future. 'After all,' she said, 'responsible adults persevere under any circumstances, don't they?'

No, Frances wasn't going to give herself any breaks, so, one day, her body literally broke down for her. She collapsed. She was unable to cope with her ill health and began a lengthy series of encounters with various physicians who could not diagnose her illness. They blamed it on a virus and – surprisingly, since they have no effect on viruses – bombarded her with numerous antibiotics. The medications made her feel worse but on doctor's orders, she continued to take them. Then, to make matters worse, Frances had a bad fall, broke her leg and dislocated her hip. At last, she had no choice but to retire to her bed encased in a massive plaster cast.

But an interesting thing happened as she was left alone with her thoughts. 'This experience gave me the opportunity to get inside my head, to really think about my life – what I had done with it and about what I could and couldn't do about my future,' she told me. After about a week, she began to feel better as far as her mystery illness was concerned and she stopped taking the antibiotics. She began to feel as if she could regain control of her situation, but exhaustion and pain still haunted her. Frances decided that, once her cast was removed, she would leave no stone unturned in the search for a diagnosis of and treatment for her persistent illness. She would also embark on a course of therapies that would show respect for her body and mind, including regular deep muscle massage and relaxation techniques as well as psychoanalysis.

Several years into her quest for mind–body awareness, Frances's condition was finally diagnosed. She had a collagen malfunction which had resulted in the deterioration of her body's connective tissue. It was no surprise,' Frances said matter of factly. 'My life had become unglued mentally, emotionally and spiritually and then physically.'

Frances actually began her healing journey when she broke her leg and took the road to self-introspection. Today, she is completely cured and claims never to have felt better.

Most of us have to reach a point of great crisis before we make a conscious effort to take better care of ourselves. I know of a number of men, for instance, who go to great lengths to take extraordinary care of their cars, but totally neglect their bodies. Imagine if the situation were reversed. A few good men would not be so hard to find . . .

MIND–BODY RELATIONSHIPS

Frances's approach to health care is a relatively new phenomenon in today's medicine. It is called psychoneuroimmunology – the study of mind–body relationships. It is a brand new science that looks at the interaction between psychology and the central nervous, immune and endocrine (hormone) systems. Medical science is discovering that the human brain is not just the seat of consciousness, but also a gland, perhaps the most prolific gland in the human body. It is certainly a most spectacular machine, which scientists claim would be taller than the World Trade Center in New York and wider than the state of Texas if they were to duplicate it as a computer.

How the mind can affect the body was put to the test by the brilliant researcher, Dr Dean Ornish. For the first time, he proved, in a landmark study of heart disease, that atherosclerosis (clogging of the arteries which leads to heart attack and stroke) can be reversed without the use of drugs or surgery. And he showed that *love* was the key component in this reversal.

He came to the conclusion that heart disease, the No. 1 killer in the UK and US, involves more than a pump in need of repair, as medical science usually views it. Dr Ornish believes that illnesses of the heart are rooted in the profound isolation experienced by great numbers of people in modern society – isolation from feelings, from other people and from a greater force in the universe. [1] This results in many people feeling spiritual and emotional pain.

We are not meant to be solitary creatures. It is vital that we cultivate a social network that meets the variety of our needs. Those who do this are much healthier, far more content and much more capable of dealing with stress than those who do not have such social support. Those who are overly preoccupied with themselves quite frequently succumb to psychological and, eventually, physical problems.

As Dr Ornish says, 'Looking out for No. 1 isn't enlightened self-interest. It's just lonely, and loneliness kills.' People who are lonely are more likely to have low levels of natural killer cell activity, an indicator of immune response. It is interesting to note, for instance, that those people who constantly use the words 'I' and 'me' in conversation are at the greatest risk of heart disease.

It appears that the closer a relationship you have with someone, the more immune you become to illness. Marriage, for instance, offers greater benefits for optimal health than friendships or group affiliations, especially for men. Today, it is known that people who have broad social contacts have the lowest mortality rates, while those who are primarily isolated have the highest rates.

A recent evaluation of 2754 adults aged between 35 and 69 showed that men without much social contact are two to three times more likely to die early.

Many of us have known people who have died shortly after they suffered the loss of a loved partner. While death is the ultimate barrier to a relationship, those who are single, divorced, widowed or otherwise isolated from others also have far higher incidences of emotional stress and physical illness. Researchers say that isolated people routinely suffer from poor health and are much more susceptible to everything from headaches and skin disorders to arthritis, heart disease and cancer. Thus, an inadequate social support system can literally mean an inadequate immune system. A positive, supportive social structure in our lives can lessen the impact of stress and help us through challenging times more efficiently. It boosts our morale and thus our stress-resistance levels. Some say that good morale is possibly the most important factor in warding off disease.

Those who have nurtured the capacity to love themselves and others are rewarded with energy, good health and love in return. But those who imprison their feelings and keep them locked up feel a sense of loss and powerlessness. Such a state paves the way to excessive stress and can lead to sickness.

For example, stress can bring on an angina attack in susceptible people. Under certain stress conditions, the adrenal glands secrete adrenaline – the hormone that causes the 'fight or flight' response. This elevates blood pressure and the heart rate, which excessively burdens the heart. While all of this is taking place, the coronary arteries, already clogged with atheroma, cannot expand enough to deliver the additional oxygen that is needed. The result: crippling angina pain.

The relationship between mind and body has been investigated for some time. For instance, researchers kept track of the health of some 1300 medical students who graduated from Johns Hopkins University in Baltimore, Maryland between 1948 and 1964. While in medical school, some of the students claimed to be emotionally removed from one or both parents. After 30 years, the investigators found, these same people suffered an unusually high incidence of mental illness, suicide and death from cancer.

SUPPRESSED HOSTILITY

It has become evident that people who are long-suffering, repress hostile feelings and possess low self-esteem are also at greater risk of disease. Some three decades ago, the public was stunned when psychologist Lawrence LeShan claimed to have discovered a 'cancer personality'. Since then, more than 1500 articles have appeared in the professional literature pontificating on the mind–body connection.

Cancer patients harbour negative emotions. When people smile on the outside and are suffocating on the inside, they are killing themselves. Nearly all of us are conditioned to respond with 'Fine' when someone enquires about our well-being, regardless of how awful we may truly feel. Such consistent numbing of emotions can destroy the body.

Cancer patients, more than most others, have trouble expressing anger. Women, especially, report having felt a build up of anger in the year or two prior to their developing cancer. Healthy women vent their anger and then get rid of it. But some choose not to reveal their rage; instead they remain outwardly calm but inwardly depressed, then fatigued, then sick. Those who remain depressed once cancer develops are twice as likely to die.

The bizarre thing about people with suppressed hostility who also develop cancer is that they appear unable to express anger only when it concerns themselves. They are perfectly capable and willing to get angry in defence of others or of a cause, but not in self-defence. Eventually, such a person begins to lose a sense of control and then soon feels helpless and hopeless. When they give up, their immune system gives up. A depressed immune system, as we already discussed, can lead to allergies, to asthma and even, in the HIV-positive, to AIDS. After all, your immune system is only acting analogously with your thoughts and actions. To maintain control, one requires a balance in life. The hopeless–helpless personality that completely gives up is just as dangerous as the Type-A personality that insists on total control. Either way, you can't reach optimal health. A realistic sense of empowerment is the only true solution.

There may, like the cancer personality, be an 'arthritis personality'. Rheumatoid arthritis sufferers are often subject to great inner turmoil and are generally overconscientious and very fearful of criticism. They are frequently depressed and without a good self-image. As a result, they are notorious people-pleasers and lock away their own problems so as not to be a burden to others.

This excessive suppression of emotions virtually eats them up. Repressed anger actually turns against the person and, under these circumstances, the immune systems mutinies against the body. What's interesting, however, is that those people who are genetically pre-disposed to rheumatoid arthritis but are emotionally healthy tend not to suffer from this disease. Women, who are generally taught to suppress emotions such as anger, develop rheumatoid arthritis four times more frequently than men.

In Dr Ornish's view, it is difficult to heal physical problems if you don't first address the cause of those disorders. He says that, to cure heart disease, for example, it's vital that the motivations for self-destructive behaviour be dealt with.

Dr Bernie Siegel gives a perfect – if slightly dramatic – example. In his outstanding book, *Peace, Love and Healing*, Dr Siegel discusses self-induced healing, and tells the story of a woman whose cancer of the cervix had spread and she was considered close to death. Her condition changed drastically, however, when her much-hated husband suddenly died: she completely recovered! The lesson we can take from this story is that, to alter the course of disease, we should alter our lifestyles. But when Dr Siegel asks his patients whether they want to change their lifestyles or undergo surgery, the majority choose the operation because 'It hurts less.'

It is evident that among the things that are most toxic to the body are excessive self-involvement, hostility and cynicism. Thus, being alone and at odds with the world can be as harmful to us as pollutants in our environment or poisons in our food. We can, given the opportunity, easily burden ourselves with unrelenting stress, but we will feel the way we think. Therefore, if we consistently view our lives in pessimistic terms, we are likely to find ourselves frequently depressed and having low self-esteem. Eventually, such negative thoughts simply wear us out. Stress-related physical problems are most commonly suffered by pessimists.

Optimists and pessimists, however, are made, not born. Being products of our environment, we mimic the behaviours and attitudes of those around us. Thus, since our perceptions are learned responses, we can also learn to abandon the self-doubt and self-criticism that we inflict upon ourselves. Otherwise, our internal critic becomes our own worst enemy.

MAKING WAVES

Dr Ornish may have proved this concept, but he certainly was not the first to make the association. Eastern thought regards mind and body as, quite simply, different manifestations of the same life force. Most people may be surprised to discover that this was also the belief held by Western societies from ancient times up through the Middle Ages. The first Westerner to make a definite connection between mind and body was the Greek philosopher Plato, who claimed that the mind exists before, during and after its occupation of the body. St Augustine wrote about the mind–body connection in his treatise *Concerning the City of God Against the Pagans* in the 4th century AD, and medical practice operated on this principle well into the 17th century – to medieval physicians, the mind and body were inseparable.

Shortly thereafter, however, the work of the French philosopher René Descartes (1596–1650) began to make waves. He said that a clear distinction between mind and body had to be made and arrived at the theory known as 'dualism'. Dualism penetrated the previously holistic art of medical practice, and Descartes' theory dominates to this day.

It wasn't until the 20th century that his assumptions began to be seriously questioned. Carl Jung (1875–1961), a pupil of Freud's and a leading figure in psychology, concluded that our emotions and thoughts are intimately intertwined with the basic life energies in our bodies.

According to Jung, 'the distinction between mind and body is an articifial dichotomy, a peculiarity of intellectual understanding than of the nature of things.'

Today, enlightened psychologists are not the only ones who share Jung's view. Illness begins at the level where people carry their belief systems and can, if not treated there, manifest in the body, according to Barbara Brennan, a former NASA physicist.

I SEE SCIENCE AS MAKING OBSERVATIONS TO TEST THEORY THAT THEN BECOMES ACCEPTED AS PHYSICAL LAW. BUT LAWS ARE LIMITED BY EQUIP- MENT THAT A SCIENTIST CAN BUILD; THEY ARE LIMITED BY THE FIVE SENSES. A TRUE SCIENTIST WOULD NOT DENY THE PHENOMENON [OF MIND– BODY CONNECTION] BUT RATHER WOULD ACKNOWLEDGE THAT WE CAN'T EXPLAIN IT YET.[2]

Some scientists are already proving this 'phenomenon', however. Re- searchers at the Ohio State University Medical Center wanted to know just how the stresses of the mind affect the body. They studied a group of people who cared for relatives with Alzheimer's disease and found that the carers had weaker immune systems than control subjects. The carers had a much lower percentage of T-cells and were prone to respiratory problems.[3]

But while negative influences can break us down, positive influences can help bring us back up. These were the conclusions of researchers at Stanford University Medical School in California, where a group of women with breast cancer were studied for up to ten years. The women who participated in psychotherapy as well as receiving standard medical treatment lived twice as long as those who received only medical treatment.[4] In another study of breast cancer, carried out at the Univer- sity of Pittsburgh School of Medicine, Dr Sandra M. Levy and her colleagues showed that 'joy' was the second leading cause of survival. The subjects who felt sadness, depression and hopelesness did not fare too well.

CHEMICAL MESSENGERS
AND CONTROLLING HEALTH

Researchers may disagree about the degree of effect the mind has over the body, but no enlightened individual today can deny that the brain and the immune system are inseparable. Let's consider a common ailment of today – allergies. Initially, it may seem odd to associate emotions with the onset of allergies – the itching, sneezing, wheezing attacks that result from an introduction to any one of the multitude of substances in the environment that act as allergy provokers. Over the years, studies have shown that animals that have been placed under stress and then exposed to an irritant always react badly, while contented animals exposed to the same irritant do not react at all. Research conducted on humans had the same results.

In most people with allergies, the white blood cells which help fight off infections confuse a normally safe substance such as milk, pollen or dust for a foreign invader, or antigen, and they mistakenly begin to create antibodies. The antibodies attach themselves to mast cells in the nose, throat and lungs, stomach, intestines or skin, and the next time the body is exposed to the antigen, the mast cells rupture, releasing histamine, which causes allergic symptoms. As a result, you've got a serious allergy problem.

The brain and the immune system constantly feed each other non-stop messages. Chemicals known as lymphokines have been isolated and are believed to be activated by the brain to help the body fight illness. Some of these chemicals actually enter the brain and affect the hypothalamus near the centre of the brain and the nearby pituitary gland (the 'master gland', which controls all the other glands), and this may contribute to the control of our emotions and stress levels. Then, the brain creates chemical messengers such as neuropeptides that help activate vital elements of the immune system such as the T-cells and B-cells. A further link between the brain and the immune system may be the extensive nerve threads found in the thymus and spleen – major organs of the immune system.

Some researchers hypothesize that such molecular links actually help us control our health. Experts have found that different emotions actually trigger different sets of messenger molecules – neuropeptides – that send a wide variety of messages that alter the metabolism of the entire body.[5] The neuropeptides which link brain cells, for example, act as direct communicators with immune cells. If you are worried or anxious, certain neuropeptides will act to depress your immune system. In other words, thought is literally responsible for how you may be feeling. It can determine whether you can tolerate toxins and resist disease. It can be the source of your contentment or depression. Did you know, for instance, that people with severe learning disabilities do not worry? As a result, they have one quarter of the cancer rate of the rest of us.

So, if negative emotions such as anger and hostility can introduce illness to our bodies, positive emotions such as joy and good will can bring about good health. In fact, at the same time that we are increasingly becoming overwhelmed by the poisons in our food, water and environment, scientists have concluded that negative emotions can actually increase the toxicity of numerous harmful substances to which we are exposed. We possess a built-in protective mechanism, directed by the mind, which can, to an extent, protect us from poisons and disease. But some researchers have gone so far as to claim that destructive emotions are actually more harmful than the toxins in our food and environment.

To believe that nothing can harm you is powerful medicine. Consequently, an optimistic thought pattern can be just about the best immunization against disease. When the mind becomes a positive influence on the immune system, we are simply better equipped to tolerate destructive forces. As positive messages are sent to the immune system by the brain, they have a healing or health-sustaining effect.

The latest medical research consistently points to on-going connections between the brain, consciousness and the body. Over and over again, researchers state that if you are philosophically willing to accept the power of positive thinking, you have to be willing to accept the punishment for negative thinking. An article in *American Medical News* said that the idea that the state of mind can influence one's medical destiny and perhaps longevity has made inroads not only into theology and psychology but into clinical medicine as well.[6]

AN INFINITE FIELD OF ENERGY

The advocates most associated with the mind–body connection are Deepak Chopra, Norman Cousins and Bernie Siegel. To some, Dr Chopra may profess the most complex or perhaps the most advanced version of this theory. He says that the connection between the mind and body arises from reality itself, a belief that is at the heart of ayurvedic medicine, of which Dr Chopra is the United States' most famous practitioner. Reality, he says, is an infinite field of energy containing all possibilities. What most of us perceive to be real is nothing but patterns imposed upon this energy by our minds. True healing, he believes, consists of a shift in consciousness in which one ceases to identify with one's quantum mechanical body – the energy field described as reality by ayurvedic medicine. As a result of this shift, according to Dr Chopra, one is no longer bound by the concept of mortality.[7]

The view of Norman Cousins – an American writer who claims that, when he was seriously ill, he laughed his way back to health by, among other things, watching Marx Brothers' films – is a bit more mainstream. Positive emotions, he says, such as festivity, purpose, determination, love, faith, hope and a strong will to live are good for the body. Negative ones such as fear are not. Hence, emotions can contribute to the development of disease. Depression, he says, can set the stage for serious illnesses such as cancer.[8]

Dr Siegel, on the other hand, gets right to the point. Heal your life, he says, and you will have a physical by-product.

None of these highly regarded individuals is claiming that positive emotions should be considered a substitute for medical care. But they are imploring you to become the master of your domain, to be in control of your mind and body to the highest degree possible.

It is important to note that psychosomatic research does not claim that psychosocial factors *cause* disease, but they do alter a person's susceptibility to it. After all, most of us are born into this world healthy and eventually acquire various illnesses, mainly as a result of lifestyle choices. Nutrition, exercise and attitude are the key determinants of good health – all within our control.

Take the example of cancer victims. As the connection between the brain and the health of the body becomes more and more evident, an increasing number of cancer patients and their families are beginning to fight this disease with their inner resources as well as with orthodox medicine. The odds are on their side. Insurance statistics published in the journal *Psychosomatic Medicine* show that people who practise meditation, for instance, have an incidence of cancer that is 55 per cent less than that of those who don't meditate. Even the conquest of cancer is a possibility. A team of scientists scoured the medical literature and found more than 400 cases of spontaneous remission. Upon closer inspection, they discovered that hope and positive feelings were the sole common factors that permitted individuals to beat the odds.

THE MIND AS DISSOLVING GELATINE

The co-existence of stress and illness is no coincidence. Whatever transpires in your mind has a rippling effect on the rest of your body. But let's consider the mind for a moment. Most of us assume that the mind is in the head and then there is the rest of the body. Not so. Although a complete definition doesn't exist yet, you could think of the mind as you might of gelatine powder dissolving in hot water – the mind is actually a whole-body phenomenon.

There is a lot of evidence in everyday life to show how the mind and body are linked. Your mind affects the body, for instance, when you see a police car light flashing in your rear-view mirror: your stomach is suddenly in your throat. Your heart feels as if it's going to pound out of your chest as you step up to the podium to make a speech. Page 3 of a certain tabloid newspaper makes most men feel real warm and friendly. When you feel the pressure of an approaching deadline, irritability, exhaustion and anxiety set in.

On the other hand, your body can influence the mind. You suffer from premenstrual syndrome and suddenly that wonderful, considerate and loving man you have been seeing becomes a total jerk who deserves to be hung at high noon in the town square. The post arrives and a welcome letter sends you over the moon. A few moments of prayer really calms you down. When you hug someone you care about, a rush of warmth and good feelings strengthens you.

What many people knew instinctively, and Eastern philosophies and biblical teachings stressed for thousands of years, medical science is proving today. At Ohio State University, for example, a study concluded that divorce can actually increase a woman's resistance to disease; it appears that women trapped in unhappy marriages had lower resistance levels than those in happy marriages. Duke University researchers concluded that people who are cynical and mistrustful of other people have more heart disease than those who don't.

'PROBLEM PATIENTS'

Associations between attitude and health appear endless. It has become common knowledge that 'problem patients' make greater and speedier recoveries than those who are submissive and passive and do not take an active role in their recovery process. I was quite delighted by what my friend Mantosh told me of her medical experience. Having suffered from arrhythmia for more than a decade and becoming increasingly dissatisfied with the lack of any progress in her medical treatment, she decided to become as knowledgeable about her condition as possible. She travelled to India and Europe and did extensive research in the United States, which eventually led to her writing a brilliant book called *Strong Women, Weak Hearts*. Mantosh receives regular treatment for her condition at a well-known and respected heart institute. The more knowledgeable she became, the more actively she participated in the management of her condition. One day, she noticed a distinctive yellow sticker on her medical file. Later, she discovered that the yellow dot meant 'problem patient'. But a health practitioner told her that being a problem patient probably saved her life: studies have shown that patients who are a bit of a pain in the neck to their physicians live longer.

Although being noncompliant is good for you, it's regarded as an inconvenience by most doctors. It has become quite evident to most of us who question our doctors that they don't particularly appreciate such an exchange. Research indicates that the patients whom doctors find most inquisitive and thus most annoying have the strongest immune systems. But the patients whom doctors consider absolutely wonderful – submissive and compliant – are the ones who are dying. So, wise patients have decided that, if their doctors are not willing to attend to their minds along with their bodies, they will find others who will. The days when patients surrender full responsibility for their health to their doctors are numbered. A patient – or medical consumer, to state it more accurately – is being deprived of the full services of a doctor if he or she does not treat that patient as a whole being. One of the most marked changes in medicine over the past decade has been the change in doctors' attitudes towards their patients.

Certain people, such as Mantosh, have immune-competent personalities – that is, they have become aware of their needs and have learned to assert them. If a part of their body is going to break down, it will have to do full battle with the mind. Experts now view personality as a crucial element to disease resistance.

Dr George Solomon, a psychiatrist, professor at the University of California at Los Angeles, and pioneer in the field of psychoneuroimmunology, says that being an immune-competent personality involves:

1 being in touch with your psychological and bodily needs.
2 being able to meet those needs by assertive action.
3 possessing coping skills, including a sense of control, which enable you to ward off depression.
4 expressing emotions, including sadness and anger.
5 being willing to ask for and accept support from loved ones.
6 having a sense of meaning and purpose in your work, daily activities and relationships.
7 having a capacity for play and pleasure.[9]

BIOPSYCHOSOCIAL MEDICINE

As apparent as all this may be, many in modern medicine still reject it flatly or simply pay it lip service but do not truly believe that the mind–body link has much validity. Aristotle accepted this link even without encouraging studies from prominent medical schools, but it is not a concept to which Marcia Angell, the executive editor of the *New England Journal of Medicine*, will subscribe. She says, 'It has not been shown unequivocally that someone's state of mind can cause or cure a specific disease,'[10] However, Dr Ronald Glaser of the Ohio State University College of Medicine views the mind–body theory quite differently. 'It's been convenient to think of these systems as separate,' he says, 'but they are clearly not, and eventually that has to change the whole of medicine.'[11]

And change is well under way. The *New York Times Magazine* has reported that American medical doctors are beginning to use such unconventional therapies as meditation, homoeopathy and acupuncture to treat patients.[12] In December 1991, the British health minister announced: 'It is now open to any family doctor to employ a complementary therapist to offer treatment on the NHS as long as the doctor remains accountable'. Later surveys showed that one third of British GPs possess a skill in one or more complementary therapies, and 34 per cent of fundholding GPs over a variety of complementary services, including acupuncture, hyprotherapy, osteopathy, homoeopathy and aromatherapy.[13] Some commentators believe that Western medicine will evolve from its narrow biochemical model to a biopsychosocial one that fully incorporates holistic techniques.

There always appears to be a time-lag between the occurrence of new stress-related illnesses and the realization that new and different approaches need to be adopted to deal with them. The current, and more sophisticated, awareness of the nature of human beings and disease has still not merged with modern medicine for the full benefit of us all.

But the mounting evidence is changing numerous beliefs that were held sacrosanct just a few years ago, and many of these are now being challenged while some are being discarded outright. The current view of psychosomatic medicine is rapidly gaining acceptance, while the field assigned to psychosomatic diseases grows by leaps and bounds.

At the turn of the century, physicians mainly focused on infection. Then, medical practice expanded to take in biochemistry, investigating particular tissues and organs. This led to a strict specialization of medical conditions, especially in the United States. More recently, however, medical literature, both for the 'trade' and for the general public, frequently speaks of the patient as a whole. Thus, disease is viewed as something more than just its local manifestation.

Take the example of the individual with a 'Type A' personality. When the emphasis in medicine was strictly biochemical, who would have given much credence to personality factors – e.g. keen ambition, anxiety, hostility and feelings of being in a constant time crunch – as key contributors to heart disease? Who would have accepted hostility as a toxic substance to the body? It took us a long time to accept that external factors such as smoking, high-fat diets and a lack of physical exercise were risk factors in heart disease. Now imagine how much more time is required for us to move on to the next phase and accept that the actions of the mind are yet another leading risk factor.

When the now-famous Type-A behaviour study was followed up by Meyer Friedman and Ray Rosenman, it was discovered that Type-As had more overt heart attacks, more silent heart attacks, more angina, more deaths and more second heart attacks if they survived the first. Recently, researchers who examined the various Type-A studies carried out over the years came to the conclusion that anger, aggression and destructive beliefs all trigger a chain of adverse biological effects that ultimately undermine our well-being and can lead to disease and death.

IMAGINED STRESS

When people are under stress, especially when they feel great mistrust towards others and turn those feelings into anger, they actually enhance the release of a wide variety of stress hormones. The extra hormones and the elevation of blood pressure and heart rate which the hormones automatically cause are a great strain on the heart. If you have the type of personality which experiences stress often and intensely enough, this chemical response can certainly contribute to illness in ways you may never have thought possible.

Therefore, you may consider the readjustment of your attitude, the control of your thoughts and emotions to be preventive medicine as much as a careful diet and proper exercise. Perhaps the Roman philosopher Epictetus (c. 55–135 AD) said it best: 'Men are disturbed not by the things that happen, but by their opinion of the things that happen.' Stress can actually be a productive force if we handle it properly. It is actually a necessary connection between us and the environment, a biological warning telling us to adapt to a new situation. It signals us to readjust, to make a change. Either we listen to those signals, make the appropriate alterations in our lives and thrive, or we merely survive. But then there is the ambiguous type of stress, which is chronic but undefined. When you are burdened by these types of stress at the same time, you never quite experience a normal mental and physiological state. You simply continue to build up a stress level until physical damage occurs.

What happens when we allow stress to take hold and don't remedy the situation? Well, a series of biochemical reactions occurs within the body to warn you that all is not well. In a seriously stressful situation, a part of your brain – the hypothalamus – sends a message via part of the automatic nervous system to the adrenal glands, which react right away by secreting extra adrenaline. All this biochemical action increases your heart rate and blood pressure, causes your blood vessels to dilate and your level of blood sugar to go up. The circulation of blood through your lungs, liver and skeletal muscles can increase by 100 per cent. The excess adrenaline interferes with digestion and reproduction. You may not have a clue about everything that is happening inside your body, but you may notice the cramps in your stomach, your clenched jaw and your tightened muscles.

What is really quite extraordinary is that, to experience all this biochemical activity, your stress can be either real or imagined. Dr Maxwell Maltz, author of *Psycho-Cybernetics*, says that 'the human nervous system cannot tell the difference between the actual experience and experience imagined vividly and in detail.' It has been determined that just thinking about a stressful situation can actually be more harmful than literally experiencing it. Studies have proved that those merely observing a sports event secreted much more adrenaline than the athletes themselves. The players, on the other hand, release more of the beneficial hormone, noradrenaline, which actually helps control stress.

Some people may not consider their stresses harmful because they are not particularly severe or because they are manageable. However, stress that you have accepted and decided to cope with simply accumulates and causes problems down the road. The majority of standard medical textbooks claim that 50 to 80 per cent of all disease has psychosomatic or stress-related origins. Holistic medical practitioners say this is likely to be 90 per cent. For a moment, think about how many people you know who suffer from frequent headaches, allergies, ulcers, insomnia, hypertension, arthritis, fatigue, alcoholism or nervous tension. Quite possibly more than you realized. People who continually worry or over-react to situations build up a warehouse of tension, fatigue and frustration which leaves them unmotivated and unproductive both to themselves and to society. Of all your family and friends, how many are completely well?

For most of us, drastically altering our lifestyle is simply not an available option. If a leading source of your stress is due to your career, partner, environment, beliefs or finances, it is certainly not very easy to make changes. After all, how many of us are bold enough, committed enough to our cause, disengaged enough from the opinions of others or capable of letting go of the security that our role in the system provides us? Not too many, unfortunately. Instead, we numb our anxieties with alcohol, medication and other, more drastic forms of self-destructive behaviour. None of these provides a single solution or alleviates a single source of our stress. We have, in fact, become very good at suppressing the debilitating symptoms of stress. Today, the norm is for society to expect and accept overwhelmingly high levels of stress.

KEEPING UP WITH YESTERDAY

Yet most of us know someone who seems to thrive on stress. Not everyone is vulnerable and passive in the face of adversity. Much can be said about our resilience, initiative and creativity. Many people survive the stress of a crisis with more vitality and energy than they had before. Like us, they are faced with stress, but at the same time, somehow they control the stress and not vice versa. Psychologists conclude that such individuals differ from the vast majority of us in several ways. They appear to be very involved in their careers and social lives, and exercise greater control over themselves. In particular they don't view potentially stressful situations as problems or obstacles but rather as challenges and new opportunities. There is tremendous exhilaration to be derived from conquering a challenge. A monotonous, non-challenged life often results in boredom and, eventually, physical and mental problems. We require challenges in order to thrive.

These stress-thrivers also tend to act forthrightly. Sometimes, the more time you give yourself to mull over a situation, the more time you have to build up anxiety. Procrastination can lead to unnecessary depression and anxiety. Frankly, the art of keeping up with yesterday is far too costly. If you wait until you have enough time to do something, you may never get started. Some people underestimate the amount of time and effort required to accomplish things; they fall behind schedule, invent a load of excuses and soon build up stress. Stress can be a positive reinforcer in our lives, but very few people have learned to benefit from it.

Some researchers refer to the concept of 'psychological hardness'. They claim that commitment, control and challenge is what keeps us at our best, and that psychological hardness, as far as our health is concerned, plays a far more crucial role than family history. Yet while some embrace change as challenge, others see it as a threat and feel alienated and helpless at any interruption in the status quo.

THE LABORATORY OF OUR OWN LIVES

As such social aspects of disease gain acceptance and preventive medicine plays a greater role, the Pasteur philosophy requires new categorization. More than 100 years ago, Louis Pasteur modernized medicine and claimed that bacteria and other 'germs' were the causes of disease. In medical schools today, this is still the only concept taught. But why is it that bacteria invade some bodies and not others? What makes some bodies strong and healthy and others weak and vulnerable?

In many instances, as we have seen, the mind plays a key role. At the same time as identifying the emotional culprits that can lead to disease, researchers point out that relaxation, optimism, happiness and friendships can help you stay well, heal and thrive. It seems as if all this confirms what many of us have discovered in the informal laboratory of our own lives. By simply having a good social network and by keeping things in perspective, our health will prosper. For us to be at our best, we really must exist in partnership with others. Experts say that a solid, close relationship can get a person through just about anything. We are fundamentally social creatures and reside in a community of which we are an integral part. Thus, we must consider ourselves in relation to our homes, work and social structures.

In psychosomatic illness, there is frequently an element of purpose in the disorder. In more cases than not, an overtaxed nervous system creates a defensive condition in order to better cope with its environment. Such a state of hyper-vigilance throws the body out of kilter as it traumatizes the mind. Some individual may develop illnesses to avoid making any kind of adjustment at all. Some experts have concluded that at least some people develop heart disease to get a break from responsibility.

Orthodox medicine does not hold the individual personally responsible for the state of his or her health. But holistic practitioners claim that people quite clearly give access to disease. They say that we do not disrupt our health unless we have given ourselves a reason and permission to do so on a subconscious level. The illness thus masks some inner conflict. It appears that the laws which govern health and the process of healing are far more complicated than most people – or medical science, for that matter – care to accept. Clearly, they are not solely a physical phenomenon and are not subject only to physical treatment.

We can say with absolute certainty that orthodox medicine has made enormous progress in healing man. But from the spiritual point of view, it has caused us to regress – to separate our state of health, from our inner selves – in favour of effecting 'instant cures'. Fortunately, the past decade has shown a promising inching forward to a point where the orthodox and the holistic may merge. Medical thinking in general is moving towards a more integrated view of illness and well-being and closer to an acceptance of the whole individual – spiritual, emotional and physical.

IN SEARCH OF HEALTH

Imagine telling a biochemist only ten years ago that a new and revolutionary science would change the very nature of the medical belief system. Now psychoneuroimmunology is doing just that. The idea of interactions between the brain's system of neurochemicals and the endocrine system of hormones and the immune system's defences against infections was thought impossible. Today, the only determination left to be made is to what extent such interactions are possible.

No time is being wasted to prove the associations. For example, scientists at the National Jewish Center for Immunology and Respiratory Medicine in Denver, Colorado have shown that toxic parents create toxic children. The ongoing study has revealed that children of asthmatic parents who continuously experience a hostile, stressful home environment develop asthma themselves.

Such evidence suggests that the recent upsurge in the popularity of psychosomatic medicine is simply putting right something that began to go wrong when, despite the words of such great minds as Socrates, Hippocrates and Plato, orthodox medicine began to reign supreme. Basically, these philosophers said that the greatest error in the treatment of sickness is to have physicians for the body and phsyicians for the mind, when, in reality, the mind and body are inseparable.

Today we are evaluating and validating one old hypothesis after another. No knowledgeable individual underestimates the integration of the emotional and physiological, but others still view disease as a defect in the mechanical body that can be probed, medicated, cut out or replaced. But such procedures cannot be applied to the all-too-many chronic illnesses we have already discussed or to those conditions for which no accurate diagnosis can be made. And because of this holistic medicine cannot help but merge with orthodox medicine. Sufferers of psychosomatic illnesses simply will never find relief in any other circumstances.

Someone once quipped that if the Spanish explorer Ponce de Leon had stopped running around the world in search of youth, he would have found it within himself. The same can be said for our health. But although most of us instinctively know that a sound mind resides in a sound body, as the Romans stated, we just don't act as if we do. When we are well, we feel good emotionally and physically. But when we are ill, we appear to be more so in the mind than in the body. A holistic physician would thus treat the whole person.

THE TRIUMPH OF ARROGANCE OVER PAIN

In the past, the psychological or psychosomatic component in chronic disease was grossly underestimated. It is obvious that many risk factors are involved in the development of an illness, and a combination of certain risk factors leads to certain diseases. A virus epidemic, for instance, can be substantial enough for you to become infected. If your diet is quite deplorable and you eat a steady supply of fats, sugar and empty calories, this infection may lead to an illness. If you smoke and/or live in a polluted environment, those are other contributing factors. If you lead a sedentary life and don't exercise, your risks mount further. If you keep to yourself and lack meaningful relationships, yet another risk factor exists. If you have a family history of one of a variety of inherited conditions – you guessed it. Similarly, if your state of mind has created chronic distress, there is a problem. Individually, one of these risk factors may not cause you to break down, but a combination of them certainly will. Hence, you can see how normal functioning can be disturbed and disease can result without any interference from outside forces. So, while you might be aware that your tension headache or backache is caused by stress, so too should you be aware that serious disease can develop in the same way.

This was certainly the case with my friend Lisa. When she developed an ulcer, in an odd sort of way she showed a certain amount of pride. The development of ulcers is often an occupational hazard for high flyers in business. A triumph of arrogance over pain is another award, the ulcer symbolizing supreme accomplishment in the competitive, cutthroat world of business today. You and I know this to be a fallacy, but Lisa, a woman in a man's world, saw it differently. Her attitude does, however, provide us with some interesting insights into psychosomatic illness. A coupling of physical and mental factors is required to develop an ulcer. It is interesting to note how the mind and body assist each other in this endeavour.

Initially, a very large quantity of impulses, created by emotional distress, travel down nerve fibres that extend from the mid-brain to the gastrointestinal tract. This part of the brain works as a maintenance centre for the automatic functioning of the body and, so far, no one has been able consciously to guide its behaviour. However, it can be affected via the automatic (i.e. unconsciously functioning) nervous system.

The nerve impulses travel to the stomach where they control the production of hydrochloric acid. It's what the impulses are supposed to do. The trouble starts when far more acid is produced than is required for digestion. So what does the stomach tell you? It's hungry. It needs food to neutralize the overabundance of acid. But the lining of the stomach or of part of the duodenum (the first part of the small intestine) has already been damaged and an ulcer is beginning to form. And the more you eat, the more acid is produced and the worse the situation becomes.

Then the smooth muscles of the digestive tract become tense, but there is nothing that you can do about it consciously. The steady rhythm of the muscles is out of sync, which may disturb the normal functioning of the muscles that convey the food from mouth to stomach. When their signals get crossed, the stomach will let you know by means of regurgitation. Excess food left in the stomach will further irritate the lining, and if all of this isn't enough, you may ingest something further troublesome to the mucus membranes that line the stomach or intestine. The stomach's hydrochloric acid and the muscle tension in unison disturb the most minute scarring of the digestive tract, and the irritated spot is then obvious, infected and painful.

Your doctor takes an X-ray and shows you your brand new ulcer. This is then treated with medication and diet, but it may eventually have to be cut out. None of this, mind you, deals with the cause of the ulcer in the first place. The stress that the mind places on the body will manifest itself one way or another. For nearly as long as medicine has been considered science, the association between the mind and gastrointestinal problems has been understood.

Back to my friend Lisa. Psychologists say that the ulcer-prone have a compulsion to assert their independence. It is Lisa's desire not to rely on others which forces her to strive for ever higher goals and has made her into what is known as a high flyer.

Overall, the likes of Lisa succeed in their worldly goals quite well, but the burning need to achieve that lies behind this type of personality is quite different from the needs of most other people. An ulcer-prone person like Lisa feels compelled to succeed beyond the dreams of the majority in order to rid herself of any suspicions of inferiority. Yet the competition is within the self and not with others – unlike that of the coronary type, for instance.

DOING THINGS FOR OURSELVES

This is only a brief outline of the mind–ulcer connection, but you get the picture. Psychological stress and physical, or somatic, reactions are not so hard to comprehend when you understand the workings of the mind–body system. The impairment of our psychological well-being as a causal factor in illness has been overshadowed by studies concerned with the impact of exposure to bacteria, viruses, noxious chemicals and physical pressures, but all these factors appear almost simple when you consider the complexity of psychosomatic stress. This involves all processes, whether originating in the external environment or within the person, which impose a demand or requirement upon the organism, the resolution or handling of which requires work or activity of the mental apparatus before any other system is involved or activated.

The rapid groundswell of public interest in and acceptance of such fields as psychosomatic and orthomolecular medicine, psychoneuroimmunology, ecology and general lifestyle awareness tells us that holistic health is an idea that's long overdue and whose time has come.

Ideally, the role of the physician today should be to examine our lifestyles carefully and teach us the principles of self-responsibility. Once again, we are reminded that the whole is greater than the sum of its parts. Hence, the physician's purpose becomes the restoration of the healing connection, which must not be completely lost in the concept of specialization. To quote an anonymous source, 'The role of specialization is getting to know more and more about less and less until we know everything about nothing.'

Dr John Knowles, former president of the Rockefeller Foundation, said that 'the next great advance in health of the American people will come not from laboratories or hospitals but from what people learn to do for themselves.'[14] After all, the science of health should always be more important than the science of curing disease. External curing will always lack permanent effect if the causes of the troubles do not receive the same care and attention.

AFTERWORD

I was still dumbstruck as I drove across the desert. I had just been to see one of the United States' top orthodontists who, over the previous two years, had been treating me for a slightly misaligned jaw. On this particular occasion, I had let the good doctor – a kindly older gentleman – know in no uncertain terms how distressed I was that my progress had been so slow. After all, when I had first gone to see him, he had told me that it would take no more than six months.

'I know the type,' he replied wearily. 'All my patients are the same. From seventeen to seventy, you're all Type-A personalities, driven perfectionists, and you're just too damn hard on yourselves.'

My orthodontist – a psychologist yet! I thought to myself, and it took a lot of self-discipline to bite back a sharp reply.

As he suggested that I 'mellow out' and take a leisurely walk every day, I was quietly plotting his murder. Then something he said caught my attention.

'I've had the same jaw disorder for the last twenty years. I also have high blood pressure, and the medication I'm taking for it is destroying my liver.' He went on to say that he suffered from frequent headaches and had severe ringing in the ears. Now that I thought of it, there had been times when I had visited him and he had looked as if he was on the verge of a nervous breakdown. 'But I don't complain!' he concluded proudly.

During the drive home across the desert, after the initial shock had passed, I became lost in thought. How was this 'expert' going to make me well if he couldn't even help himself? Would I go to an obese nutritionist, or a terribly out-of-shape fitness expert? Would I go to a mechanic whose own car continually broke down? Of course not!

Most of us can come up with examples of how we knew instinctively that we were not being adequately treated by health professionals, or were simply being humoured by the 'experts'. And most of us, in these circumstances, felt helpless.

Theoretically, government, science and health-care professionals should be able to help us all live healthy and productive lives. Yet the system has not only failed to achieve this aim of making total health possible, it has often – albeit mostly unknowingly – propelled us in the opposite direction. Many of us are now taking matters into our own hands. We are at last questioning just what 'modern living' means and examining its effects on us as a whole. Adulterated food, frantic lifestyles and a rapidly deteriorating environment are quickly becoming an unacceptable price to pay for this way of life.

We are no longer shocked to hear that people have cancer, heart disease or some other chronic condition. We write it off as unfortunate, perhaps fated, and wonder how much longer they'll be around. These thoughts are terrible enough, but what is tragic is our passive or helpless attitude towards our own well-being.

A few years ago, I thought that diseases such as cancer and AIDS were *the* great mysteries of medicine. Imagine my surprise when I found out that the causes of and effective treatments for simple muscle spasm were equally unknown. All that the orthodox medical profession can do for back pain caused by muscle spasm is relieve the symptoms with drugs such as muscle relaxants, anti-inflammatories and painkillers. Never mind that this course of action doesn't get rid of the problem, may produce undesirable side-effects and may actually slow down your body's natural recovery process.

I was concerned that I was suffering this kind of back pain, and rather than taking it lying down – as many medical authorities would have us do – I began to read up on the subject. I eventually concluded that, because my life had become increasingly sedentary, I was beginning to break down physically – even though I was still in my 20s. So I decided to try and cure myself through walking (seven to ten miles a day now), stretching exercises, weight training and deep tissue massages. Although it took more than a year of all this for the pain to subside, I can honestly say that my back – and the rest of me – never felt stronger. Now my exercising and so on has become a daily habit and I could not live without my workouts.

All around me, I see people simply surviving rather than enjoying optimal health. My younger friends are fatigued, stressed, worried about ageing prematurely. Many of the business executives I know are working on their second and third heart attacks. Other acquaintances have accepted the fact that they are going to have to live with conditions such as arthritis and ulcers and a variety of other chronic ailments. I'm amazed at how few actually radiate high energy, enthusiasm and basic good health.

But the tide is slowly turning. Too many people are, as one author has put it, 'sick and tired of being sick and tired'. From fatigue to cancer,

orthodox medicine has yet to alleviate the suffering of millions. Consequently, people the world over are seeking other healing options in the
hope of better health. Over the past century, preventive medicine has
become alternative, then complementary, and is now nearly mainstream.

Optimal health is entirely possible for those who know how to make
the right choices and are willing to make the effort. Although the length
and convenience of our lives have improved considerably, the quality of
our lives is lagging behind drastically. But as *Life Force* has pointed out,
you can change this.

I recently had lunch with a 37-year-old friend who, in his short life,
has managed to accumulate more than $200 million (£133 million) of
commercial real estate. But what's the point? He's in fairly poor health –
ulcers, anxiety attacks, very low energy, and general depression. Besides real estate and Monty Python movies, nothing much interests him.
He wishes things weren't this way, but, he says, they just are and he can't
do anything about it. Really?

He proclaimed that the secret of his success was knowing exactly
when to sell and when to buy. But he didn't know the first thing about
lunch.

You, of course, know better.

NOTES

Chapter 1: The Modern Diet Myth

1   Quoted in Sarah Glazer, 'How America Eats', *Research Reports*, vol. 1, April 1988, pp. 218–30.
2   S. Boyd Eaton, Marjorie Shostake & Melvin Konner, *The Paleolithic Prescription: A program of diet & exercise & a design for living*, Harper & Row (US), 1989.
3   Department of Health, *Dietary Reference Values for Food Energy and Nutrients for the United Kingdom* (Report on Health and Social Subjects 41), HMSO, 1991.
4   'Stretching Your Nutrition Dollar', *Ostomly Quarterly*, vol. 27, summer 1990, p. 33. Sue Dibb, 'Sweet Messages: selling food to kids', *Eat Up*, Channel 4 Television, October/November 1993.
5   'A Pyramid Topples at the USDA', *Consumer Reports*, October 1991, pp. 663–66.
6   'The Crunching Truth: You're eating insects', *Palm Beach Post*, 15 August 1990.
7   *Summary of Labelling Particulars Required by the Food Safety Act 1990: The Food Labelling Regulations 1984 (SI No. 1305) (As Amended)*, Consumer Protection Division, Ministry of Agriculture, Fisheries & Food, January 1992, pp. 5–6.
8   Peter Burney, 'Asthma and Epidemiology', *Asthma News*, December 1989.
9   Glazer, *op. cit.*
10 Chris W. Lecos, 'Food Labels: Test your knowledge', *FDA Consumer*, March 1988, pp. 16–20.
11 *Summary of Labelling Particulars . . . .*, *op. cit.*, p. 3.
12 Earl Mindell, *Unsafe at Any Meal*, Warner Books (US), 1987.
13 *Look Before You Eat! Food Additives: A shopper's guide*, Channel 4 Television, 1992. *Report of the European Community's Scientific Committee for Food*, 16th series, 1985.
14 John Yudkin, *The Penguin Encyclopaedia of Nutrition*, Penguin Books, 1985, p. 331.
15 Janny Scott, 'Cancer, Calories and Controversy', *Los Angeles Times Magazine*, 7 October 1990, p. 14.
16 'Longer Lives for the Japanese', *Which? Way to Health*, February 1990, p. 4.
17 Glazer, *op. cit.*
18 News release, National Dairy Council, 11 November 1993.
19 *Summary of Labelling Particulars . . .*, *op. cit.*, p. 2.
20 Dr Denis Burkitt, 'Relationship as a Clue to Causation', *Lancet*, 12 December 1970.
21 'Fibre', *Which? Way to Health*, February 1991, p. 20. Adrienne Mayes, *The A–Z of Nutritional Health*, Thorsons, revised ed. 1991.
22 Laurence Sombke, 'How Our Meals Have Changed', *USA Today*, 11–13 November 1988. Microwave Association (UK), 1993.
23 John Naisbitt, 'The Healing Power of Food', *New Age Journal*, September/October 1988, p. 24.
24 Linus Pauling, 'Orthomolecular Psychiatry', *Science*, vol. 160, April 1968, pp. 265–71.

Chapter 2: The Food Crisis

1   'MSG Alert', *Glamour*, March 1992.
2   *Report of the European Community's Scientific Committee for Food*, 21st series, 1989.
3   *Look Before You Eat! Food Additives: A shopper's guide*, Channel 4 Television, 1992. 'Artificial Sweeteners', *Which? Way to Health*, December 1991, pp. 200–203. Laura Flynn McCarthy, 'The Fake Food Diet', *Harper's Bazaar*, March 1992, p. 190.

4 US Food & Drug Administration, 'How Safe Is Safe?', *FDA Consumer*, September 1988, pp. 16–19.
5 General Accounting Office, *Pesticides: Need to enhance FDA's ability to protect the public from illegal residues*, 1986.
6 Working Party on Pesticide Residues, *Annual Report*, Ministry of Agriculture, Fisheries & Food, November 1992.
7 Greenpeace, 'The Pesticides Debate', *Which? Way to Health*, October 1992.
8 *Bioscience*, vol. 28, 1978, p. 772.
9 Testimony of EPA Assistant Administrator John A. Moore to the Subcommittee on Department Operations, Research and Foreign Agriculture of the House Committee on Agriculture, 7 April 1987.
10 Laurie Mott & Martha Broad, *Pesticides in Food*, Natural Resource Defense Council Inc., 1985.
11 Sheila Kaplan, 'The Food Chain Gang', *Common Cause*, September/October 1987, pp. 12–15.
12 'Risks of Radiation: Too many questions about food safety', *USA Today*, 22 January 1992.
13 C. Bhaskaram & G. Sadasivan, 'Effects of feeding irradiated wheat to malnourished children', *American Journal of Clinical Nutrition*, vol. 28, 1975, pp. 130–35.
14 Shirley Swede, 'Nuclear Food: How can it be safe?', *Better Nutrition for Today's Living*, May 1988, p. 13.
15 Donald B. Louria, 'Zapping the Food Supply', *Bulletin of the Atomic Scientists*, September 1990, p. 34.
16 Richard Piccioni, 'Food Irradiation: Contaminating our food', *The Ecologist*, vol. 18, no. 2, April 1988, p. 48.
17 'Irradiation in the Processing and Handling of Food', *Federal Register*, April 1986, p. 13,376.
18 J. R. Hickman, L. A. McLean & F. J. Ley, 'Rat Feeding Studies on Wheat Treated with Gamma Radiation', *Food and Cosmetic Toxicity*, vol. 2, no. 2, 1964, pp. 175–80. J. L. Radomski *et al.*, 'Chronic Toxicity Studies in Irradiated Beef Stew and Evaporated Milk', *Toxicology and Applied Pharmacology*, vol. 7, no. 1, 1965, pp. 113–21.
19 H. W. Renner & D. Reichelt, 'Zur Frage der gesundheitlichen Unbedenklichkeit hoher Konzentrationen von freien Radikalen in Bestrahlten Lebesmitteln', *Zentralblatt fur Veterina Medizi*, vol. 20, no. 8, 1973, pp. 648–60.
20 E. Weirbicki *et al.*, *Ionizing Energy in Food Processing and Pest Control*, Part 1, Council for Agricultural Science and Technology, July 1986. A. B. Khattak & C. F. Klopfenstein, 'Effects of Gamma Irradiation on the Nutritional Quality of Grains and Legumes', *Cereal Chemistry*, vol. 66, no. 3, 1989, pp. 171–72. N. Raica Jnr, J. Scott & N. Nielson, 'Nutritional Quality of Irradiated Foods', *Radiation Research Review*, vol. 3, no. 4, 1972, pp. 447–57.
21 Tim Lang & Tony Webb, 'Should Our Food Be Irradiated?', *Which? Way to Health*, March 1988, p. 27.
22 *Summary of Labelling Particulars Required by the Food Safety Act 1990: The Food Labelling Regulations 1984 (SI No. 1305) (As Amended)*, Consumer Protection Division, Ministry of Agriculture, Fisheries & Food, January 1992, p. 2.
23 K. Terry, 'Why is DoE for Food Irradiation?, *The Nation*, 7 February 1987, pp. 142–56.
24 Richard Piccioni, *op. cit.* K. Terry, *op. cit.*
25 Sharon Begley & Elizabeth Roberts, 'Dishing Up Gamma Rays', *Newsweek*, 27 January 1992.
26 Georgia Department of Natural Resources, US Department of Energy & Nuclear Regulatory Commission, *First Interim Report of the RSI Incident Evaluation Task Force*, June 1989.
27 Marion Burros, 'Irradiated Foods Meet Resistance', *New York Times*, 26 August 1992.
28 'Coming Soon to a Salad near You', *Time*, 8 June 1992, p. 31.
29 Walter Truett Anderson, 'Food without Farms', *Futurist*, January/February 1990, pp. 16–21.
30 Wade Roush, 'Who Decides about Biotech?' *Technology Review*, July 1991, pp. 28–36.
31 *Ibid.*
32 Interviewed on *Food File*, a Stephens Kerr production for Channel 4 Television, February 1993.
33 R. A. Holman, 'The Answer to Cancer', *Journal of the Soil Association*, vol. 11, no. 4, October 1960, p. 371.
34 Arnold S. Lehman, 'Procedures for the Appraisal of Toxicity of Chemicals in Foods', *Food, Drug and Law Quarterly*, vol. 4, 1959, p. 73.
35 ECAS 'EC Non-policy on Food and Health', *European Citizen*, September 1991.
36 Committee on Medical Aspects of Food Policy, *Dietary Reference Values for Food Energy and Nutrients for the United Kingdom*, HMSO, 1991.
37 Secretary of State for Health, *The Health of the Nation*, HMSO, 1991.
38 William Ogilvy Kermack & Philip Eggleton, *Stuff We're Made Of: A biochemical survey of life for the general reader*, Longmans Green, 1948, p. 226.

Chapter 3: Living Dangerously

1 Anita Gordon & David Suzuki, *It's a Matter of Survival*, Harvard University Press, 1991.
2 Edgar Wayburn, 'Human Health and Human Environment', *Western Journal of Medicine*, vol. 154, March 1991, p. 341.
3 Albert Gore, *Earth in the Balance*, Houghton Mifflin (US), 1992.
4 Gordon & Suzuki, *op. cit.*
5 Joseph L. Jacobsen *et al.*, 'Determinants of polychlorinated biphenyls (PLBs), polybrominated biphenyls (PBBs) and dicholrodipheryl trichloroethane (DDT) levels in the sera of young children', *American Journal of Public Health*, vol. 79, October 1989, p. 1401.
6 Linda Mason Hunter, *The Healthy Home*, Rodale Press (US), 1989.
7 Wayburn, *op. cit.*
8 Fiona Godlee & Alison Walker, 'Importance of a Healthy Environment', *British Medical Journal*, vol. 303, November 1991, p. 1124.
9 Lee Niedringhaus Davis, *Corporate Alchemists: Profit takers and problem makers in the chemical industry*, William Morrow & Co. (US), 1984.
10 William J. Cunliffe, *A Pocket Guide to Acne*, Science Press, 1988, p. 51.
11 *New England Journal of Medicine*, 24 January 1991, p. 212.
12 Boly Williams, 'Downwind from the Cold War', *In Health*, July/August 1990, p. 58.
13 Quoted in Judith Cook, *Red Alert: The worldwide dangers of nuclear power*, New English Library, 1986.
14 Cook, *op. cit.*, p. 3.
15 House of Commons Select Committee on the Environment, *First Report on Radioactive Waste, 1985–86*, HMSO, 1986.
16 Marilynne Robinson, *Mother Country: Britain, the welfare state and nuclear pollution*, Farrar, Straus & Giroux (US), 1989.
17 'Energy News', *Private Eye*, 1 December 1993, p. 14.
18 Hunter, *op. cit.*
19 'Unanswered Prayers and Questions', *New Times*, 7–13 October 1992, p. 18.
20 Cynthia P. Green, 'The Environment and Population Growth: Decade for action', *Population Reports*, May 1992, p. 1.
21 Frank Murray, 'Fluoridation Fears Gaining Credence', *Better Nutrition for Today's Living*, vol. 52, April 1990, p. 6.
22 H. J. Roberts, 'Fluoridation: The controversy continues', *Nutrition Health Review*, spring 1992, p. 8.
23 Gordon & Suzuki, *op. cit.*
24 Earl Randall Dunford & Kevin G. May, *Your Health and the Indoor Environment*, NuDawn Publishing (US), 1991.
25 Andrew Skonick, 'Even air in the home is not entirely free of potent pollutants', *Journal of the American Medical Association*, vol. 26, December 1989, p. 3102.
26 John Bower, 'Are You Chemically Sensitive? What to do when everything makes you sick', *East West*, vol. 21, March 1991, p. 22.
27 Dunford & May, *op. cit.*
28 *Ibid.*
29 'Passive Smoking', *Which? Way to Health*, February 1991, p. 12.
30 Hunter, *op. cit.*
31 *Ibid.*
32 Dunford & May, *op. cit.*
33 Hunter, *op. cit.*
34 Geoff Scott, 'Your Environment and Your Health', *Current Health*, 18 April 1992, p. 7.
35 Kim C. Flodin, 'Now Hear This', *American Health*, January/February 1992, p. 58.
36 Hunter, *op. cit.*
37 Flodin, *op. cit.*
38 Hunter, *op. cit.*
39 Robert O. Becker, *Cross Currents*, Jeremy P. Tarcher Inc. (US), 1990.
40 *Working with VDUs*, Health & Safety Executive, May 1993.
41 Becker, *op. cit.*
42 Michael J. Hodgson, 'Do Buildings Make You Sick? *Executive Health's Good Health Report*, vol. 27, August 1991, p. 1.
43 *Ibid.*
44 John Mitchell, 'Experts Assess Ills of 1990s and Medical Advances to Combat Them', *Health News and Review*, vol. 7, November/December 1989, p. 1.

45   Kaye H. Kilburn, 'Is the Human Nervous System Most Sensitive to Environmental Toxins?' *Archives of Environmental Health*, vol. 44, November/December 1989, p. 343.
46   House Committee on Energy and Commerce, 'Indoor Air Pollution', 102nd US Congress, 1st Session, vol. 144, 1991, pp. 150–51.
47   Bower, *op. cit.*
48   G. R. Oberg, 'An Overview of the Philosophy of the American Academy of Environmental Medicine', AAEM Official Philosophy Paper, 1991.
49   Keith Mumby, *The Complete Guide to Food Allergies and Environmental Illness*, Thorsons, 1993, pp. 77–78.

Chapter 4: The Quest for Optimal Health

1   *Mosby's Medical and Nursing Dictionary*, C. V. Mosby Co. (US), 2nd ed. 1986.
2   *Ibid.*
3   'Homeopathic Remedies: Safe, inexpensive . . . and they seem to work', *Health Facts*, vol. 16, April 1991, p. 1.
4   Louis W. Sullivan, US Department of Health Services/Public Health Services, *Healthy People 2000*, DHSS Publication no. (PHS)91-50212 (US), 1990.
5   T. A. Hodgson & D. P. Rice, 'Economic Impact of Cancer in the United States', *Cancer Epidemiology and Prevention*, forthcoming. Public Health Services, *Promoting Health/Preventing Disease: Objectives for the nation*, US Department of Health and Human Services (US), 1980.
6   'Preventive Care: From self-care to lab tests', *University of California, Berkeley, Wellness Letter*, vol. 7, May 1991, p. 4.
7   John A. McDougal, 'Do You Need a Yearly Physical?' *Vegetarian Times*, October 1989, p. 72.
8   Kate J. Thomas *et al.*, 'Use of Non-orthodox and Conventional Health Care in Great Britain', *British Medical Journal*, vol. 302, 26 January 1991, p. 20.
9   Sharon Begley, 'Alternative Medicine: A cure for what ails us?' *American Health*, April 1992, p. 40.
10   Kleijnen *et al.*, 'Clinical Trials of Homoeopathy', *British Medical Journal*, vol. 302, 26 January 1991, pp. 316–23.
11   Maggie Garb, 'Non-traditional Appeal: Alternative doctors tell why some patients favor their practices', *American Medical News*, vol. 34, 25 November 1991, p. 13.
12   *Ibid.*
13   H. Zaman, 'The South-east Asian Region', in R. H. Bannerman (ed.), *Traditional Medicine*, World Health Organization (Geneva), 1974, pp. 231-39.
14   Hari M. Sharma *et al.*, 'Maharishi Ayur-Veda: Modern insights into ancient medicine', *Journal of the American Medical Association*, vol. 265, 22 May 1991, p. 2633.
15   *Ibid.*
16   *Ibid.*
17   H. M. Sharma *et al.*, 'Antineoplastic Properties of Maharishi-4 against DMBA-induced Mammary Tumours in Rats', *Pharmacology Biochemical Behaviour*, vol. 35, 1990, pp. 767–73. H. M. Sharma *et al.*, 'Antineoplastic Properties of Dietary Maharishi-4 and Maharishi Amrit Kalash Ayurvedic Food Supplements', *European Journal of Pharmacology*, vol. 183, 1990, p. 193.
18   S. S Harris *et al.*, 'Physical Activity Counseling for Healthy Adults as a Primary Preventive Intervention in the Clinical Setting', *Journal of the American Medical Association*, vol. 261, 1989, pp. 3590–98.
19   K. E. Powell *et al.*, 'Physical Activity and Chronic Disease', *American Journal of Clinical Nutrition*, vol. 49, 1989, pp. 999–1006. J. T. Salonen & J. Tuomilehto, 'Physical Activity and Risk of Myocardial Infarction, Cerebral Stroke and Death: A longitudinal study in eastern Finland', *American Journal of Epidemiology*, vol. 115, 1982, pp. 526–37. L. D. Cady *et al.*, 'Strength and Fitness and Subsequent Back Injuries in Firefighters', *Journal of Occupational Medicine*, vol. 21, 1979, pp. 269–72. R. S. Paffenberger *et al.*, 'Physical Activity, All-cause Mortality, and Longevity of College Alumni', *New England Journal of Medicine*, vol. 314, 1986, pp. 605–13. S. Katz *et al.*, 'Active Life Expectancy', *New England Journal of Medicine*, vol. 309, 1983, pp. 1218–24.
20   Robert L. Smith, 'European Alternative Health Specialist Dr Jan DeVries', *Total Health*, vol. 12, December 1990, p. 12.
21   Shelby Tyson, 'Herbs for the '90s: Experts pick top 10', *Health News & Review*, March/April 1990, p. 1.
22   'Many Points to Needle: Acupuncture to treat alcoholism' (editorial), *Lancet*, vol. 335, 6 January 1990, p. 20.

23 'Acupuncture as a Treatment of AIDS-related Stress', *AIDS Weekly*, 4 November 1991, p. 14.
24 Begley, *op. cit.*
25 *Ibid.*
26 Larry Beresford, 'Is It Time to Back Chiropractic?' *Business and Health*, vol. 9, December 1991, p. 50.
27 *British Medical Journal*, vol. 300, 1990, pp. 1431–37.
28 British Medical Journal Council, 'Back to Basics', *Medical Update*, December 1990, p. 4.
29 *British Medical Journal*, vol. 303, 1991, pp. 1298–1303.

Chapter 5: The Vitamin Revolution

1 Anastasia Toufexis, 'The New Scoop on Vitamins', *Time*, 6 April 1992, p. 54.
2 *Ibid.*
3 Deborah Seymour Taylor, 'Food and Mood: Can nutrition affect your mental health?' *Today's Living*, vol. 20, December 1989, p. 12.
4 Carl C. Pfeiffer, *Mental and Elemental Nutrients*, Keats Publishing (US), 1975.
5 Patrick Quillin, *Healing Nutrients*, Contemporary Books (US), 1987.
6 'Psychiatric Disorders that Can Stimulate Dementia', *Nutrition Health Review*, winter 1990, p. 5.
7 Iris R. Bell *et al.*, 'B-complex Vitamin Patterns in Geriatric and Young Adult Inpatients with Major Depression', *Journal of American Geriatrics Society*, vol. 39, March 1991, pp. 252–57.
8 Donald R. Miller *et al.*, 'Vitamin B_{12} Status in a Macrobiotic Community', *American Journal of Clinical Nutrition*, vol. 53, February 1991, p. 524.
9 Mark N. Mead, 'Are You B_{12} Deficient? How to recognize symptoms and find solutions', *East West*, vol. 19, October 1989, p. 42.
10. Gregory L. Clementz & Stanley G. Schade, 'The Spectrum of Vitamin B_{12} Deficiency', *American Family Physician*, vol. 41, January 1990, p. 150.
11 G. Vreugdenhil *et al.*, 'Anaemia in Rheumatoid Arthritis: The role of iron, vitamin B_{12} and folic acid', *Annals of Rheumatic Diseases*, vol. 49, February 1990, p. 93.
12 E. H. Reynolds *et al.*, 'Multiple Sclerosis Associated with Vitamin B_{12} Deficiency', *Archives of neurology*, vol. 48, August 1991, p. 808.
13 I. S. Dokal *et al.*, 'Vitamin B_{12} and Folate Deficiency Presenting as Leukaemia', *British Medical Journal*, vol. 300, 12 May 1990, p. 1263.
14 Frank Murray, 'Bone Up on B Vitamins', *Better Nutrition for Today's Living*, vol. 51, October 1989, p. 8.
15 *Ibid.*
16 H. C. T. van Zaanen & J. van der Lelie, 'Thiamine Deficiency in Hematologic Malignant Tumors', *Cancer*, vol. 69, 1 April 1992, p. 1710.
17 Hanna Seligmann *et al.*, 'Thiamine Deficiency in Patients with Congestive Heart Failure Receiving Long-term Furosemide Therapy: A pilot study', *American Journal of Medicine*, vol. 91, August 1991, p. 151.
18 Ronald G. Munger *et al.*, 'Prolonged QT Interval and Risk of Sudden Death in South-east Asian Men', *Lancet*, vol. 338, 3 August 1991, p. 280.
19 Marie T. Fanelli-Kuczmarski *et al.*, 'Folate Status of Mexican-American, Cuban and Puerto Rican Women', *American Journal of Clinical Nutrition*, vol. 52, August 1990, p. 368.
20 Amy F. Subar *et al.*, 'Folate Intake and Food Sources in the United States Population', *American Journal of Clinical Nutrition*, vol. 50, September 1989, p. 508.
21 Paula Kurtzweil & Theresa A. Young, 'Folate', *FDA Consumer*, vol. 25, July/August 1991, p. 41.
22 Frank Murray, 'Bone Up on B Vitamins', *op. cit.*
23 'More on Folic Acid and Neural Tube Defects: Vitamins and minerals in health and disease', *Nutrition Research Newsletter*, vol. 11, 1992, p. 48.
24 Subar *et al.*, *op. cit.*
25 Dokal *et al.*, *op. cit.*
26 Frank Murray, 'Bone Up on B Vitamins', *op. cit.*
27 Helio Vannucchi & Fernando Salvador Moreno, 'Interaction of Niacin and Zinc Metabolism in Patients with Alcoholic Pellagra', *American Journal of Clinical Nutrition*, vol. 50, August 1989, p. 364.
28 Frank Murray, 'Nutrient Therapy Relieves Skin Ailments: B-complex vitamins, omega-3 fish oils, vitamin C and zinc help alleviate psoriasis and eczema', *Better Nutrition*, vol. 52, April 1990, p. 10.
29 Ashima K. Kant & Gladys Block, 'Dietary Vitamin B_6 Intake and Food Sources in the United

States Population: NHANES II, 1976–1980', *American Journal of Clinical Nutrition*, vol. 52, October 1990, p. 707.

30 Judith R. Turnlund *et al.*, 'A Stable-isotope Study of Zinc, Copper and Iron Absorption and Retention by Young Women Fed Vitamin B_6-deficient Diets', *American Journal of Clinical Nutrition*, vol. 54, December 1991, p. 105.

31 Frank Murray, 'Bone Up on B Vitamins', *op. cit.*

32 Bradley R. Straatsma *et al.*, 'Lens Capsule and Epithelium in Age-related Cataract', *American Journal of Ophthalmology*, vol. 112, 15 September 1991, p. 283.

33 'Prenatal Vitamin K', *Prevention*, vol. 42, January 1990, p. 9.

34 Andrew W. McNinch & John H. Tripp, 'Haemorrhagic Disease of the Newborn in the British Isles: Two-year prospective study', *British Medical Journal*, vol. 303, 2 November 1991, p. 1105.

35 Mary Ann Howkins, 'The Nutrient Gap', *Glamour*, April 1992.

36 'Vitamins and Cancer Prevention', *Health Facts*, vol. 17, January 1992, p. 5.

37 'Free Radicals and Antioxidants: Finding the key to heart disease, cancer, and the aging process', *University of California, Berkeley, Wellness Letter*, vol. 8, October 1991, p. 4.

38 Stanley Fahn, 'An Open Trial of High-dosage Antioxidants in Early Parkinson's Disease', *American Journal of Clinical Nutrition*, vol. 53, January 1991, p. 3805.

39 'Vitamin E Supplementation and Exercise', *Nutrition Today*, vol. 25, September/October 1990, p. 5.

40 Mary Ellen Hettinger, 'Research Shows Roles for Vitamin E in Ills from Cataracts to Cancer', *Health News & Review*, vol. 1, April 1991, p. 1.

41 'Free Radicals and Antioxidants', *op. cit.*

42 R. B. Shekelle *et al.*, 'Dietary Vitamin A and Risk of Cancer', *Lancet*, vol. 2, 1981, p. 1185.

43 R. Petro *et al.*, 'Can Dietary Beta-carotene Reduce Human Cancer Risk?', *Nature*, vol. 290, 1981, p. 201.

44 M. Jurin & I. F. Tannock, 'Influence of Vitamin A on Immunological Responses', *Immunology*, vol. 23, 1974, p. 283.

45 R. L. Gross & P. M. Newberne, 'The Role of Nutrition in Immunological Function', *Physiological Reviews*, vol. 60, 1980, p. 188.

46 E. Seifter *et al.*, 'Impaired Wound Healing in Diabetes: Prevention by supplemental vitamin A', *Annals of Surgery*, vol. 194, 1981, p. 42.

47 'Vitamin A Therapy for Measles', *American Family Physician*, vol. 42, December 1990, p. 1635.

48 *New England Journal of Medicine*, vol. 323, 19 July 1990, p. 160.

49 'Vitamin A and Malnutrition/Infection Complex in Developing Countries', *Lancet*, 1 December 1990, p. 1349.

50 Shelby Tyson, 'Numerous Studies, International Congress Confirm: Vitamin C is still a wonder worker and more', *Health News & Review*, vol. 1, July/August 1991, p. 1.

51 Peter Jaret, 'Vitamin C Vindicated', *Allure*, July 1992.

52 Sandra Goodman, 'Vitamin C: The master nutrient', *Health News & Review*, December 1991, p. 20.

53 *Ibid.*

54 *Ibid.*

55 'Vitamin C and Cataract Prevention', Department of Epidemiology, University of Western Ontario, Canada.

56 *American Journal of Clinical Nutrition*, vol. 53, January 1991, pp. 3465–3515.

57 *Ernahrungswiss*, March 1989, pp. 56–75.

58 *Journal of American Podiatry*, August 1990, pp. 414–18.

59 *Indian Journal of Medical Sciences*, vol. 6, 1952, pp. 252–55.

60 *American Journal of Clinical Nutrition*, December 1991, pp. 1310S–1314S.

61 Cathy Perlmutter, 'Vitamin C against Cancer', *Prevention*, vol. 43, March 1991, p. 62.

62 C. Alan Clemetson, 'Vitamin C and Multifactorial Disease', *Nutrition Health Review*, spring 1992, p. 19.

63 Willa Vae Bowles *et al.*, 'Total Health's Vitamin Supplement Guide', *Total Health*, vol. 13, December 1991, p. 34.

64 Stephen Langer, 'Chronic Fatigue Syndrome', *Better Nutrition for Today's Living*, vol. 52, June 1990, p. 14.

65 Willa Vae Bowles *et al.*, *op. cit.*

66 Shelby Tyson, *op. cit.*

67 'AIDS Virus May Be Inhibited by Vitamin C', *Nutrition Health Review*, spring 1992, p. 4.

68 Marianna K. Baum *et al.*, 'Association of Vitamin B_6 Status with Parameters of Immune Function

in Early HIV-1 Infection', *Journal of Acquired Immune Deficiency Syndrome*, November 1991, p. 1122.
69   Daniel J. DeNoon, 'Diet, Immunity and Nutritional Therapies', *AIDS Weekly*, 23 July 1990, p. 15.
70   Daniel J. DeNoon, 'Nutritional Aspects of HIV Infection', *AIDS Weekly*, 23 July 1990, p. 3.
71   Frank Murray, 'Are the FDA and FTC Trying to Harm Us?' *Better Nutrition for Today's Living*, March 1992, p. 10.
72   Richard A. Passwater, 'FDA to Ban Vitamin Supplements', *Health News & Review*, vol. 1, December 1991, p. 2.

Chapter 6: Mineral Values

1   Willa Vae Bowles, 'Minerals Essential to Health', *Total Health*, vol. 13, April 1991, p. 14.
2   *Ibid.*
3   'Maximizing Your Minerals', *University of California, Berkeley, Wellness Letter*, vol. 8, August 1991, p. 3.
4   Department of Health, *Dietary Reference Values for Food Energy and Nutrients for the United Kingdom* (Report on Health and Social Subjects 41), HMSO, 1991.
5   'Dietary Minerals and Sudden Cardiac Death', *Nutrition Research Newsletter*, vol. 9, August 1990, p. 87.
6   Dorothy West, 'How Junk Food, Pollution Are Hurting Women's Health', *Health News & Review*, vol. 7, September/October 1989, p. 5.
7   'NOS Calls for Urgent Review of Recommended Daily Calcium Intake', National Osteoporosis Society press release, 3 August 1993.
8   Susan M. Kleiner, 'Mineral and Your Bones', *Executive Health Report*, vol. 27, December 1990, p. 7.
9   Stephen Langer, 'The Multidimensional Role of Calcium', *Better Nutrition For Today's Living*, vol. 52, January 1990, p. 15.
10   Deborah S. Taylor, 'Sports Nutrition: Boost your performance naturally', *Better Nutrition for Today's Living*, vol. 52, July 1990, p. 24.
11   John Mitchell, 'Forget Gold – Here's Real Mineral Value: Calcium, zinc, chromium', *Health News & Review*, vol. 2, winter 1992, p. 7.
12   Ralph Myerson, 'Magnesium Maximizes Heart Health', *Better Nutrition for Today's Living*, vol. 51, December 1989. p. 18.
13   Mark Bricklin, 'New Respect for Nutritional Healing', *Prevention*, vol. 44, February 1992, p. 31.
14   Liz Applegate, 'Mineral Deposits: Minerals needed by runners and which foods contain them', *Runner's World*, vol. 24, October 1989, p. 18.
15   Frank Murray, 'Potassium Can Lower Blood Pressure', *Better Nutrition for Today's Living*, vol. 52, January 1990, p. 6.
16   Liz Applegate, *op. cit.*
17   *Ibid.*
18   Charlotte Pratt, *The Nutrition Report*, July 1991.
19   D. Baley *et al.*, *Journal of Nutrition*, vol. 120, 1990.
20   C. James Chuong, *Science News*, 17 October 1991.
21   Mark Bricklin, *op. cit.*
22   Frank Murray, 'Zinc Helps the Immune System', *Better Nutrition for Today's Living*, vol. 53, May 1991, p. 10.
23   Frank Murray, 'Chromium Is Intimately Related to Blood Sugar', *Better Nutrition for Today's Living*, vol. 20, October 1989, p. 10.
24   *Ibid.*
25   James F. Scheer, 'The Nutritional Approach to Hypertension', *Better Nutrition for Today's Living*, vol. 52, July 1990, p. 14.
26   *Ibid.*
27   James F. Scheer, 'Selenium: Cancer fighter', *Better Nutrition for Today's Living*, vol. 54, June 1992, p. 15.
28   Kathy Feld Berkowitz, 'Mining for Toxic Minerals Hidden in Our Diets', *Environmental Nutrition*, vol. 15, March 1992, p. 1.

Chapter 7: New Age Stress

1   Vicki Brower, 'Think "Seed", Not "Weed": Visualization therapy paints positive picture', *American Health: Fitness of Body and Mind*, vol. 9, July/August 1990, p. 34.

2 'A Workout that's No Sweat', *Edell Health Newsletter*, vol. 10, November 1991, p. 5.
3 Quoted in Steven Underleider, 'Visions of Victory: Using imagery visualization', *Psychology Today*, vol. 25, July/August 1992, p. 46.
4 Ed Rehbein, 'Discovering the Power of the Right Brain', *Total Health*, vol. 12, October 1990, p. 12.
5 'Aerobics and Relaxation May Equal AZT in Slowing HIV', *AIDS Weekly*, 17 February 1992, p. 2.
6 'Researcher Advises Meditation to Relieve Back Pain', *The Back Letter*, vol. 4, September 1990, p. 6.
7 *Ibid.*
8 Dean Ornish, 'The Drug-free, Surgery-free Heart Health Program', *Men's Health*, vol. 6, July 1990, p. 12.
9 *Ibid.*
10 Barbara K. Bailey, 'Biofeedback: A way to counter stress effects', *Diabetes in the News*, vol. 10, March/April 1991, p. 6.
11 Quoted in Lisa Delany, 'Dictionary of Healing Techniques and Remedies', *Prevention*, vol. 43, August 1991, p. 123.
12 'Can Hypnosis Put Grinding to a Halt?' *In Health*, vol. 5, September/October 1991, p. 2.

Chapter 8: Revitalizing Your Body

1 'Rx: Exercise', *Medical Update*, vol. 15, November 1991, p. 1.
2 'Is Exercise the Cure for High Blood Pressure?' *University of California, Berkeley, Wellness Letter*, vol. 6, August 1990, p. 1.
3 Keith Johnsgard *et al.*, 'Peace of Mind', *Runner's World*, vol. 25, April 1990, p. 73.
4 *Monthly Index of Medical Specialities*, December 1993.
5 Nancy N. Bell, 'Oh, My Aching Back!', *Business and Health*, vol. 9, April 1991, p. 63.
6 *Ibid.*
7 A. Bhalla *et al.*, 'Prevention of Osteoporosis: Current strategies' (editorial), *Osteoporosis Review*, July 1992.
8 *Lancet*, 28 September 1991, p. 774.
9 Marvin E. Levin, 'Living Off the Fat of the Land', *Clinical Diabetes*, vol. 9, March/April 1991, p. 18.
10 'Does Exercise Protect Against Cancer?' *University of California, Berkeley, Wellness Letter*, vol. 9, November 1992, p. 6.
11 *Ibid.*
12 'Study Shows Positive Effects of Stress Management and Exercise in AIDS Patients', *AIDS Weekly*, 1 April 1991, p. 8.
13 'Walk Away Those Blues', *Executive Health's Good Health Report*, vol. 28, November 1991, p. 8.
14 'Walking Helps Dementic Patients to Communicate', *Brown University Long-term Care Letter*, vol. 3, 10 September 1991, p. 4.
15 'Walk Your Way to Health', *Edell Health Letter*, vol. 9, November 1990, p. 1.
16 'Walk Out PMS', *Prevention*, vol. 42, July 1990, p. 10.
17 Ethan A. Bergman and Janice C. Bovungs, 'Indoor Walking Programs Increase Lean Body Composition in Older Women', *Journal of the American Dietetic Association*, 1991, p. 1433.
18 'The New Fat-burning Bench', *US News & World Report*, vol. 108, 18 June 1990, p. 69.
19 'Step Aerobics: Don't over do it', *Which? Way to Health*, June 1993, p. 76.
20 Joe Barks & E. J. Muller, 'Sports Yoga', *Men's Health*, February 1992, p. 48.
21 Ernest Wood, *Seven Schools of Yoga*, Theosophical Publishing House (US), 1976.
22 Bob Howells, 'Moving Meditation: T'ai Chi Chih', *Women's Sports and Fitness*, vol. 13, January/February 1991, p. 10.
23 'What's the Best Way to Relax?', *Edell Health Letter*, vol. 11, November 1992, p. 3.
24 Phil Dunphy, 'Balance Body and Spirit with T'ai Chi Ch'uan', *East West*, vol. 22, September/October 1992, p. 32.
25 Phyllis White & Robert White, 'Soft Fist Fitness', *American Fitness*, September/October 1992, p. 46.

Chapter 9: Knowing Your Mind

1 Bill Thompson, 'Prescription for a Failing Heart', *East West*, vol. 21, July/August 1991, p. 46.
2 Jean Marie Angelo, 'Auric Healer Barbara Brennan', *East West*, vol. 20, October 1990, p. 24.

3   Stephen Phillip Policoff, 'The Mind/Body Link', *Ladies' Home Journal*, vol. 107, October 1990, p. 126.
4   *Ibid.*
5   *Ibid.*
6   Arthur D. Silk, 'Is Positive Thinking as Medicine Really Powerful?', *American Medical News*, vol. 33, 27 July 1990, p. 25.
7   Flora Johnson Skelly, 'Mind, Body and Miracles', *American Medical News*, vol. 33, 27 July 1990, p. 18.
8   *Ibid.*
9   Henry Dreher, 'Are You Immune-competent?', *East West*, vol. 22, January/February 1992, p. 52.
10 Steven Findlay & Shannon Brownlee, 'The Delicate Dance of Body and Mind', *US News & World Report*, vol. 109, 2 July 1990, p. 54.
11 *Ibid.*
12 Douglas S. Barasch, 'The Mainstreaming of Alternative Medicine', *New York Times Magazine*, 4 October 1992, p. S6.
13 Candace Burch, 'Alternatives on the NHS', *Which?Way to Health*, August 1993, p. 125.
14 Irving Oyle, *The New American Medicine Show*, Unity Press (US), 1979.

INDEX

supplements, 129
value of, 129

waking dream therapy, 182
walking, 211–16
    water, in, 218–20
walls and furniture, fumes from, 83–4
water pollution
    deliberate, 72–3
    nitrates, by, 70
    pesticides and herbicides, by, 70
    petrol, from, 69
    refuse, from, 68
    sewage, by, 70
    toxic waste, from, 69

yoga
    athletes practising, 229–30
    basic postures, 231–3
    breathing, 230, 232

circulation, improving, 229
concentration, 233
hatha, 227–8
postures, 227–8
practising, 231
sexual performance, improving, 231
teaching, 228
tension, releasing, 232
types of, 228

zinc
    absorption, 167
    AIDS, treatment of, 168
    deficiency of, 168–9
    head injuries, treatment of, 168
    importance of, 166
    premenstrual syndrome, treatment of,
        167–8
    sources of, 167
    therapeutic use of, 168